Health Informatics: Integrating Healthcare and Information Technology

Health Informatics: Integrating Healthcare and Information Technology

Editor: Leonidas Waugh

FOSTER ACADEMICS

www.fosteracademics.com

www.fosteracademics.com

FOSTER ACADEMICS

Cataloging-in-Publication Data

Health informatics : integrating healthcare and information technology / edited by Leonidas Waugh.
p. cm.
Includes bibliographical references and index.
ISBN 978-1-63242-878-3
1. Medical informatics. 2. Medicine--Data processing. 3. Health--Data processing.
4. Medical care--Data processing. 5. Information technology. I. Waugh, Leonidas.
R858 .H43 2020
610.28--dc23

Foster Academics,
118-35 Queens Blvd., Suite 400,
Forest Hills, NY 11375, USA

ISBN 978-1-63242-878-3 (Hardback)

Contents

Preface

Health informatics is the field that integrates information technology, healthcare and communications for improving the quality and safety of patient care. It uses health information technology to improve healthcare through a combination of higher efficiency, higher quality and improved opportunities. Health informatics tools include information and communication systems, computers, clinical guidelines, formal medical terminologies, etc. for improving the effectiveness of patient care delivery. For designing a robust information system, it is imperative to identify changing requirements and improve system design. This facilitates health information, improved quality of care, and decentralized planning and management. This book elucidates the concepts and innovative models around prospective developments with respect to health informatics. While understanding the long-term perspectives of the topics, it makes an effort in highlighting their impact as a modern tool for the growth of the discipline. It attempts to assist those with a goal of delving into this field.

All of the data presented henceforth, was collaborated in the wake of recent advancements in the field. The aim of this book is to present the diversified developments from across the globe in a comprehensible manner. The opinions expressed in each chapter belong solely to the contributing authors. Their interpretations of the topics are the integral part of this book, which I have carefully compiled for a better understanding of the readers.

At the end, I would like to thank all those who dedicated their time and efforts for the successful completion of this book. I also wish to convey my gratitude towards my friends and family who supported me at every step.

Editor

1

A pattern learning-based method for temporal expression extraction and normalization from multi-lingual heterogeneous clinical texts

Tianyong Hao[1,2], Xiaoyi Pan[1], Zhiying Gu[1], Yingying Qu[3*] and Heng Weng[4*]

Abstract

Background: Temporal expression extraction and normalization is a fundamental and essential step in clinical text processing and analyzing. Though a variety of commonly used NLP tools are available for medical temporal information extraction, few work is satisfactory for multi-lingual heterogeneous clinical texts.

Methods: A novel method called TEER is proposed for both multi-lingual temporal expression extraction and normalization from various types of narrative clinical texts including clinical data requests, clinical notes, and clinical trial summaries. TEER is characterized as temporal feature summarization, heuristic rule generation, and automatic pattern learning. By representing a temporal expression as a triple <*M*, *A*, *N*>, TEER identifies temporal mentions *M*, assigns type attributes *A* to *M*, and normalizes the values of *M* into formal representations *N*.

Results: Based on two heterogeneous clinical text datasets: 400 actual clinical requests in English and 1459 clinical discharge summaries in Chinese. TEER was compared with six state-of-the-art baselines. The results showed that TEER achieved a precision of 0.948 and a recall of 0.877 on the English clinical requests, while a precision of 0.941 and a recall of 0.932 on the Chinese discharge summaries.

Conclusions: An automated method TEER for multi-lingual temporal expression extraction was presented. Based on the two datasets containing heterogeneous clinical texts, the comparison results demonstrated the effectiveness of the TEER method in multi-lingual temporal expression extraction from heterogeneous narrative clinical texts.

Keywords: Temporal expression identification, Heuristic rule, Pattern generation, Clinical texts, Heterogeneous

Background

The popularity of Electronic Medical Record (EMR) provides opportunities and challenges to accelerate clinical science using large scale of practical clinical data in less expense [1]. As a result, a large amount of unstructured clinical texts is generated such as clinical discharge summaries and progress notes, which contain a variety of temporal expressions and medical concepts [2]. Taking a clinical discharge summary as an example, it is a type of clinical reports by physicians or other medical professionals at the end of a hospital stay or series of treatments. A summary text outlines a patient's admitting diagnosis, diagnostic findings, diagnostic procedures performed, therapy received while hospitalized, and clinical course during hospitalization, prognosis, and plan of action upon discharge with stated time to follow up [3]. Consequently, temporal expressions usually are involved in sequential events and patients' phenotype value variations with time. Therefore, it is highly meaningful to extract temporal expressions and their associated diagnosis procedure actions

* Correspondence: jessie.qu@gdufs.edu.cn; ww128@qq.com
[3]School of Business, Guangdong University of Foreign Studies, Guangzhou, China
[4]The Second Affiliated Hospital, Guangzhou University of Chinese Medicine, Guangzhou, China
Full list of author information is available at the end of the article

as well as patient phenotypes for deep analysis [4]. Similarly, automatic processing and formulation of clinical data requests is desired to improve the labor-intensive, time-consuming process of data requests translation into executable database requests [5, 6]. However, the identification of temporal expressions is one of major bottlenecks to the automatic data request formulation. Our previous analysis on 400 actual data requests submitted to the Columbia University Medical Center (CUMC)'s clinical data warehouse showed that about 64% of the data requests contain temporal expressions [1].

Temporal expression extraction is also essential to an extensive scope of Natural Language Processing (NLP) applications, e.g., question understanding and text comprehension, since the extraction plays an unique role in the analysis of chronological events [7, 8]. Narrative clinical texts are different from other types of unstructured texts. They commonly contain a large number of International Classification of Diseases (ICD), Admit Discharge Transfers (ADT), Current Procedural Terminology (CPT) codes, concept abbreviations, etc., increasing the complexity of texts dramatically [1]. For example, the ICD code "*002.2*" may cause a confusion with a temporal expression "*2002.2*". A large amount of quantitative expressions exist and may also incur wrong identification [9, 10]. Moreover, a wide range of representations in particularly special temporal expression formats, e.g., "*May 30 = 04*" and "2 + 月", causing the texts even more difficult to process. In addition, the texts frequently contain noise data, e.g., incorrect spelling "*2 moths*". As a result, a number of commonly used NLP tools have been applied for medical temporal expression extraction, but few work works well for multi-lingual heterogeneous narrative clinical texts.

To that end, we develop a new method – Temporal Expression ExtractoR (TEER). TEER integrates heuristic rule generation and automatic pattern learning to extract temporal expressions from various types of narrative clinical texts, e.g., clinical data requests, discharge summary texts, etc. In TEER, a list of structural patterns are automatically learned from a part of annotated texts. After that, the patterns are validated by calculating their confidence values through matching with more annotated texts. Eventually, TEER utilizes achieved patterns with summarized heuristic rules to extract candidate temporal expressions and filter out irrelevant ones.

Our experiments used two datasets: 1) 400 actual clinical data requests from CUMC's data warehouse. The requests were labelled by three human annotators. 100 request texts were used for training and the other 300 were used for testing. 2) The unstructured discharge summaries from the electronic medical records (EMR) of 1459 actual patients with breast cancer disease, who received medical treatment (operation) from a 3A hospital in mainland China. These discharge summaries were also manually labelled by three human annotators. 276 patient records were randomly selected and used for training and 134 records were used for testing. We used 6 baseline methods including CMedTEX, GUTime, and HeidelTime for performance comparison. The results presented that our method TEER outperformed all the baselines and demonstrated that the TEER method was effective in extracting temporal expressions from multi-lingual heterogeneous clinical texts.

Related work

In response to the need of temporal expression extraction, an open evaluation challenge-TempEval for temporal expression identification, was held in 2007 [8], 2010 [11], 2013 [12], 2015 [13], 2017 [14], resulting in the wide adoption of a number of systems. HeidelTime [7], an instance of the systems, outperformed the other systems the English temporal expression identification and normalization task of the TempEval 2 challenge. TempEval challenge released official guidelines for annotating temporal expressions in the challenges. For example, the guideline for English text annotation in TempEval 2010 consisted of nouns, proper nouns, noun phrases, adjectives, adjective phrases, adverbs, and adverb phrases.

Targeting at temporal expression extraction, TempEx recognized temporal expressions and normalized them using the TIMEX2 standard. Both absolute time (e.g., *May 7, 2017*) and relative time (e.g., *last weekend*) could be identified by TempEx through the way of local context. GUTime further enhanced the capabilities. Based on the idea of utilizing a reference time, the method identified and annotated lexical triggers such as *yesterday* and phrase triggers such as *last year.* Temporal extraction gained more attention since 2010. As the result, more progressive methods about temporal expression extraction were developed, e.g., HeidelTime. Nevertheless, all the methods focused on newspaper and narrative texts primarily, without testing on medical texts [1].

For clinical temporal expression extraction, Informatics for Integrating Biology & the Bedside (i2b2) NLP Challenge devoted on temporal relation identification in medical narratives for EMR data records. The challenge also offered a corpus containing clinical discharge summaries with human annotations of events and temporal expressions for research communities. The corpus was widely applied to the development and evaluation of temporal expression and event identification methods [15]. The challenge tried to evaluate different submitted methods on: 1) temporal expressions including date, time, duration, or frequency types, 2) clinical events containing medical concepts such as treatments, and events related to the clinical timeline of patients, e.g., admissions, transfers among departments, and 3) temporal relations between temporal expressions and clinical events.

Clinical TempEval 2015 concentrated on the method competition for timeline extraction and annotation for the medical domain. The challenge included six different tasks.

The Task 12 (clinical TempEval) of SemEval-2017 succeeded Clinical TempEval [16] and the past i2b2 temporal challenge [17] directly. The Clinical TempEval focused on clinical timeline extraction and understanding for clinical narratives, basing on the THYME corpus with temporal annotations [18]. 16 teams participated in TempEval 2017 [19].

There are a number of research and systems for English temporal expression extraction from clinical texts. Sohn et al. reported a hybrid method to detect temporal information using regular expression matching and matching learning [15]. A comprehensive system for extracting temporal information from clinical texts was proposed by Tang et al. [20]. Tao et al. presented a method for identifying temporal representations of vaccine adverse events using ontology for temporal analysis [21]. Li & Patrick [22] addressed a statistical model using linguistic, contextual and semantic features for extracting temporal expressions from an extremely noisy clinical corpus. Xu et al. [23] introduced an end-to-end temporal relation system including a temporal extraction sub-system based on a Conditional Random Fields (CRF) for name entity extraction and context-free grammar-based normalization. Luo et al. [24] extracted temporal constraints from the eligibility criteria texts of clinical trials using CRF. Chang et al. [25] proposed a hybrid method TEMPTING to identify temporal links among entities combining a rule-based method and a maximum entropy model. Nevertheless, comparing and evaluating the performance of the systems could be difficult due to lack of system open source codes. Moreover, only a few of these systems processed complexity clinical texts, such as user-generated clinical notes. Most of them still focused on the process of the relatively formal clinical texts.

Moreover, there was research on Chinese temporal expression extraction. Li et al. [26] proposed a Chinese temporal tagging (extraction and normalization) method by developing Chinese HeidelTime resources. Shen et al. [27] constructed a temporal expression extraction model based on Tsinghua Chinese Treebank. Zhou et al. [28] proposed a method for the recognition of Chinese temporal expressions using regular expression matching and a temporal relationship extraction approach based on CRF. Yan and Ji [29] proposed a Chinese temporal information identification method using CRF and a semi-supervised learning method. Wu et al. [30] built a Chinese temporal parser for the extraction and normalization of temporal information utilizing grammar rules and constraint rules. Zhu et al. [31] presented a CRF-based approach for temporal phrases recognition. Liu et al. [32] proposed a new Chinese time expression recognition method combined with common features plus semantic role features according to the characteristics of Chinese time expression and CRF.

In the standardization of temporal annotation, TimeML is a robust specification markup language for annotating temporal expressions in texts [33]. It deals with four different issues in labelling temporal and event expressions including time stamping of events and reasoning with contextually underspecified temporal expressions. With respect to TimeML specifications [34], we use TIMEX3 for annotating temporal expressions throughout the paper. All the attributes of TIMEX3 are inherited from the THYME annotations [18].

Methods

Aiming at automatically identifying temporal expressions from narrative multi-lingual clinical texts, TEER is proposed by leveraging temporal features, heuristic rules and automated learned patterns. In TEER, a temporal expression is represented as a triple $TE = <M, A, N>$, where M is a collection of temporal mentions, A represents the type attributes of the mentions M, and N is the normalized temporal values of the mentions M. The normalized values represent the temporal semantics of temporal expressions as specified using TimeML. Therefore, the purpose of TEER is to: 1) identify temporal mentions M, 2) assign M with type attributes A, and 3) normalize the values of mentions M into formal representations N.

Initially, we summarize a list of heuristic rules representing a group of selected temporal features observed from temporal expression annotations for matching temporal expression candidates. After that, an algorithm is applied to automatically generate temporal structural patterns from clinical texts containing temporal expression annotations. Then the learned candidate patterns are matched to original texts for calculating matching confidence scores. The patterns evaluated by comparing with a confidence threshold are ranked and kept as final patterns. Eventually, the heuristic rules and the ranked patterns are combined to be applied to temporal extraction for newly coming clinical texts. The overall framework of the TEER is shown as Fig. 1.

In addition to English clinical texts. Temporal expressions in Chinese EMR have certain special representation features. We extract temporal expressions from manually annotated datasets and observe their features. Table 1 shows part of the identified features from training dataset. We further summarize a list of heuristic rules by analyzing the features of a list of training temporal expressions with human annotations. These heuristic rules in Chinese and English, as shown in Table 2, are used to identify temporal expressions for a given new clinical text.

Using solely heuristic rules may cause incorrect matching. For example, *"1/17"* in *"左腋窝淋巴结(1/17)"* is wrongly matched by a heuristic rule as it is similar to a date representation *"January 17"*. Moreover, in clinical texts, some temporal expressions may be contextually connected, e.g., *"from Feb. 2016 to May 2016"*. A list of contextual relationships thus can be defined as patterns for extracting these types of temporal expressions. However, the summarized patterns without effective validation can cause wrong

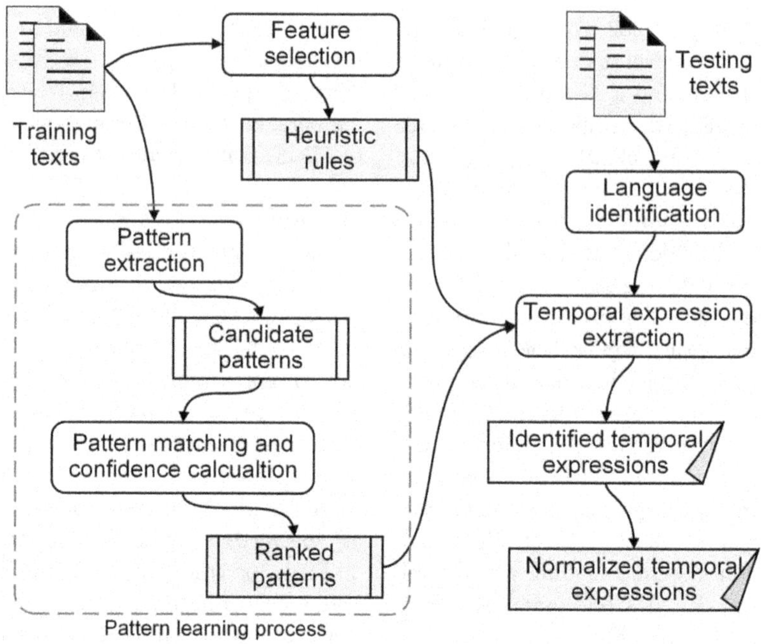

Fig. 1 The overall framework of TEER incorporating heuristic rule generation and pattern learning

identifications of temporal expressions, e.g., the incorrect extraction of the ICD9 codes *"321.0"* and *"322.9"* in *"unspecified meningitis 321.0–322.9"* as temporal expressions. Consequently, an algorithm incorporating with automatic temporal pattern learning is more preferred.

Our method TEER automatically generates a group of temporal patterns from a manually annotated training dataset and validates the generated patterns. The core idea of the pattern learning is to extract all pattern candidates with high accuracy confidence in matching original annotated texts. Those patterns with a confidence lower than a threshold are filtered out and the patterns are applied to verify temporal expression candidates that cannot be determined by solely heuristic rules. Finally, TEER normalizes the extracted temporal expressions and represented them using TimeML.

Table 1 A list of identified temporal features in Chinese as examples

Types		Features
Unit		年, 月, 日, 天, 周期, 星期, 周, 小时, 时, 分钟, 秒, 毫秒..
Numeric		半, 一, 二, 三, 四, 五, 六, 七, 八, 九, 十, 百, 千, 万, 兆, 亿
Explicit	Day	年-月-日, 月-日, 日..
	Day-time	上午, 下午, 早上, 白天, 傍晚, 晚上..
	Week	星期一, 星期二, 星期三, 星期四, 星期五, 星期六, 星期日, 星期天..
	Month	一月, 正月, 二月, 三月, ...
Referred	Current	现在, 现, 今, 今日, 当日, 本年, 今年, 本月..
	Current-referred	昨日, 昨天, 明日, 去年, 前年, 上年, 明年, 上个月, 下个月
	Other-referred	*x*后*y*天, *x*前*y*星期..
Frequency		第, 每..
Implicit		大概, 近期, 近, 约, 前, 后, 余前, 余, 来...

As shown in Algorithm 1, the detailed automatic pattern learning algorithm mainly contains the following five steps: 1) sentence boundary detection. This is to split discharge summary texts into sentences. We use both the widely used NLTK sentence boundary identifier and our defined rules to correct the splitting since some incorrect sentences may be obtained such as "e.g.," symbols; 2) tag replacement. This is to replace the original annotation temporal expression tags with a specified tag for the purpose of context extraction; 3) extract candidate patterns. By setting a word window length, we can extract all possible candidate patterns that containing the specified tag and their surrounding words, as shown from line 7 to 11. We empirically choose 8 as the word window size; 4) calculate pattern confidence. Each candidate pattern is matched back to original texts to calculate its support and confidence values. Support metric is defined as the count of correct matches and confidence metric is defined as the rate of correct expression matches among all matches; 5) final pattern generation. By comparing with a confidence threshold, the candidates with confidence greater than or equal to the threshold are kept as final learned patterns.

Algorithm 1 Automatic Temporal Pattern Learning

```
Input a clinical discharge summaries group G containing n discharge summary texts
Pattern set patts ← 0; candidate pattern set c_patts ← 0
ForEach record g in G
    sentences ←NLTK sentence boundary identification(g)
    ForEach (sentence in sentences)
        sentence ← Tag relabelling(sentence, original tags, specified tag)
        word window size wl ← 8
        ForEach (word_window in windows from sentence with size wl)
            generate structures as candidate patterns from word_window
            add the patterns to c_patts iff they are >= two words
        EndFor
    EndFor
EndFor
ForEach (c_patt in c_patts)
    match(c_patt, G)
    If number of correct match m >= support threshold α
        confid ← # of correct matchs / # of matchs
        If confid >= confidence threshold β
            Add (c_patt, confid) to patts
        EndIf
    EndIf
EndFor
Output patts
```

For example, there is a sentence "入院后完善相关检查,未见明显手术禁忌症,遂于 < T > *22/9*</T > 行右乳癌改良根治术 + 右腋窝前哨淋巴结活检 + 腋窝清扫术,术后病理未回", where "<T > </T>" is a temporal annotation tag defined by annotators. Our algorithm replaces the whole temporal expression annotations with a [TE] tag. With the setting of word window length, a list of pattern candidates are extracted, as shown in Table 3. After that, all the pattern candidates are matched to all training texts to calculate their support and confidence values. For example, "于[TE]行" is matched with "于 < T > *2014–9-30*</T > 行右乳癌根治性保乳术", "于 < T > *2014年10月5日*</T > 行腹腔镜探查术", and "于门诊行". Only those candidate patterns with both support and confidence values larger than predefined thresholds are considered as validated patterns for applying to a testing dataset. We empirically set support threshold $\alpha = 3$ and confidence threshold $\beta = 0.6$ to enlarge their matching coverage.

Table 3 A list of pattern candidates with their support and confidence values generated by the algorithm for the example sentence

Pattern candidates	Support	Confidence	Keep
遂于[TE]行右乳癌	3	1	YES
遂于[TE]行右	3	1	YES
遂于[TE]行	4	1	YES
遂于[TE]	5	0.83	YES
于[TE]行	8	0.4	NO
于[TE]	34	0.52	NO
[TE]行	9	0.06	NO

Eventually, the extracted temporal expressions need to be formally represented. Based on our previous experience on English clinical text annotation [1], we continually apply the temporal expression schema TimeML and use TimeX3 as the annotation format standard. Using the markup language, a temporal expression can be annotated in a XML-based format, e.g., <TIMEX3 tid = "*t5*" Type = "*Duration*" Value = "*P3D*" > *3 days*</TIMEX3>. In the TimeX3 representation, each expression is labelled with one of the four types: "Date", "Time", "Duration", and "Set". The representations of the types are formally defined in the TimeX3. For example, the "Duration" type starts with letter *'P'* as duration usually denotes a period of time. In TEER, we classify the extracted temporal expressions into the types and normalize them using commonly used normalized value representations. For example, "<T > 今日</T > 出院" is labelled and normalized as "<TIMEX3 tid = "*t2*" Type = "*Date*" Value = "*2014–10-7*" > 今日</TIMEX3>出院",

Table 2 Examples of generated heuristic rules from Chinese clinical texts

<table>
<tr><th>Language</th><th>Expression</th><th>Representation format</th><th>Heuristic rule</th></tr>
<tr><td>Chinese</td><td>约10天</td><td>[SLOT: prefix][SLOT: num][SLOT: day]</td><td>('+prefix+')(\d{1,6})('+ dmy+')</td></tr>
<tr><td></td><td>2014年10月5日</td><td>[SLOT: num][SLOT: year][SLOT: num][SLOT: month][SLOT: num] [SLOT: day]</td><td>(\d{1,4}[年]\d{1,2}[月]\d{1,2}[日])</td></tr>
<tr><td></td><td>约一个周期</td><td>[SLOT: prefix](LIST: 半|一|二|两|三|四|五|六|七|八|九|十|十一|十二|十三|十四|十五|二十|三十) < S: 个 > [SLOT: day]</td><td>('+prefix+')('+num+')(个)('+dmy+')</td></tr>
<tr><td></td><td>第7、9、14天</td><td>[SLOT: prefix][SLOT: num] < SM: 、 > [SLOT: num] < SM: 、 > [SLOT: num][SLOT: day]</td><td>('+prefix+')(((\d{1,6})('+u'、'+')){1,5}(\d{1,6})('+dmy+'))</td></tr>
<tr><td>English</td><td>2014–11-04</td><td>[SLOT: year] < SM: - > [SLOT: month] < SM: - > [SLOT: day]</td><td>d{1,4}) r'(– |-| -|- |)('+[month] + r'(– |-| -|- |)\ d{1,2}</td></tr>
<tr><td></td><td>November 2nd, 2016</td><td>[SLOT: month] < SM: >[SLOT: day](LIST: st, nd, rd, th) < SM:,> < SM: > [SLOT: year]</td><td>('+[month]+'(– |-| -|- |)\ d{1,2}(st|nd|rd|th)(, |,|)\ d{1,4})</td></tr>
<tr><td></td><td>May 3–5, 2013</td><td>[SLOT: month] < SM: >[SLOT: day] < SM:- > [SLOT: day] < SM:,> < SM: > [SLOT: year]</td><td>('+[month] + r' \d{1,2}(– |-| -|-)\ d{1,2}(, |,|)\ d{2,4})</td></tr>
<tr><td></td><td>37 years old</td><td><RULE: negative></td><td>If context_distance([SLOT: num], [SLOT: age]) < n; Then filter out</td></tr>
</table>

where *"Date"* is a type and *"2014–10-7"* is the normalized value of "今日" *(today)* corresponding to its reference date of "出院"*(discharge date)*.

Results

Datasets

For English clinical texts, we used the same 400 real free-text clinical requests, as used in [1], submitted to the data warehouse of Columbia University Medical Center (CUMC). Three human annotators including two clinical researchers and one IT scientist labelled all the request texts. The overlap among the annotators was calculated as 87%. All the disagreements were recorded and further manually classified as "minor", "partial", and "distinct". Most of the disagreements (92%) were minor (e.g., *"the* < T > *last month*</T>" versus "<T > *the last month*</T>") and partial (e.g. *"through* < T > *May 11 = 02*</T>" versus *"through* < T > *May 11*</T > *=02*"). All the disagreements were eventually resolved through discussions. All annotations followed the TimeML annotation guideline. Among the 400 annotated request texts, 100 were randomly selected as a training dataset and the remaining 300 requests were used as a testing dataset. The 400 request texts contained 1044 sentences (2.61 sentences per request on average) and 2397 tokens in total. There were in total 553 temporal expressions identified and annotated (1.38 temporal expressions per request text on average).

For Chinese clinical texts, the EMR records of 1459 real patients with breast cancer, acquired from a 3A hospital in mainland China, were used. We randomly selected 400 narrative discharge summary texts considering manageable human annotation workload with 276 as a training dataset, and 134 as a testing dataset. The 400 EMR texts contained 11,943 sentences (29.86 sentences per record on average) and 35,250 clauses in total. A total of 5303 temporal expressions were annotated (13.26 temporal expressions per record text). Please note each temporal expression had been labeled with date type, e.g., <T Type = *"Time"* > *2014/10/8 9:16:34*</T>, <T Type = *"Date"* > *5月26日*</T>, <T Type = *"Duration"* > 一个月</T>, <T Type = *"Set"* > 第*7*、*9*、*14*天</T>, etc. A summary of the two datasets is reported in Table 4.

Table 4 The data summary of the training and testing datasets

Language	Dataset	#texts	#sentences	#clauses	#temp. Exp.	#ave. temp. exp. /text
Chinese	Training	276	7747	23,423	3525	12.77
	Testing	134	4196	11,827	1778	13.27
	Total	400	11,943	35,250	5303	13.26
English	Training	100	257	694	155	1.55
	Testing	300	787	1703	398	1.33
	Total	400	1044	2397	553	1.38

Baselines

We use the following six publicly available temporal expression extraction systems as baseline methods for performance comparison:

1) HeidelTime [35] is a domain-sensitive temporal expression tagger supporting multi-languages developed by the Dataset Systems Research Group at Heidelberg University. It uses a group of rules and adopts different strategies, according to the domain texts that are to be processed. It utilizes hand-crafted resources and currently supports 13 languages including Chinese. It is used to automatically create resources for more than 200 languages.
2) IllinoisTemporalExtractor (The Illinois Temporal Extractor) [36] extracts temporal expressions as well as optionally associate the expressions to reference dates. The method can be applied programmatically. A number of rudimentary command-line functions are provided to enable users reuse and evaluate its capability locally. It also provided an online version. The method currently works for English plain texts only.
3) GUTime [37] utilizes the TimeML TIMEX3 as the standard for temporal expression annotation. It extends TempEx and allows using functional styles of encoding offsets in temporal expressions. The method also can handles a variety of temporal expressions that are not covered by TempEx, including varieties of temporal modifiers and date formats in different countries.
4) SUTime [38] is a part of the Stanford CoreNLP pipeline. It uses a rule-based temporal tagging strategy to annotate temporal information in free texts. SUTime outperformed a list of baseline methods on the TempEval-2 evaluation challenge.
5) NLTK Timex [39] is a library belongs to NLTK Contrib repository. It contains a module named as timex.py for identifying temporal expressions. The Timex library is open source and widely applied to general natural language processing tasks. The library provides a general way to annotate and normalize English temporal expressions.
6) CMedTEX [40] is a rule-based system for extracting and normalizing temporal expressions for Chinese electronic medical records. It can identify four types of temporal expressions including Date, Time, Duration and Frequency. It normalizes temporal values with TIMEX3 standard. The CMedTEX has been applied to annotate Chinese clinical texts and has reported a good performance of temporal expression extraction and normalization.

Results

Based on the two training datasets, TEER generated 21 heuristic rules and 65 structural patterns in total for English data request texts, while generated 26 heuristic rules and 58 structural patterns for Chinese EMR record texts. Table 5 shows some example patterns with an example of their matched texts.

In the evaluation, CMedTEX had a different temporal annotation standard with us on Chinese clinical texts. For example, it annotated "后*1*年余" as "后 <T> *1*年余 </T>" while our method annotated it as "<T> 后*1*年余 </T>". To compare the methods with the same annotation standard, we intentionally revised our TEER method to adapt to the annotation standard of CMedTEX. For example, "[*temporal expression*] 后" and "后 [*temporal expression*]" were labeled as "<T> [*temporal expression*]</T> 后" and "后 <T> [*temporal expression*]</T>", respectively. We named the revised method as TEER_C, which was used for Chinese clinical text processing only.

After that, we applied both TEER and TEER_C to test the scalability of our method on various numbers of temporal expressions randomly selected from the training dataset. We tested a different number of expressions from the Chinese EMR record text data with the increasing number from 10 to 1700. The results, as shown in Fig. 2, presented that the performances of both TEER and TEER_C were relatively stable when the number of temporal expressions was larger than 200. After that, the performance changed slightly in terms of F1 score with the increasing number of testing temporal expressions.

After training TEER and TEER_C on the two training datasets, all the testing datasets containing 1778 Chinese temporal expressions and 398 English expressions were applied to each of the baseline methods for performance comparison. The results are shown as Table 6. For Chinese text annotation, GUTime had a F1 score of 0.375 only, while Heideltime had a F1 score of 0.603. Though CMedTEX obtained a lower precision as 0.717, it significantly improved the recall to 0.925, achieving an overall F1 of 0.808. Our method TEER_C achieved a recall of 0.907 while a higher precision of 0.916, increasing the F1 to 0.912. The TEER further improved the performance into a F1 of 0.936. For English text annotation, NLTK Timex, GUTime, and IllionisTExtractor acquired F1 scores as 0.242, 0.353, and 0.765, respectively. Heideltime obtained a precision of 0.828 and a recall of 0.822. One of our previous work named as TEXer, as reported in [1], achieved a F1 score of 0.897. Our TEER achieved a precision of 0.948, a recall of 0.877, and a F1 score of 0.911, outperforming all the baseline methods.

Table 5 The examples of learned patterns that are categorized into four types

Language	Type	Structural pattern	Matching text
English	Time	with [TE] prior to	*starting with 24 h prior to the patients admission*
	Date	discharged in [TE]	*surgery patients discharged in 2015*
	Duration	study period [TE] - [TE]	*study period May 1st, 2016 - May 21th, 2016*
	Set	issued on a [TE] basis	*issued on a weekly basis*
Chinese	Time	后[TE]内	在入院后 24小时内
	Date	[TE]返院化疗	*2014.11.3*返院化疗
	Duration	[TE]/次	*3–5*天/次
	Set	[TE]检查	每三个月检查一次

Discussion

We analyzed all extraction errors by our TEER and the baseline methods. For the English temporal expression extraction, some errors were brought by special clinical codes in the clinical data requests in the representation of numerical values, e.g., ICD9, CPT codes, etc. For example, "*between 2005 - 2007 with one of the following DRG codes 291.0 Alcohol Withdrawal, 303.0 Acute Alcoholic Intoxication, or 305.0 Alcohol Abuse*". NLTK Timex labelled most of the codes as temporal expressions incorrectly, dramatically lowering its performance. The requests also contained a large number of quantitative expressions, which frequently caused errors using NLTK Timex, GUTime, and IllionisTExtractor. For example, IllinoisTExtractor incorrectly annotated "*2000*" as a date in "*2000 mg per ml*". Moreover, some user-defined temporal expressions with special representation format frequently caused unexpected errors. For instance, the texts "*May 22 = 02*" and "*patient started HD 2/00*" were in uncommon representation formats. As a result, TEER and the baseline systems only labelled them partially. Finally, noise data, such as incorrect spellings affected the performance of the methods, e.g., "*1995-pr!esent*" ("*present*" was expected) and "*2 moths*" ("*months*" was expected). The processing of clinical request texts commonly suffered from the above types of errors. Therefore, the design of new methods need to tolerate the texts as much as possible. TEER showed improvement on this particular point.

In addition to the errors caused by the complexity of the texts, some errors were incurred by the methods themselves. The GUTime heavily relied on Part-of-Speech tagging thus it incorrectly annotated some texts. For example, the "*2/3/1999*" was incorrectly tagged into "2/3/ <TIMEX3 tid = "*t1*" Type = "*Date*" Value = "*1999*" > <lex pos = "*CD*" > *1999* </lex></TIMEX3>". The method incorrectly tagged "*the current*" as EVENT type rather than temporal expression based on POS tags. The Heideltime wrongly ignored some special temporal terms and abbreviations, e.g., "current", "weekly", and "*12 h*". The IllinoisTemporalExtractor incorrectly

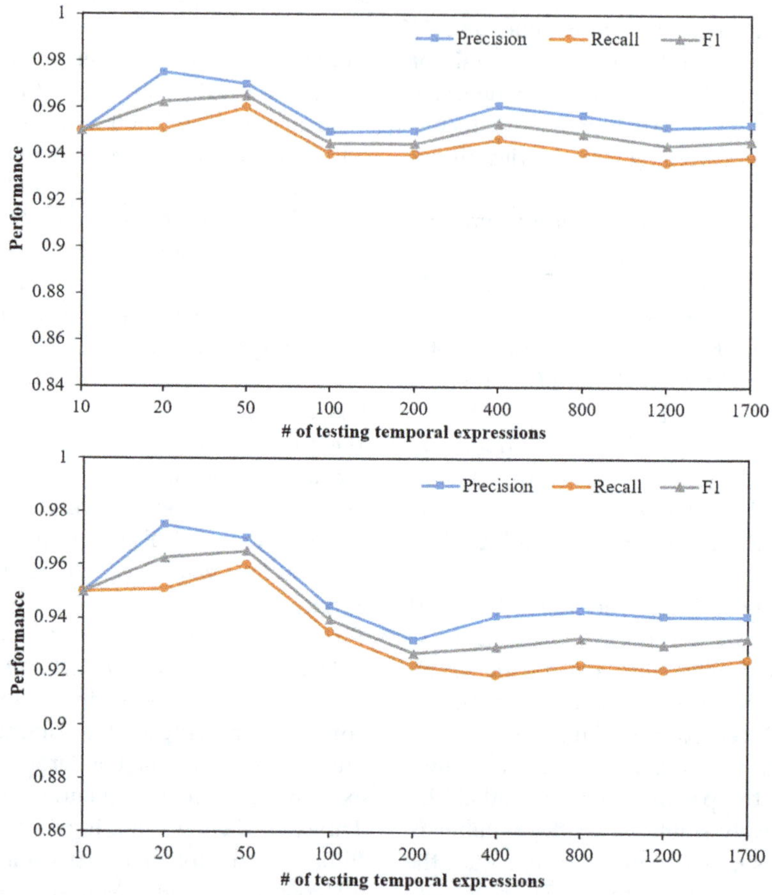

Fig. 2 An implemented graphical user interface of TEER for temporal expression extraction

labelled all *"fall"* words as temporal expressions but none was truly temporal expression, e.g., *"falling down"*. The method also missed some short representations, e.g., *"present"*, and minute type, e.g., *"2 mins"*. NLTK Timex performed worst on the identification of month and year abbreviations, e.g., only *"2015"* was identified in *"Feb. 2015"*. Moreover, all the baseline methods labelled age-related expressions as temporal expression, while the age information should be independently annotated and distinguished from temporal information. TEER had errors on the identification of some certain abbreviations. For instance, it incorrectly annotated *"MAR"* as a date type in *"MAR info tables"*.

Table 6 The performance comparison of our method with baseline methods

Language	Method	# exp.	# correct	Precision	Recall	F1
Chinese	GUTime	512	429	0.838	0.241	0.375
	HeidelTime	954	824	0.864	0.463	0.603
	CMedTEX	2293	1645	0.717	0.925	0.808
	TEER_C	1761	1613	0.916	0.907	0.912
	TEER	1761	1657	0.941	0.932	0.936
English	NLTK Timex	106	61	0.575	0.153	0.242
	GUTime	101	88	0.871	0.221	0.353
	IllinoisTExtractor	352	287	0.815	0.721	0.765
	Heideltime	395	327	0.828	0.822	0.825
	TEXer	360	340	0.944	0.854	0.897
	TEER	368	349	0.948	0.877	0.911

For the Chinese temporal expression extraction, GUTime only identified two types of temporal expressions: Date and Time. According to our evaluation, it was not suitable for Chinese clinical texts due to its very limited language-specified rules. Heideltime correctly identified most of common and simple temporal expressions but it missed complex expressions. For example, it tagged *"5月"* in *"5月余"* and *"1月"* in *"1月后"* only and wrongly missed their modifiers "余" and "后". CMedTEX correctly extracted these frequently used expressions such as "三次" and "随诊". However, it incorrectly tagged hospital admission numbers and patient ages as temporal expressions. For example, the *"1258年"* in *"住院号: 761258 年龄:52岁"* was annotated as a temporal expression. In addition, CMedTEX incorrectly tagged some of the mentioned medical codes (e.g., ICD9, ADT, and CPT codes) as temporal expressions. In TEER, the learned patterns were able to use contextual relations to eliminate the interference of these codes. From the results, the pattern learning was tested to be an effective strategy in temporal expression identification.

Nevertheless, we identified a number of error cases by TEER method. The errors and their potential reasons were summarized as follows: 1) Errors by heuristic rule and pattern coverage. Since the heuristic rules and patterns were either summarized or automated learned from the limited number of annotated training dataset, some necessary rules and patterns were missing for the testing dataset. For example, a new temporal expression *"1 + 月"* was found in the testing dataset but was incorrectly annotated due to the lack of matched patterns. 2) Errors caused by informal representations or typos. Clinical discharge summary texts contained a number of informal representations or even typos, causing unexpected errors. For example, the text *"2013..07"* contained a punctuation typo ".." and *"2014–09-2014/10/11"* was an complex informal representation, causing wrong annotations by TEER. These informal cases and typos were unpredictable and inevitable as they may come from clinicians themselves.

The TEER method was programmed using Python and a graphical user-interface was implemented using C#. As shown in Fig. 3, TEER can annotate the raw texts in the left side panel automatically and output the annotated results in the right side panel. The identified temporal expressions are marked in green color, starting with "<T>". Users can select the "Use TimeML" option to output results in TimeML annotation format. In addition to the TimeX3 format, it also supports other types of annotation formats including user specifically defined annotation tags. The annotation output is visualized using different colors, where green color denotes temporal expressions and bule color denotes events. The system also provides a tool for quick manual annotation on raw texts as well as a standard evaluation tool for comparing the system output with gold stand annotations or the outputs from other baseline methods. TEER can be used in the ways of graphical user-interface, library integration, Web-based, and command line-based interface. TEER can be potentially applied to a variety of natural language processing libraries for clinical text processing. The python code was publically available on Github (https://github.com/Tony-Hao/TEER).

Conclusions

Temporal expression extraction is a fundamental and essential step in the processing of clinical texts. This paper proposed an automated method TEER for multi-lingual temporal expression extraction through the learning of temporal features, heuristic rules, and patterns. Based on the two datasets including 400 actual clinical data requests in English and 1459 EMR records in Chinese, we conducted the comparison of TEER with six baseline methods. The experiment results presented that the TEER method achieved the best performance, demonstrating its effectiveness in the temporal expression extraction from multi-lingual heterogeneous clinical texts. We will continue to improve the performance of TEER on temporal abbreviation identification, temporal value normalization, and event identification in the future.

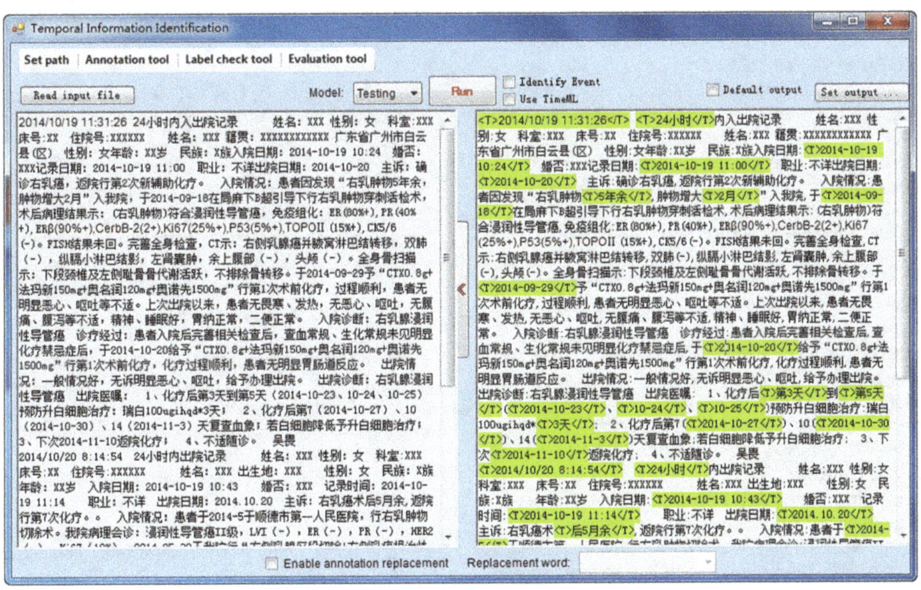

Fig. 3 The scalability evaluation of TEER (the first) and TEER_C (the second) using the increasing number of temporal expressions randomly selected from the testing datasets

Abbreviations

ADT: Admit Discharge Transfers; CPT: Current Procedural Terminology; CRF: Conditional Random Fields; CUMC: Columbia University Medical Center; EMR: Electronic Medical Record; i2b2: Informatics for Integrating Biology & the Bedside; ICD: International Classification of Diseases; IllinoisTemporalExtractor: The Illinois Temporal Extractor; NLP: Natural Language Processing; TEER: Temporal Expression ExtractoR

Funding

Publication of the article is supported by the grants from National Natural Science Foundation of China (No. 61772146) and the Innovative School Project in Higher Education of Guangdong Province (No.YQ2015062).

Authors' contributions

HTY provided theoretical guidance and leaded the method design. He also participated in result analysis and paper revision. XYP and ZYG participated in method development, data preprocessing, experiment design, result analysis, and manuscript revision. YYQ and HW participated in method design, result analysis, and manuscript revision. All authors read and approved the final manuscript.

Competing interests

The authors declare that they have no competing interests.

Author details

[1]School of Information Science and Technology, Guangdong University of Foreign Studies, Guangzhou, China. [2]School of Computer, South China Normal University, Guangzhou, China. [3]School of Business, Guangdong University of Foreign Studies, Guangzhou, China. [4]The Second Affiliated Hospital, Guangzhou University of Chinese Medicine, Guangzhou, China.

References

1. Hao T, Rusanov A, Weng C. Extracting and normalizing temporal expressions in clinical data requests from researchers. Lect Notes Comput Sci. 2013;8040:41–51.
2. Rink B, Harabagiu S, Roberts K. Automatic extraction of relations between medical concepts in clinical texts. J Am Med Inform Assoc. 2011;18(5):594–600.
3. Simpson A, Lakkol S, Alnaib M. Discharge summaries: a guide for foundation doctors. Br J Hosp Med. 2010;71(9):M142–3.
4. Madkour M, Benhaddou D, Tao C. Temporal data representation, normalization, extraction, and reasoning: a review from clinical domain. Comput Methods Prog Biomed. 2016;128:52–68.
5. Lonsdale DW, Tustison C, Parker CG, Embley DW. Assessing clinical trial eligibility with logic expression queries. Data Knowl Eng. 2008;66(1):3–17.
6. Hruby GW, Boland MR, Cimino JJ, Gao J, Wilcox AB, Hirschberg J, et al.: Characterization of the Biomedical Query Mediation Process. In: Proc. of AMIA 2013 Clinical Research Informatics Summit. 2013; San Francisco, CA, 2013: 89–93.
7. Strötgen J, Gertz M. HeidelTime: high quality rule-based extraction and normalization of temporal expressions. In: Proc. of ACL; 2010. p. 321–4.
8. Pustejovsky J, Verhagen M. Semeval-2010 task 13: evaluating events, time expressions, and temporal relations (tempeval-2). In: Proc of ACL; 2009. p. 112–6.
9. Hao T, Liu H, Weng C. Valx: a system for extracting and structuring numeric lab test comparison statements from text. Methods Inf Med. 2016;55(3):266–75.
10. Hao T, Wei Y, Qiang J, Wang H, Lee K. The representation and extraction of quantitative information. In: Proc. of 13th Joint ISO - ACL Workshop Interoperable Semantic Annotation; 2017. p. 74–83.
11. Verhagen M, Sauri R, Caselli T, Pustejovsky J. Semeval-2010 Task 13: Tempeval-2. In: Proc. of the workshop on semantic evaluation, ACL; 2010. p. 57–62.
12. UzZaman N, Llorens H, Allen J, Derczynski L, Verhagen M, Pustejovsky J. Tempeval-3: Evaluating events, time expressions, and temporal relations. arXiv preprint arXiv. 2012;1206:5333.
13. Bethard S, Derczynski L, Savova G, Pustejovsky J, Verhagen M. SemEval-2015 task 6: clinical TempEval. In: Proc. of the 9th international workshop on semantic evaluation (SemEval-2015); 2015. p. 806–14.
14. Huang P, Huang H, Wang Y, Huang C, Chen H. NTU-1 at SemEval-2017 task 12: detection and classification of temporal events in clinical data with domain adaptation. In: Proc. of 11th international workshop on semantic evaluation (SemEval-2017); 2017. p. 1010–3.
15. Sohn S, Wagholikar K, Li D, Jonnalagadda SR, Tao C, Komandur ER, et al. Comprehensive temporal information detection from clinical text: medical events, time, and Tlink identification. J Am Med Inform Assoc. 2013;20(5): 836–42. https://doi.org/10.1136/amiajnl-2013-001622. Epub 2013 Apr 4
16. Sun W, Rumshisky A, Uzuner O. Evaluating temporal relations in clinical text: 2012 i2b2 challenge. J Am Med Inform Assoc. 2013;20(5):806–13.
17. Sun W, Rumshisky A, Uzuner O: Annotating temporal information in clinical narratives. J Biomed Inform. 2013;46:S5-12.
18. Styler IV, William F. THYME annotation guidelines. Technical report. 2014b;34
19. Bethard S, Savova G, Chen WT, Derczynski L, Pustejovsky J, Verhagen M. SemEval-2016 task 12: clinical TempEval. In: Proc. of 10th international workshop on semantic evaluation (SemEval-2016); 2016. p. 1052–62.
20. Tang B, Wu Y, Jiang M, Chen Y, Denny JC, Xu H. A hybrid system for temporal information extraction from clinical text. J Am Med Inform Assoc. 2013;20(5): 828–35. https://doi.org/10.1136/amiajnl-2013-001635. Epub 2013 Apr 9
21. Tao C, He Y, Poland G, Chute C, Yang H. Ontology-based time information representation of vaccine adverse events in Vaers for temporal analysis. Journal of Biomedical Semantics. 2012;3(1):13.
22. Li M, Patrick J. Extracting temporal information from electronic patient records. Proc. of AMIA Annu Symp Proc. 2012;2012:542–51.
23. Xu Y, Wang Y, Liu T, Tsujii J, Chang EI. An end-to-end system to identify temporal relation in discharge summaries: 2012 i2b2 challenge. J Am Med Inform Assoc. 2013;20(5):849–58. https://doi.org/10.1136/amiajnl-2012-001607. Epub 2013 Mar 6
24. Luo Z, Johnson S, Lai A, Weng C. Extracting temporal constraints from clinical research eligibility criteria using conditional random fields. In: Proc. of AMIA annual symposium; 2011. p. 843–52.
25. Chang YC, Dai HJ, Wu JC, Chen JM, Tsai RT, Hsu WL. TEMPTING system: a hybrid method of rule and machine learning for temporal relation extraction in patient discharge summaries. J Biomed Inform. 2013;46(Suppl): S54–62. https://doi.org/10.1016/j.jbi.2013.09.007. Epub 2013 Sep 20
26. Li H, Strotgen J, Zell J, Gertz M. Chinese temporal tagging with HeidelTime. In: Proc. of the 14th Conference of the European Chapter of the Association for Computational Linguistics. Gothenburg: ACL; 2014. p. 133–7.
27. Shen S, Su XN, Xie J, Wang DB. Construction of temporal expression extraction model based on Tsinghua Chinese treebank. Library and Information Service. 2012;6(18):127–32.
28. Zhou X, Li HLX, Duan H. Temporal expression recognition and temporal relationship extraction from Chinese narrative medical records. In: Proc of 5th International Conference on Bioinformatics and Biomedical Engineering; 2011. p. 1–4.
29. Yan Z, Ji D. Exploration of Chinese temporal information extraction based on CRF and semi-supervised learning. Computer Engineering and Design. 2015;36(6):1242–6.
30. Wu M, Li W, Lu Q, Li B. CTEMP: a Chinese temporal parser for extracting and normalizing temporal information. Lect Notes Comput Sci. 2005;3651:694–706.
31. Zhu S, Liu Z, Fu J, Zhu F. Chinese temporal phrase recognition based on conditional random fields. Computer Engineering and Design. 2011;37(15):164–7.
32. Liu L, He Z, Xing X, Mao X. Chinese time expression recognition based on semantic role. Application Research of Computers. 2011;28(7):2543–5.
33. Pustejovsky J, Castaño JM, Ingria R, Sauri R, Gaizauskas RJ, et al. Timeml: robust specification of event and temporal expressions in text. New directions in question answering. 2003;3:28–34.
34. Pustejovsky J, Castano J, Ingria R, Saurı R, Gaizauskas R, et al. Timeml: A specification language for temporal and event expressions. In: Proc. of the International Workshop of Computational Semantics; 2003. p. 193.
35. HeidelTime. https://code.google.com/p/heideltime/ (Accessed 15 June 2017).
36. IllinoisTemporalExtractor. http://cogcomp.org/page/software_view/illinois-time. (Accessed 15 June 2017).
37. GUTime. http://www.timeml.org/tarsqi/modules/gutime/index.html. (Accessed 15 June 2017).
38. SUTime. http://nlp.stanford.edu:8080/sutime/process (Accessed 15 June 2017).
39. NLTK Timex. https://github.com/nltk/nltk_contrib/tree/master/nltk_contrib (Accessed 15 June 2017).
40. CMedTEX. http://icrc.hitsz.edu.cn:8096/CMedTEX/ (Accessed 15 June 2017).

2

Patient facing decision support system for interpretation of laboratory test results

Georgy Kopanitsa[1,2*] and Ilia Semenov[3]

Abstract

Background: In some healthcare systems, it is common that patients address laboratory test centers directly without a physician's recommendation. This practice is widely spread in Russia with about 28% of patients who visiting laboratory test centers for diagnostics. This causes an issue when patients get no help from the physician in understanding the results.

Computer decision support systems proved to efficiently solve a resource consuming task of interpretation of the test results. So, a decision support system can be implemented to rise motivation and empower the patients who visit a laboratory service without a doctor's referral.

Methods: We have developed a clinical decision support system for patients that solves a classification task and finds a set of diagnoses for the provided laboratory tests results.

The Wilson and Lankton's assessment model was applied to measure patients' acceptance of the solution.

Results: A first order predicates-based decision support system has been implemented to analyze laboratory test results and deliver reports in natural language to patients. The evaluation of the system showed a high acceptance of the decision support system and of the reports that it generates.

Conclusions: Detailed notification of the laboratory service patients with elements of the decision support is significant for the laboratory data management, and for patients' empowerment and safety.

Keywords: Decision support, Laboratory information system, Telemedicine, First order predicates, User acceptance

Background

In some healthcare systems, it is common that patients address laboratory test centers directly without a physician's recommendation [1]. This practice is widely spread in Russia with about 28% of patients who visiting laboratory test centers for diagnostics [2]. This causes an issue when patients get no help from the physician in understanding the results. Patients face a problem when they need to decide how to continue the diagnostics and treatment process. A possible solution to this problem could be that a laboratory test center not only delivers the test results but also their explanation to the patients. This, however, should be done automatically, or at least semi-automatically, to exclude a critical load on the test centers. Clinical decision support systems can become a good technology for an automatic interpretation of test results [3, 4]. The experience in implementation of decision support systems for health care professionals shows their efficiency for medical diagnostics. However, patients require a different approach in data presentation and interpretation [5–11].

Studies [12–15] have demonstrated that many providers do not have systems that can ensure that the test results are reliably communicated to patients. As shown in [16, 17] normal and abnormal test results are commonly missed, even when a health care system widely uses electronic health records (EHRs), and providers miss 1–10% of abnormal test results. It would not be an exaggeration to say that we do not have sufficient mechanisms to ensure that test results are consistently delivered to patients and understood by them.

As a problem importance is recognized, a number of potential solutions has been studied [18–23]. The first approach originates from the development of computerized

* Correspondence: georgy.kopanitsa@gmail.com
[1]Institute Cybernetic Center, Tomsk Polytechnic University, Lenina 30, 634050 Tomsk, Russia
[2]Tomsk State University for Architecture and Building, Tomsk, Russia
Full list of author information is available at the end of the article

decision support systems that support test centers in reviewing results and notifying patients in case of abnormal results [18, 19, 21, 23]. Another approach has involved implementation of such testing processes where test centers consistently deliver test results directly to patients. Such systems vary from sending each piece of the test results by mail to complex patient web portals, where they can have access to the history of test results [20, 24].

Interpretation of the test results is a resource consuming task that delays the results and increases costs of each test [25, 26]. However, the computer decision support systems proved to solve such tasks efficiently. To increase motivation and support the patients who refer to a test center without a doctor's referral in making better informed decisions, a computer decision support system can be designed and implemented.

The goal of this study is to develop and evaluate a decision support system for patients, which:

a) provides a personalized tool to inform patients on the results of the laboratory tests
b) empowers patients to form opinions on how to continue or not to continue with a treatment
c) prepares patients to have an informed discussion with their doctor.

To support patients, we have implemented and evaluated a decision support system that automatically generates interpretations for laboratory test results:

This paper focuses on the evaluation of correctness and user acceptance of a decision support system for patients of a test center in Saint-Petersburg, Russia.

Methods

Implementation

We have developed a clinical decision support system for the patients that solves a classification problem by connecting test results to a list of diagnoses. The decision support is based on a classification algorithm, which produces the following conclusions:

- Located a list of diagnoses that can be related to the test results;
- Found no fitting diagnoses;

To enable a definition of inference rules we have developed a knowledge representation language that is based on the predicate calculus [27] and a user interface to allow medical professionals defining the system rules. For the pilot project, we have chosen a limited set of laboratory tests that could be automatically interpreted by the system. We have interviewed 3 laboratory physicians and 3 specialist physicians (gynecologist, urologist and general practitioner) to define the inference rules for the system.

The decision support system has been implemented and operating in the Helix laboratory center in Saint-Petersburg, Russia.

The system has been implemented using the following technologies:

1. User interfaces and a back-end are based on the. NET Core 2.0
2. Data storage is based on PostgreSQL

Evaluation

Accuracy of the decision support

To evaluate accuracy of the results produced by the system, we have performed a validation of 1000 randomly generated reports. The reports were generated in a way to allow validating all of 89 decision support algorithms. The reports were given to two independent pathology experts to be reviewed independently. The results of the expert review were used to calculate the following criteria [28]:

1. Error rate as an average classification error
2. Accuracy as an average effectiveness of a classifier
3. Precision ((All terms – Mistakes)/All terms),
4. Recall (ratio of true positives to (true positives + false negatives)), and
5. F-measure ($2\cdot\frac{recall\cdot precision}{recall+precision}$).

The reviewers' disagreements were settled by consensus. Cohen's kappa was calculated to rate the disagreement between reviewers [29].

User acceptance

To assess the user acceptance of the system, a Wilson and Lankton's model of patients' acceptance of electronic health solutions was applied [30]. The model allowed measuring the following criteria: behavioral intention (BI) to use, intrinsic motivation (IM), perceived ease-of-use (PEOU), and perceived usefulness (PU) of the decision support system.

BI represents the intention to utilize the system and to rely on the decision support that it provides; IM represents the willingness to use the system provided that no direct compensation is available; PEOU represents the extent to which the provided reports are clearly presented and comprehended by users; and PU denotes the degree to which the patients believe that the utilization of the decision support system will improve their experience with laboratory tests.

We have applied a Wilson's and Lankton [30] revision of the Davis's et al. [31] method to measure BI, PEOU, and PU. Intrinsic motivation was measured by utilizing the Davis's et al. method [31].

Questionnaire

We started with detection of possible items for the questionnaire by collecting a large list of acceptance test questions. The questions were collected from preceding internal studies, from the literature and from brainstorming. The list was then reviewed by the study team to eliminate the items that do not help to reach the goals of the study and duplicate questions. The remaining items were simplified and worded as clear to the potential participants as possible.

BI measure consisted of 2 objects whereas IM, PEOU, and PU consisted of 3 objects each. Russian translation of the questionnaires made by the research team was used during the study. To rate each item a Likert scale from 1 (not at all) to 7 (very much) was applied [32].

Recruitment

The recruitment of the study participants was done in Saint-Petersburg, Russia. The patients were eligible to be invited if they had experience using the system with a minimum of 5 reports on the test outcomes. The recruitment was done by sending invitations to the 500 eligible patients. Later, we have formed a group of 120 patients based on the first responded – first included principal with a recruitment rate of 24%.

Demographic characteristics of the study participants are shown in Table 1. We assessed Information technology (IT) literacy of the patients based on how frequently they use smartphones or personal computer. We assessed IT literacy on the scale from beginners – patients who started using computer or smartphone maximum 6 months before the study begin; intermediate – computer or smartphone users who do it at least 2 times a week; and advanced – daily users of a computer or a smartphone.

Data collection and analysis

All the study participants were given individual access to the online questionnaire, which they were asked to fill in (please see Additional file 1 for the questionnaire details). All the patients received a written detailed instruction on how to operate with a questionnaire and the sense of the rating scale.

GNU Octave [33] version 4.0.2 was applied to calculate the statistics of the participants' general characteristics and user acceptance measurements.

Ethics commission approval

The study was approved by the ethics commission of the committee of healthcare of Saint-Petersburg, Russia. All the study participants were informed in written form about the goals of the study and about the meaning of the questionnaires. We assured in written form every participant of their rights to anonymity and confidentiality. Written consent was obtained from every participant. Every participant was informed in written form about a right to withdraw personal data from the study record for up to 3 months after their approval.

Results

Implementation

The clinical decision support system consists of the following modules, which provide the main features of the system (Fig. 1):

- A Data extraction system receives data from external sources, such as hospital or laboratory information systems. It checks the syntax validity of data and sends it to a Database
- A Data base receives and saves facts from an external laboratory information system.
- A Knowledge base editor (see section "User acceptance".1) provides an interface to experts to define inference rules that are sent to a Knowledge base.
- A Knowledge base stores inference rules.
- Inference engine applies rules from the knowledge base to the facts from the Database to conclude the results and sends them to the explanation system and report generator.
- Explanation system scrutinizes the sequence of the applied inference rules to demonstrate how the result has been achieved.
- Report generator creates a readable report from the inference results and sends it to the report storage.

The example of how the system operates is presented in section "Inference example".

Table 1 Demographic characteristics of the study participants

Gender	Average age	Age > 60	Education			IT habits		
			Higher	Secondary	Below secondary	Beginners	Intermediate	Advanced
56 Males	41.3	16	18	28	10	6	34	16
64 Females	42.3	12	22	36	6	16	8	0
Total 120		28	30	64	16	22	42	16

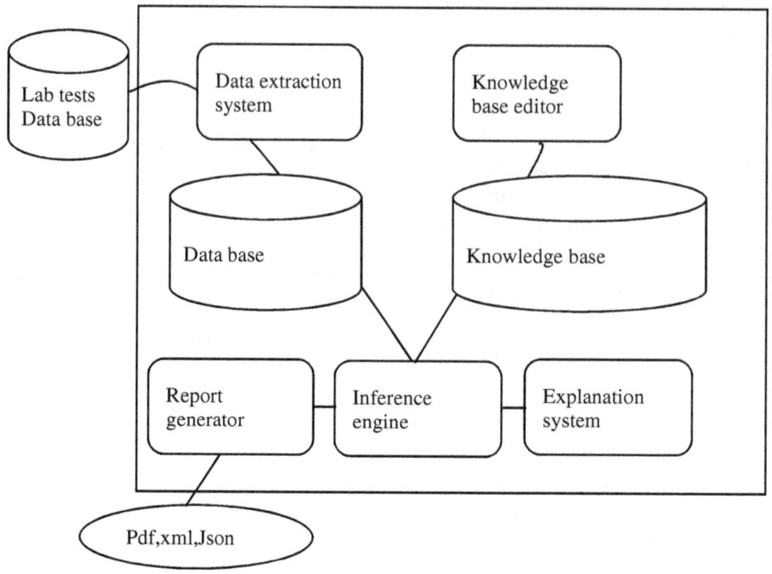

Fig. 1 Structural scheme of the decision support system

The knowledge representation language of the system is built upon a first order predicate logic. The scheme of the knowledge base is shown in Fig. 2.

- The main object that the system processes is a laboratory test configuration that consists a laboratory test object and of a list of direct inference rules that can be related to this object.
- Laboratory test object is a model that comprises a list of atomic components of the test e.g. a complete blood count test includes 22 atomic components.
- For each component of a test, we define a list of direct inference rules that have conditions for including this components in the inference. The conditions are represented as comparison operators: =, <>, includes (> = or = <), excludes (> = and = <).

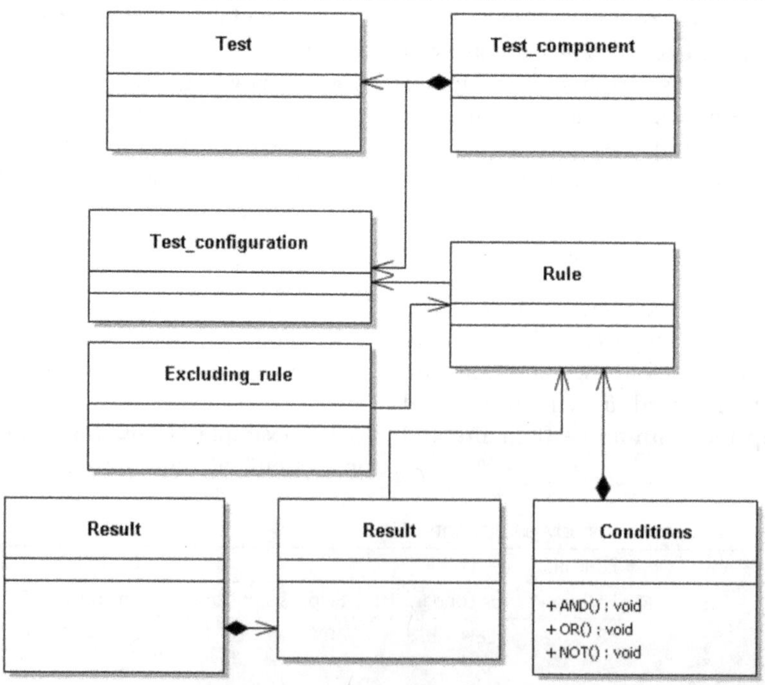

Fig. 2 Object model of the system

Within a rule, the conditions are related by logical operators "and", "or" and "not".

- For each direct rule, an expert can model a list of exclusion rules to exclude a direct rule from an inference process if the exclusion conditions are met.
- An order the object groups laboratory tests reflect the commercial orders that patients actually make.

General inference process is divided into the following steps:

1. When the system receives an order bundle from a laboratory information system, the tests in the order are being analyzed to generate a list of tests, configurations for which are available in the knowledge base.
2. Actual test results are loaded to the Database of the system and become available for an inference process.
3. The inference engine receives the list of tests and selects proper direct inference rules and exclusion rules in the proper sequence, which can be applied to the received facts.
4. If a direct rule has been successfully applied and no exclusion rule is effective, the inference engine adds a text artefact to the resulting json file (Fig. 3).
5. After the inference has been completed, the resulting json file is sent to the reporting service to generate a pdf report.

The decision support system has been implemented in the Helix laboratory service in Saint-Petersburg, Russia. The system is in commercial production now generating about 20,000 reports a day.

The system has inference algorithms for the following International Statistical Classification of Diseases and Related Health Problems (ICD) 10 groups:

1. Kidney:
   1.1. N30 Cystitis
   1.2. N04 Nephrotic syndrome
   1.3. N39 Other disorders of urinary system
   1.4. N10 Acute pyelonephritis
2. Liver:
   2.1. K75 Other inflammatory liver diseases
   2.2. K72 Hepatic failure, not elsewhere classified

[
{
"Id": 107201,
"GroupName": "ESR Level",
"Severity": 148,
"Text": "The CBC determined your erythrocyte sedimentation rate (ESR). \n ESR is most impacted by the count, shape, and size of red blood cells (RBCs), and physicochemical properties of the blood. Changes in ESR levels may be caused by various conditions and are often non-specific, which means they do not help identify the cause.\n You have a normal ESR."
},
{
"Id": 107116,
"GroupName": "WBC differential count",
"Severity": 61,
"Text": "The CBC assessed the following parameters: total WBC count (blood cells involved in protection of the body against infections and foreign agents) and WBC differential count (relative numbers of each type of WBC).\n Your test result suggests that you have eosinophilia – elevated counts of eosinophils in the blood (eosinophils are WBCs that are involved in developing allergic reactions and fighting parasitic infections). Changes of this type are most commonly seen in various allergic reactions or parasitic infections. Less often, similar changes in the CBC may be found in a range of various pathologic conditions, including some autoimmune diseases. Eosinophil counts may also be elevated by some medications.\n You should consult your physician to specify the cause of the change in your eosinophil count."
},
{
"Id": 107106,
"GroupName": "Platelet Hemostasis",
"Severity": 51,
"Text": "The CBC assessed the following parameters: platelets, platelet indices.\n You do not have signs of impaired platelet hemostasis, platelet counts are normal, major platelet indices are not changed."
},
{
"Id": 107089,
"GroupName": "Signs of Anemia and General Erythropoiesis Status",
"Severity": 33,
"Text": "The CBC assessed the following parameters: RBC count, hemoglobin level, RBC indices (size and shape of RBCs, hemoglobin concentration in RBCs).\Your test result shows that you have signs of erythrocytosis – a condition in which blood RBC counts are elevated.\n the most common cause of an elevated RBC count is long-term hypoxia (inadequate oxygen supply). It is found in chronic lung diseases, in alpine sickness (in individuals who live in the mountains, in mountaineers), in smokers. Erythrocytosis may also be found in other diseases, including polycythemia vera.\n You should consult your physician or hematologist to determine the cause of your erythrocytosis."
}
]

Fig. 3 Results of the inference in a json format

2.3. K71 Toxic liver disease
2.4. K81 Cholecystitis
3. Pancreas:
3.1. K85 Acute pancreatitis
4. Thyroid gland
4.1. E05 Thyrotoxicosis
4.2. E03 Other hypothyroidism
5. Red blood cells:
5.1. D50 Iron deficiency anemia
6. White blood cells:
6.1. D72 Other disorders of white blood cells
7. Prostate:
7.1. N41 Inflammatory diseases of prostate

Inference example

The full json code of rules and artefacts for the blood sugar testis presented in Additional file 2. The input of the inference is a bundle of resources that has been extracted from a laboratory tests database and were added to the decision support system database (Fig. 1):

1. Patient
2. Observation: Concentration of HbA1C, mmol/mol
3. Observation: Concentration of HbA1C, %
4. Observation: Concentration of Hb, mmol/mol
5. Observation: Concentration of Glucose in Plasma, mmol/L
6. Observation: Concentration of C-Peptide, pmol/L

After the system receives the actual values, an inference engine starts building an inference sequence (see Additional file 2. Inference sequence for the rules details and Fig. 4 for the graphical representation of the sequence) based on the available rules from the knowledge base (Fig. 1).

The inference ends up with the conclusion id = 4785 with the artefact id = 4786. The found artefact is added to the generated report, which is then sent to the report generator to create a human readable pdf file. The resulting rules sequence is being visualized by the explanation system (Fig. 1).

User interaction

The decision support system consists of 2 main interfaces: for experts to model knowledge and inference rules and for patients to have access to the test results and their interpretation.

Expert's interface

We have developed a web knowledge management application that provides the following features:

- Create and edit inference rules
- Group inference rules
- Create and edit artefacts with doctor's recommendations that form a decision support report as a result of a logical inference.

Fig. 5 shows an inference rule creation screen. A rule consists of several conditions connected by logical operators and a resulting artefact, which represents a text

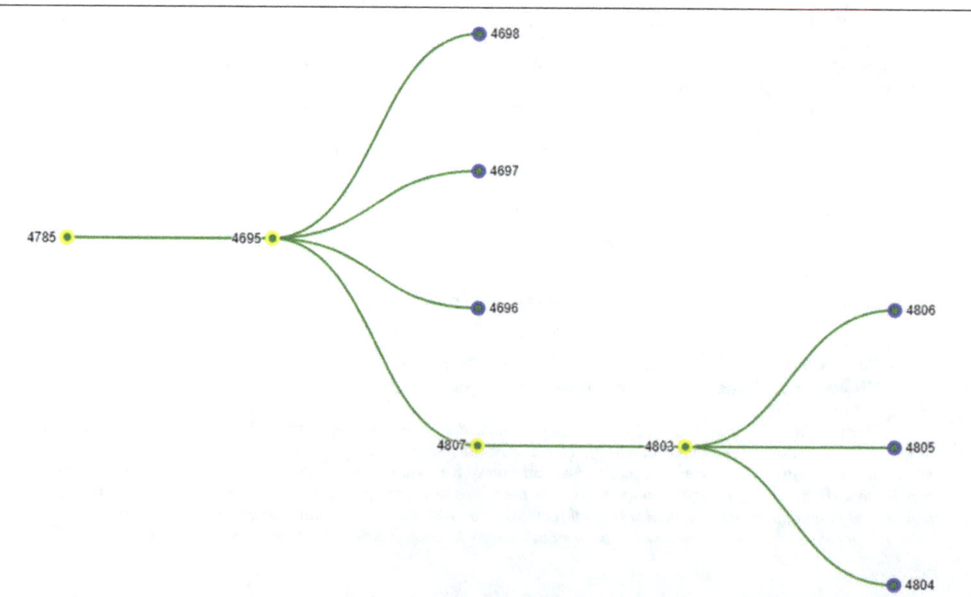

Fig. 4 Inference rules sequence

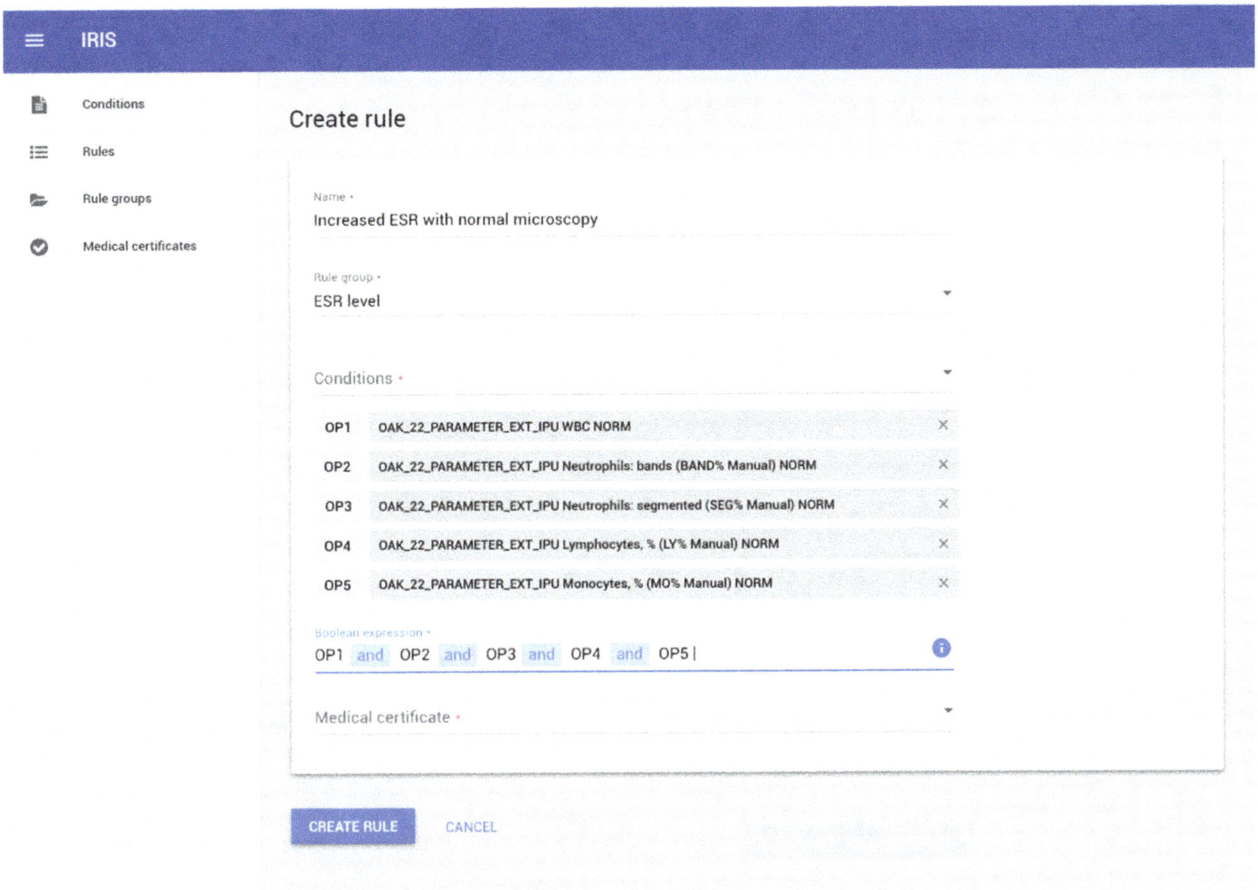

Fig. 5 Create rule interface for an expert

with recommendations to the patient. The artefacts can be created using an interface from Fig. 6.

Patient's user interface

Patient has access to the test results through a web portal, where a list of available tests is provided. For each test, a patient can have an overview of the results (Fig. 7). The results are presented in the table form with the following columns: Parameter name, My Results and a Reference interval. A patient can click on the "Generate report" button (second button from the left with a doctor icon on the Fig. 7) to open a decision support report (Fig. 8).

Evaluation

Correctness

A sample of 1000 reports was independently assessed by two independent pathology experts. The results of assessment for each criterion are shown in Table 2. The experts revealed disagreement in the assessment of 2 reports.

Acceptance

The mean values for BI, IM, PEOU, and PU (5.9, 6.2, 5.7, and 5.9 respectively) showed a high acceptance of the decision support system and the reports that it generates (Table 3).

Discussion

The paper describes a development of a patient facing clinical decision support system, which provides interpretation of the test results in the natural language.

Notification ethics

We need to be very cautious when providing test results to the patients by e-mail or on a web portal. We should assume that the patients may not fully and properly comprehend the interpretation of the results. So, the capability to deliver results and their interpretation in a manner they are understood by a patient is essential for a motivation to refer to a health care professional, particularly when test results are abnormal. Our decision support system only interprets and sends test results that do not need a humane communication according to the standards of the laboratory service. Test results that

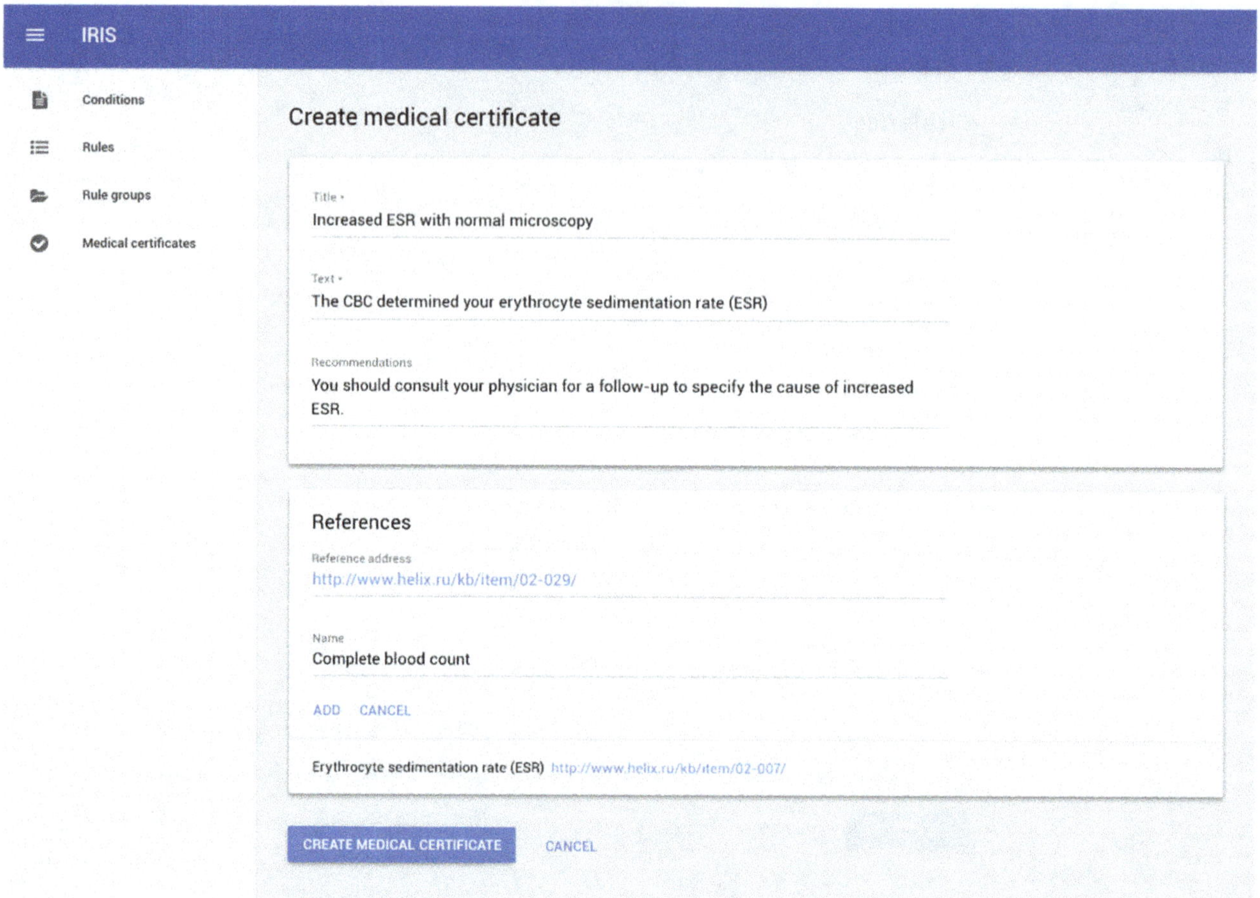

Fig. 6 Expert's interface for recommendations

can be communicated only in person include positive HIV test, all kinds of hepatitis and all kind of positive cancer tests.

The decision support system never intended to be prescriptive and communicate a single possible clinical decision to a patient. To follow this approach, we have implemented the reports in a way that they are descriptive and informative rather than prescriptive.

Correctness

Rules definition process shall be controlled and always reviewed. The evaluation showed that the correctness of the generated reports is high. Seven mistakes out of 1000 analyzed reports were caused by a human factor. The mistakes that were detected by the experts during the assessment were caused by the inaccuracies of the experts when modelling inference rules. This led to a change of rules' definition procedure, where we apply 4 eyes principle [34]. Now, when each rule goes to production only after a review and acceptance of a second expert.

Use acceptance

One of the measures of feasibility was the percent of patients who agreed to take part in the testing of the decision support tool. The rate of 86% of patients who agreed to take part in the study shows high interest and motivation, which is supported by quantitative measurements that were done within the study.

The user acceptance of the system was evaluated after 2 months of operation. Acceptance scores were high, all of them above 5.7 out of 7. Among elder users (60+) the results were a little worse in comparison to the younger users. The maximum difference was 0.7 (10%) for the PU. Elder people felt less motivated about storing their medical data in electronic format (5.0 versus 5.7 for the younger participants). Maximum rates were similar for each statement and age group, and a high median value also indicates a positive attitude to the system. Minimum rates of 4 show an encouragement towards the system, as all the rates were in the positive part of the scale. This is true for all age groups. This indicates high acceptance of the solution and the way the notifications are being delivered.

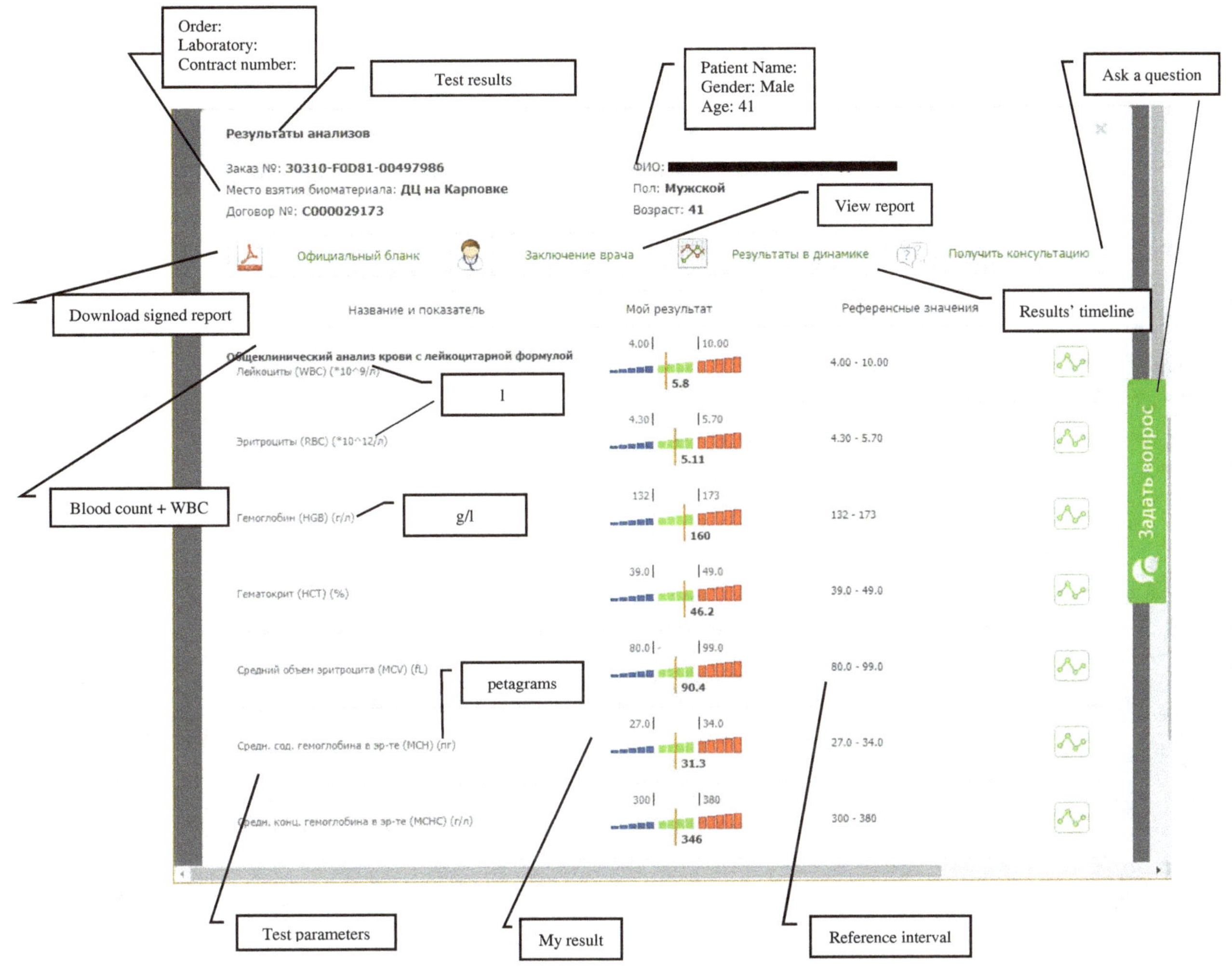

Fig. 7 Personal space for a patient on the online portal

Partial correlations calculated using scales derived for these dimensions suggested that Ease of Use and Usefulness impact one another in a way that enhancements in Ease of Use increase the scores of Usefulness and the other way round. Whereas both Ease of Use and Usefulness steer Satisfaction with Usefulness having comparatively less significant influence. Users are more flexible in their Usefulness scores when they have only reduced experience with a system.

Unfortunately, we could not compare them to the similar studies, as we did not find a patient-oriented decision support system, for which a user acceptance was evaluated. However, we tried to compare the results with similar systems that were not patient oriented.

Acceptance scores were relatively high compared to the results of evaluation results of previous studies [35–38] management smartphone app. This can be explained by the fact that most of the study participants had average or above average IT skills. This is in a contrast with the previous studies on the patients' acceptance of decision support tools and can be explained by the increased computer literacy and changing IT habits. Our results mean that the health care providers and EHR developers can move in the direction of electronic notifications of the patients. This will facilitate communication and decrease its costs.

Implications

The results of our study support other literature suggesting that patients want timely and detailed information and they want to be notified of all laboratory test results, even if they are normal [39, 40]. However, our results contradict the previous ones in regards to the patients preferring phone calls and sealed letters to the web based notification methods [40].

The findings of this research have valuable inferences for the design and implementation of patient notification

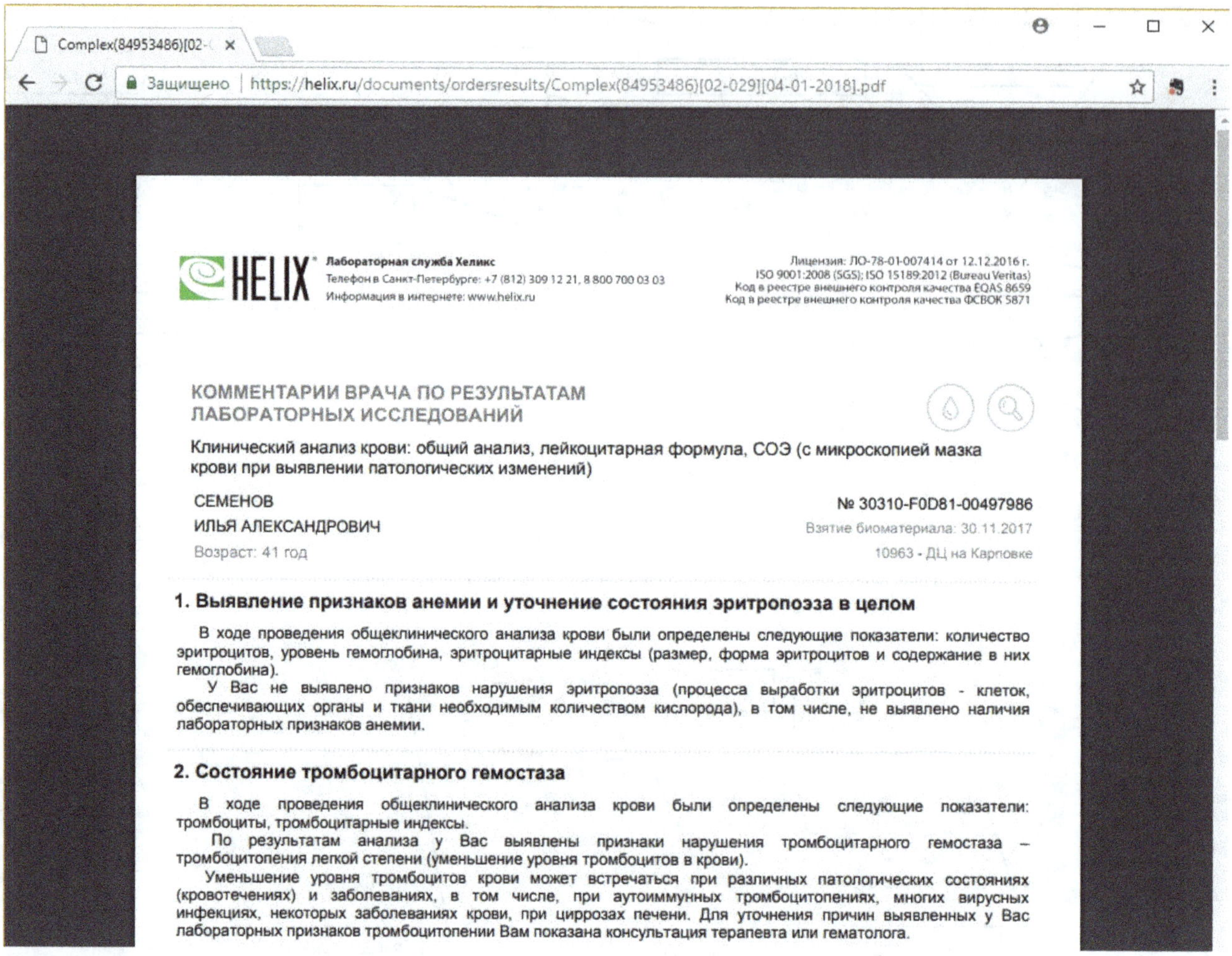
Complex(84953486)[02-
Защищено | https://helix.ru/documents/ordersresults/Complex(84953486)[02-029][04-01-2018].pdf

HELIX Лабораторная служба Хеликс
Телефон в Санкт-Петербурге: +7 (812) 309 12 21, 8 800 700 03 03
Информация в интернете: www.helix.ru

Лицензия: ЛО-78-01-007414 от 12.12.2016 г.
ISO 9001:2008 (SGS); ISO 15189:2012 (Bureau Veritas)
Код в реестре внешнего контроля качества EQAS 8659
Код в реестре внешнего контроля качества ФСВОК 5871

КОММЕНТАРИИ ВРАЧА ПО РЕЗУЛЬТАТАМ ЛАБОРАТОРНЫХ ИССЛЕДОВАНИЙ

Клинический анализ крови: общий анализ, лейкоцитарная формула, СОЭ (с микроскопией мазка крови при выявлении патологических изменений)

СЕМЕНОВ
ИЛЬЯ АЛЕКСАНДРОВИЧ
Возраст: 41 год

№ 30310-F0D81-00497986
Взятие биоматериала: 30.11.2017
10963 - ДЦ на Карповке

1. Выявление признаков анемии и уточнение состояния эритропоэза в целом

В ходе проведения общеклинического анализа крови были определены следующие показатели: количество эритроцитов, уровень гемоглобина, эритроцитарные индексы (размер, форма эритроцитов и содержание в них гемоглобина).

У Вас не выявлено признаков нарушения эритропоэза (процесса выработки эритроцитов - клеток, обеспечивающих органы и ткани необходимым количеством кислорода), в том числе, не выявлено наличия лабораторных признаков анемии.

2. Состояние тромбоцитарного гемостаза

В ходе проведения общеклинического анализа крови были определены следующие показатели: тромбоциты, тромбоцитарные индексы.

По результатам анализа у Вас выявлены признаки нарушения тромбоцитарного гемостаза – тромбоцитопения легкой степени (уменьшение уровня тромбоцитов в крови).

Уменьшение уровня тромбоцитов крови может встречаться при различных патологических состояниях (кровотечениях) и заболеваниях, в том числе, при аутоиммунных тромбоцитопениях, многих вирусных инфекциях, некоторых заболеваниях крови, при циррозах печени. Для уточнения причин выявленных у Вас лабораторных признаков тромбоцитопении Вам показана консультация терапевта или гематолога.

Translation from Russian:
Doctor's comments on the results of the laboratory test
Clinical Blood Test: blood count, white blood cells, Erythrocyte Sedimentation Rate

1. **Anemia and a state of erythropoiesis.**
   During the general blood test, the following parameters were measured: the number of erythrocytes, the level of hemoglobin, erythrocyte indices (the size of the form of erythrocytes and the content of hemoglobin in them). You have no signs of disturbance of erythropoiesis (the process of producing erythrocytes - cells that provide organs and tissues with the necessary amount of oxygen), including the absence of laboratory signs of anemia.
2. **The state of thrombocytic hemostasis**
   During the general blood analysis, the following parameters were measured: platelets, platelet indices. On the results of the analysis, you showed signs of a disorder of platelet hemostasis -thrombocytopenia of mild degree (decrease in the level of platelets in the blood). This can be caused by various pathological conditions (bleeding) and diseases including autoimmune thrombocytopenia, many viral infections, in some cases of cirrhosis of the liver. To clarify the reasons for the laboratory signs of thrombocytopenia revealed by the test, you are advised a consultation of a therapist or hematologist.

Fig. 8 Report, produced by a decision support system

systems. We found that patients in general find the detailed notifications useful, are motivated to use them and don't face significant difficulties to adopt such solutions. It is very important when designing and implementing patients' notification systems to make them valid, easy and simple to use. To achieve this, we advise that a pilot application of the decision support system is tested by the experts for verification and validation of the rules and potential users for the user acceptance, so that corrections can be made during the implementation phase to increase the system's reliability and acceptance.

The results of our study suggest that there is a major impact of patients' habits on the test results notification

Table 2 Reports' quality evaluation

Analyzed reports	Error rate	Accuracy	Precision	Recall	F-measure	Cohen's kappa
1000	7 (0.7%)	0.	0.99	0.99	0.99	0.99

utilization. In addition to the unswerving and natural effect of habit on IT use, a habit also functions as a stowed purpose trail to affect behavior. Promotion of electronic test results notifications still demands major communication effort to strengthen both the stowed intention and its relation to behavior.

Legal

It is important to mention that in Russia laboratory ervices are legally obliged to provide results of laboratory tests to patients. Providing not only the results but the explanations of their meaning will enhance the notifications and make them more valuable for patients.

Limitations of the study and future work

Tool's impact on patients' decision-making

We did not thoroughly gather data on participants' decision to follow up or not laboratory tests especially for the tests with abnormal results. This will become a major part of our next study where we will investigate how the patients decide to follow up or not laboratory tests. A systematic review by Callen et al. found that, across 19 published studies, 6.8–62% of lab tests were not followed up on [41, 42]. We think that this rate will increase for the patients that receive detailed information about the test results and their possible implications.

Evolving the decision support system

We are evolving the decision support system every day by adding new inference rules and optimizing its architecture. The next steps would be to add a possibility of working with fuzzy rules [43] to make the inference more flexible. Also, we are redesigning a data storage architecture to move from relational data base to a graph data base, that in our mind is more suitable for modeling knowledge and inference rules.

Mobile application for the patients is also under development now. This can potentially involve younger users to the system.

Conclusions

The findings of the research provide us with a better understanding of how patients experience detailed notification of laboratory tests without health care professional participating in the process. Detailed notification of laboratory service patients with the elements of decision support is significant for laboratory data

Table 3 Acceptance criteria

Criterion, Item	Entire group (120 participants)				> 60 (28 participants)				< 60 (92 participants)			
	Mean	Median	Max	Min	Mean	Median	Max	Min	Mean	Median	Max	Min
Behavioral intention to use	5.9				5.6				6.1			
I intend to use the tool to understand my test results	5.7	5	7	4	5.5	5.5	6	4	5.8	6	7	5
I feel like I will use it in the future	6.1	5.5	7	5	5.7	5.5	7	5	6.3	6	7	5
Intrinsic motivation	6.2				6.1				6.2			
I find the system useful for me	6.2	6	7	6	6.0	6	7	6	6.2	6	7	6
The system helps me to make more informed decisions	5.9	5.5	7	4	5.7	5.5	6	4	6.0	6	7	5
The system is reliable and I trust it	6.4	6	7	5	6.3	6	6	5	6.4	6	7	5
Perceived ease of use	5.7				5.6				6.1			
The reports are clear and understandable	6.3	6	7	6	6.2	6	7	6	6.4	6.5	7	6
It is easy to access the reports	5.7	6	7	5	5.5	5.5	7	5	5.8	6	7	6
I like that I can keep all my reports in the electronic format	5.4	5.5	7	4	5.0	5	6	4	5.7	6	7	5
Perceived usefulness	5.9				5.5				6.2			
Using the system enhances the effectiveness of managing my health conditions	5.7	5.5	7	5	5.0	5	6	5	6.0	6	7	6
It explains me what my health status is	6.1	6	7	5	5.9	5.5	6	5	6.3	6.5	7	6
I can provide all the information about my test results to any doctor I visit	5.9	6	7	5	5.9	6	7	5	5.9	6	7	5

management, and for patients' empowerment and safety. We suppose that patients empowered in such way can play a significant role in the process of delivering test results to the physicians, which positively affects the efficiently of a diagnostics and treatment process.

Abbreviations

BI: Behavioral intention to use; EHR: Electronic health record; ICD: International Statistical Classification of Diseases and Related Health Problems; IM: Intrinsic motivation,; IT: Information technology; LIS: Laboratory information system; PC: Personal computer; PEOU: Perceived ease-of-use; PU: Perceived usefulness

Acknowledgements

Preliminary results of this work have been presented at a conference at Tomsk Polytechnic University.

Funding

The research is funded from Russian Science Foundation (RSF), The research was at Tomsk Polytechnic University within the framework of Tomsk Polytechnic University Competitiveness Enhancement Program grant.
The funding bodies did not play any roles in the design of the study and collection, analysis, and interpretation of data and in writing the manuscript.

Authors' contributions

GK was responsible for a literature review, setting up the concept and methods and writing the manuscript. IS was responsible for the implementation and evaluation of the system. Both authors read and approved the final version of the manuscript.

Competing interests

The authors declare that they have no competing interests.

Author details

[1]Institute Cybernetic Center, Tomsk Polytechnic University, Lenina 30, 634050 Tomsk, Russia. [2]Tomsk State University for Architecture and Building, Tomsk, Russia. [3]Medlinx LLC, Saint-Petersburg, Russia.

References

1. Semenov I, Kopanitsa G. Development of a clinical decision support system for the patients of a laboratory service. Stud Health Technol Inform. 2016;228:90–4.
2. Arhangelskaya E. Laboratory services, how to enter the business, that grows 20–45% a year. In. https://www.rbc.ru/magazine/2016/09/57bc29549a794702a314361f: rbc 2016.
3. Ahmadian L, van Engen-Verheul M, Bakhshi-Raiez F, et al. The role of standardized data and terminological systems in computerized clinical decision support systems: literature review and survey. Int J Med Inform. 2011;80:81–93.
4. Jo S, Park HA. Development and evaluation of a smartphone application for managing gestational diabetes mellitus. Healthc Inform Res. 2016;22:11–21.
5. Kopanitsa G. Standard based multiclient medical data visualization. Stud Health Technol Inform. 2012;180:199–203.
6. Kopanitsa G. Evaluation study for a multi-user oriented medical data visualization method. Stud Health Technol Inform. 2014;200:158–60.
7. Kopanitsa G, Tsvetkova Z, Veseli H. Analysis of metrics for the usability evaluation of EHR management systems. Stud Health Technol Inform. 2012;180:358–62.
8. Kopanitsa G, Tsvetkova Z, Veseli H. Analysis of metrics for the usability evaluation of electronic health record systems. Stud Health Technol Inform. 2012;174:129–33.
9. Lin YL, Guerguerian AM, Tomasi J, et al. Usability of data integration and visualization software for multidisciplinary pediatric intensive care: a human factors approach to assessing technology. BMC Med Inform Decis Mak. 2017;17:122.
10. Skyttberg N, Vicente J, Chen R, et al. How to improve vital sign data quality for use in clinical decision support systems? A qualitative study in nine Swedish emergency departments. BMC Med Inform Decis Mak. 2016;16
11. Madkour M, Benhaddou D, Tao C. Temporal data representation, normalization, extraction, and reasoning: a review from clinical domain. Comput Methods Prog Biomed. 2016;128:52–68.
12. Murff HJ, Gandhi TK, Karson AK, et al. Primary care physician attitudes concerning follow-up of abnormal test results and ambulatory decision support systems. Int J Med Inform. 2003;71:137–49.
13. Poon EG, Gandhi TK, Sequist TD, et al. "I wish I had seen this test result earlier!": dissatisfaction with test result management systems in primary care. Arch Intern Med. 2004;164:2223–8.
14. Montes A, Francis M, Ciulla AP. Assessing the delivery of patient critical laboratory results to primary care providers. Clin Lab Sci. 2014;27:139–42.
15. Litchfield IJ, Bentham LM, Lilford RJ, et al. Adaption, implementation and evaluation of collaborative service improvements in the testing and result communication process in primary care from patient and staff perspectives: a qualitative study. BMC Health Serv Res. 2017;17:615.
16. Casalino LP, Dunham D, Chin MH, et al. Frequency of failure to inform patients of clinically significant outpatient test results. Arch Intern Med. 2009;169:1123–9.
17. Sung S, Forman-Hoffman V, Wilson MC, Cram P. Direct reporting of laboratory test results to patients by mail to enhance patient safety. J Gen Intern Med. 2006;21:1075–8.
18. Matheny ME, Gandhi TK, Orav EJ, et al. Impact of an automated test results management system on patients' satisfaction about test result communication. Arch Intern Med. 2007;167:2233–9.
19. Laxmisan A, Sittig DF, Pietz K, et al. Effectiveness of an electronic health record-based intervention to improve follow-up of abnormal pathology results: a retrospective record analysis. Med Care. 2012;50:898–904.
20. Edmonds SW, Wolinsky FD, Christensen AJ, et al. The PAADRN study: a design for a randomized controlled practical clinical trial to improve bone health. Contemp Clin Trials. 2013;34:90–100.
21. Main C, Moxham T, Wyatt JC, et al. Computerised decision support systems in order communication for diagnostic, screening or monitoring test ordering: systematic reviews of the effects and cost-effectiveness of systems. England: NHS R & D HTA Programme (Great Britain); National Co-ordinating Centre for HTA (Great Britain), NIHR Health Technology Assessment Programme; 2010. p. 1–227.
22. Carmona-Cejudo JM, Hortas ML, Baena-García M, et al. DB4US: a decision support system for laboratory information management. Interact J Med Res. 2012;1:e16.
23. Sepulveda JL, Young DS, Carmona-Cejudo JM, et al. The ideal laboratory information system DB4US: A decision support system for laboratory information management. Arch Pathol Lab Med. 2013;137:1129–40.
24. Wald JS, Burk K, Gardner K, et al. Sharing electronic laboratory results in a patient portal–a feasibility pilot. Stud Health Technol Inform. 2007;129:18–22.
25. Haeckel R, Wosniok W, Arzideh F. Proposed classification of various limit values (guide values) used in assisting the interpretation of quantitative laboratory test results. Clin Chem Lab Med. 2009;47:494–7.
26. Romatowski J. Problems in interpretation of clinical laboratory test results. J Am Vet Med Assoc. 1994;205:1186–8.
27. Michalski RS. Pattern recognition as rule-guided inductive inference. IEEE Trans Pattern Anal Mach Intell. 1980;2:349–61.
28. Kawada T. Sample size in receiver-operating characteristic (ROC) curve analysis. Circ J. 2012;76:768. author reply 769
29. Berry KJ, Johnston JE, Mielke PW, Jr. Weighted kappa for multiple raters. Percept Mot Skills 2008; 107: 837–848.
30. Wilson EV, Lankton NK. Modeling patients' acceptance of provider-delivered e-health. J Am Med Inform Assoc. 2004;11:241–8.
31. Davis FD, Bagozzi RP, Warshaw PR. User acceptance of computer technology: a comparison of two theoretical models. Manag Sci. 1989;35:982_1003.
32. Drinkwater BL. A comparison of the direction-of-perception technique with the Likert method in the measurement of attitudes. J Soc Psychol. 1965;67:189–96.
33. Rogel-Salazar J. Essential MATLAB and octave. Boca Raton: Taylor & Francis, CRC Press; 2015.
34. HM RW. Applying the four-eyes principle to management decisions in the manufacturing sector: are large family firms one-eye blind? Manag Res Rev. 2015;38:264–82.
35. Kuo KM, Liu CF, Ma CC. An investigation of the effect of nurses' technology readiness on the acceptance of mobile electronic medical record systems. BMC Med Inform Decis Mak. 2013;13:88.

36. Chen IJ, Yang KF, Tang FI, et al. Applying the technology acceptance model to explore public health nurses' intentions towards web-based learning: a cross-sectional questionnaire survey. Int J Nurs Stud. 2008;45:869–78.
37. Guo SH, Lin YH, Chen RR, et al. Development and evaluation of theory-based diabetes support services. Comput Inform Nurs. 2013;31:17–26. quiz 27–18
38. Vallance JK, Courneya KS, Taylor LM, et al. Development and evaluation of a theory-based physical activity guidebook for breast cancer survivors. Health Educ Behav. 2008;35:174–89.
39. Campbell L, Watkins RM, Teasdale C. Communicating the result of breast biopsy by telephone or in person. Br J Surg. 1997;84:1381.
40. Baldwin DM, Quintela J, Duclos C, et al. Patient preferences for notification of normal laboratory test results: a report from the ASIPS collaborative. BMC Fam Pract. 2005;6:11.
41. Callen JL, Westbrook JI, Georgiou A, Li J. Failure to follow-up test results for ambulatory patients: a systematic review. J Gen Intern Med. 2012;27:1334–48.
42. Semenov I, Kopanitsa G, Karpov A, et al. Implementation of a clinical decision support system for interpretation of laboratory tests for patients. Stud Health Technol Inform. 2016;224:184–8.
43. Boegl K, Adlassnig KP, Hayashi Y, et al. Knowledge acquisition in the fuzzy knowledge representation framework of a medical consultation system. Artif Intell Med. 2004;30:1–26.

3

Utility of social media and crowd-intelligence data for pharmacovigilance

Andrea C. Tricco[1,2*], Wasifa Zarin[1], Erin Lillie[1], Serena Jeblee[3], Rachel Warren[1], Paul A. Khan[1], Reid Robson[1], Ba' Pham[1], Graeme Hirst[3] and Sharon E. Straus[1,4]

Abstract

Background: A scoping review to characterize the literature on the use of conversations in social media as a potential source of data for detecting adverse events (AEs) related to health products.

Methods: Our specific research questions were (1) What social media listening platforms exist to detect adverse events related to health products, and what are their capabilities and characteristics? (2) What is the validity and reliability of data from social media for detecting these adverse events? MEDLINE, EMBASE, Cochrane Library, and relevant websites were searched from inception to May 2016. Any type of document (e.g., manuscripts, reports) that described the use of social media data for detecting health product AEs was included. Two reviewers independently screened citations and full-texts, and one reviewer and one verifier performed data abstraction. Descriptive synthesis was conducted.

Results: After screening 3631 citations and 321 full-texts, 70 unique documents with 7 companion reports available from 2001 to 2016 were included. Forty-six documents (66%) described an automated or semi-automated information extraction system to detect health product AEs from social media conversations (in the developmental phase). Seven pre-existing information extraction systems to mine social media data were identified in eight documents. Nineteen documents compared AEs reported in social media data with validated data and found consistent AE discovery in all except two documents. None of the documents reported the validity and reliability of the overall system, but some reported on the performance of individual steps in processing the data. The validity and reliability results were found for the following steps in the data processing pipeline: data de-identification ($n = 1$), concept identification ($n = 3$), concept normalization ($n = 2$), and relation extraction ($n = 8$). The methods varied widely, and some approaches yielded better results than others.

Conclusions: Our results suggest that the use of social media conversations for pharmacovigilance is in its infancy. Although social media data has the potential to supplement data from regulatory agency databases; is able to capture less frequently reported AEs; and can identify AEs earlier than official alerts or regulatory changes, the utility and validity of the data source remains under-studied.

Keywords: Surveillance, Adverse event, Drug safety, Social media, Data analytics, Knowledge synthesis

* Correspondence: triccoa@smh.ca
[1]Li Ka Shing Knowledge Institute of St. Michael's Hospital, 209 Victoria Street, East Building, Toronto, ON M5B 1W8, Canada
[2]Epidemiology Division, Dalla Lana School of Public Health, University of Toronto, 6th Floor, 155 College St, Toronto, ON M5T 3M7, Canada
Full list of author information is available at the end of the article

Background

Each year, thousands of people die from an *adverse drug reaction*, defined as an undesirable health effect that occurs when medication is used as prescribed [1]. Adverse drug reactions can vary from a simple rash to more severe effects, such as heart failure, acute liver injury, arrhythmias, and even death [1]. These events have a significant impact on both patients and the health care system in terms of cost and health service utilization (e.g., frequent visits to physicians and emergency departments, hospitalizations) [2].

Post-marketing adverse drug reaction surveillance in most countries is suboptimal and consists largely of spontaneous reporting. It is estimated that spontaneous reporting systems only capture 1–10% of all adverse drug reactions. For example, one out of every five physicians reports an adverse drug reaction using the Canada Vigilance Database [3].

In order to advance *pharmacovigilance* (defined as the science and activities related to detection, comprehension and prevention of adverse drug events) [4], monitoring and analysis of data collected from social media sources (i.e., social media listening) is being researched as a potential to supplement traditional drug safety surveillance systems. Three reviews [5–7] have been recently published to explore the breadth of evidence on the methods and use of social media data for pharmacovigilance; however, none of the reviews found rigorous evaluations of the reliability and validity of the data.

As this is a rapidly evolving field, we conducted a comprehensive scoping review to assess the utility of social media data for detecting adverse events related to health products, including pharmaceuticals, medical devices, and natural health products.

Methods

Research questions

The specific research questions were:

(1) Which social media listening platforms exist to detect adverse events related to health products, and what are their capabilities and characteristics?

(2) What is the validity and reliability of data from social media for detecting these adverse events?

Study design

We used a scoping review method to map the concepts and types of evidence that exist on pharmacovigilance using social media data [8]. Our approach followed the rigorous scoping review methods manual by the Joanna Briggs Institute [9].

Protocol

The Preferred Reporting Items for Systematic Reviews and Meta-analysis Protocols (PRISMA-P) [10] guideline was used to develop our protocol, which we registered with the Open Science Framework [11] and published in a peer-reviewed journal [12]. The protocol was developed by the research team and approved by members of the Health Canada Health Products and Food Branch, the commissioning agency of this review. Since the full methods have been published in the protocol [12], they are briefly outlined below.

Eligibility criteria

The eligibility criteria were any type of document (e.g., journal article, editorial, book, webpage) that described listening to social media data for detecting adverse events associated with health products (see Additional file 1: Appendix 1). The following interventions were excluded from our review: programs of care, health services, organization of care, as well as public health programs and services. Documents related to the mining of social media data to detect prescription drug misuse and abuse were eligible for inclusion. *Social media listening* was defined as mining and monitoring of user-generated and crowd-intelligence data from online conversations in blogs, medical forums, and other social networking sites to identify trends and themes of the conversation on a topic (see Additional file 1: Appendix 2). We included documents that reported on at least one of the following outcomes: social media listening approaches, utility of social media data for pharmacovigilance and their performance capabilities, validity and reliability of user-generated data from social media for pharmacovigilance, and author's perception of utility and challenges of using social media data.

Information sources and search strategy

Comprehensive literature searches were conducted in MEDLINE, EMBASE, and the Cochrane Library by an experienced librarian. The MEDLINE search strategy was peer-reviewed by another librarian using the PRESS checklist [13], which has been published in our protocol [12], and also available in Additional file 1: Appendix 3. In addition, we searched grey literature (i.e., difficult to locate, unpublished documents) sources outlined in Additional file 1: Appendix 4 using the Canadian Agency for Drugs and Technologies in Health guide [14], and scanned the reference lists of relevant reviews [5, 6, 15].

Study selection process

After the team achieved 75% agreement on a pilot-test of 50 random citations, each citation was independently screened by reviewer pairs (WZ, EL, RW, PK, RR, FY, BP) using Synthesi.SR; an online application developed by the Knowledge Translation Program [16]. Potentially relevant full-text documents were obtained and the same process (described above) was followed for full-text screening.

Data items and data abstraction process

Data were abstracted on document characteristics (e.g., type of document), population characteristics of social media users (e.g., disease), characteristics of social media data (e.g., social media source), characteristics of social media listening approaches (e.g., pre-processing), and performance of the different approaches (e.g., validity and reliability of social media data). After the team pilot-tested the data abstraction form using a random sample of 5 included documents, each document was abstracted by one reviewer (WZ, EL, RW, PK, RR, FY, BP) and verified by a second reviewer (WZ, EL). The data were cleaned by a third reviewer (WZ, EL) and confirmed by the content expert (SJ, GH).

Risk of bias assessment or quality appraisal

Risk of bias or quality appraisal was not conducted, which is consistent with the Joanna Briggs Institute methods manual [9], and those documented in scoping reviews on health-related topics [17].

Synthesis of results

To characterize the health conditions studied, the World Health Organization version of the International Statistical Classification of Diseases and Related Health Problems (10th Revision, ICD-10) was used [18]. The social media system characteristics were described and categorized according to the steps typically involved in a social media data processing pipeline [19]. In addition, the social media systems were classified according to whether they were manual systems (i.e., coded by hand, without computer assistance), experimental/developmental stage systems (i.e., automatic information extraction systems being developed by researchers), or fully developed systems (i.e., automatic information extraction systems that are either commercially available or being used by regulatory agencies).

Descriptive statistics were performed (e.g., frequencies, measures of central tendency) using Excel 2010. Thematic analysis of open-text data was performed by two reviewers (WZ, EL) and verified by a third reviewer (ACT or SJ) to categorize the author perception of utility and challenges of using social media data for pharmacovigilance [20].

Results

Study flow

A total of 3631 citations from electronic databases and grey literature and other sources (e.g., reference scanning) were screened (Fig. 1). Of these, 321 potentially relevant full-text records were screened and 70 unique records with an additional 7 companion reports were included in our scoping review. The full list of included documents and companion reports can be found in Additional file 1: Appendix 5.

Document characteristics

The documents were dated between 2001 and 2016 with 78% of the relevant documents being from 2013 onwards (Table 1). The most common document types were journal articles (57%) and conference papers (33%). Most of the corresponding authors were from North America (73%) and Europe (17%). Public sources of funding were the most common (40%). Most of the papers (66%) described an experimental/developmental automated information extraction system to mine data from social media for drug safety surveillance.

Social media data characteristics

The commonly mined sources of social media platforms were Twitter (33%), MedHelp (13%), DailyStrength (11%), and AskaPatient (9%) (Fig. 2). The majority of the documents mined only one social media site to obtain user-generated data (54%) (Table 2). The user types included patients from health forums, such as BreastCancer.org (50%); the general population on micro-blogging sites, such as Twitter (39%); or both (10%). The geographic location of the social media users was seldom reported (17%). When it was reported, the users were from high-income countries as per the World Bank classification [21]. The social media posts were mostly in English (86%), followed by Spanish, French, and multiple languages (3% each). A small fraction (1% each) of posts was written in German and Serbian.

The posts were collected for a median duration of 1.13 years (i.e., the investigators "listened" to social media conversations for this duration), with an interquartile range of 6 months to 7 years. A median of 42,594 posts were included in the documents, with an interquartile range of 4608 to 711,562 posts. A variety of techniques were used to identify relevant social media posts, such as web crawlers or spiders (27%, i.e., an automated program that scans the social media source to identify posts about adverse events), application programming interfaces (APIs) of the host site (20%, i.e., a set of applications, rules, and definitions used to build the data set) and keyword search of social media sites (10%). Four papers (6%) used a combination of the above methods. Other approaches included using browser add-ons to monitor search query activities, using a pre-existing database of social media conversations, and

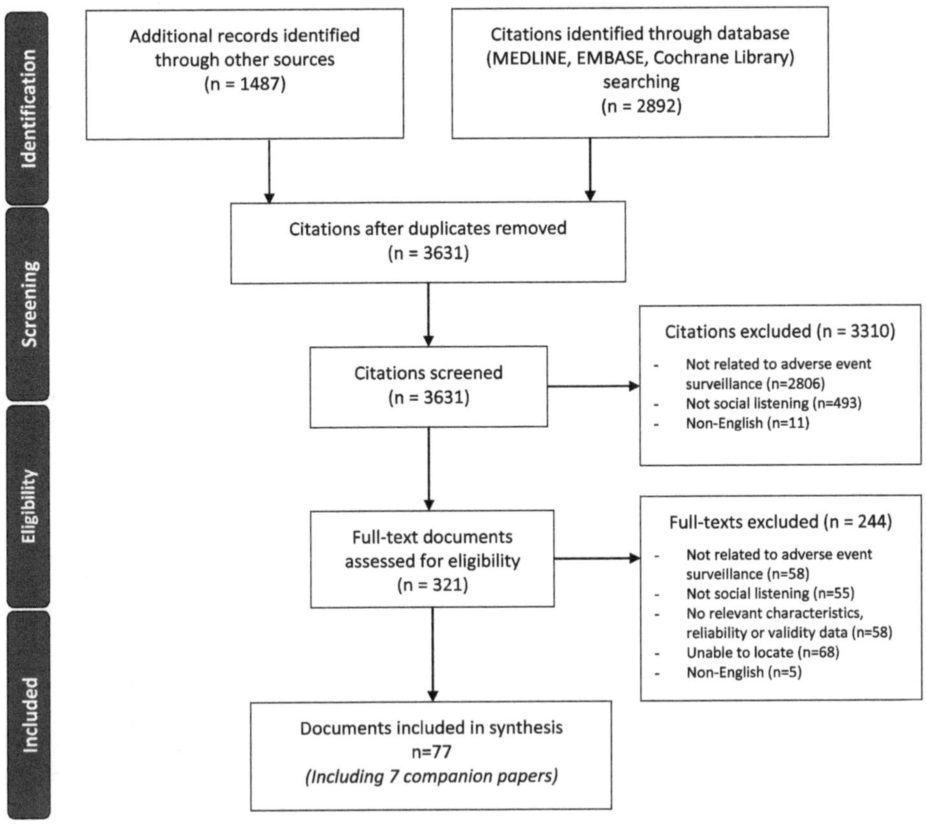

Fig. 1 Study flow diagram

requesting processed database from the social media site system administrators.

Health conditions, types of surveillance, and types of health products

The majority of the documents applied their social media listening approach to the study of a specific health condition (Table 3). According to the ICD-10 classification system, almost half (46%) included patients with health conditions from more than one disease system, 13% included patients with neoplasms, and 11% included patients with mental illness and behavioural disorders. The focus of surveillance was most commonly any adverse event (74%), and the type of health products examined were mostly pharmaceutical drugs (98.6%).

Social media data processing pipeline

A variety of data processing approaches were identified (Additional file 1: Appendix 6):

- supervised learning (21%, i.e., a machine learning approach that is trained from a set of labeled data that has been coded typically by humans)
- rule-based learning (9%, i.e., a learning algorithm that allows automatic identification of useful rules, rather than a human needing to apply prior domain knowledge to manually constructed rules and curate a rule set)
- semi-supervised learning (7%, i.e., a machine learning method that uses both labeled and unlabeled data for training)
- unsupervised learning (6%, i.e., machine learns patterns in the data without any labels given by humans)

After the social media dataset was created, the following steps were typically used to process the social media data (Fig. 3):

1) pre-processing (e.g., removing punctuations and stop words; breaking text into words, phrases, and symbols or tokens; reducing words to the root; and correcting spelling mistakes)
2) de-identification (e.g., removing identifiable information, such as user names and addresses)
3) de-duplication (e.g., removing duplicate and related posts)
4) concept identification (e.g., identifying adverse drug reactions and other events from a sequence text)

Table 1 Document characteristics

Document characteristics (*n* = 70)		Count (%)
Year of dissemination	2001–2004	1 (1.4%)
	2005–2008	1 (1.4%)
	2009–2012	13 (18.6%)
	2013–2016	55 (78.6%)
Document type	Blog	1 (1.4%)
	Dissertation	1 (1.4%)
	Book section	2 (2.9%)
	Report	3 (4.3%)
	Conference paper/poster	23 (32.9%)
	Journal article	40 (57.1%)
Geographic region of publication	Asia	2 (2.9%)
	Australia & New Zealand	5 (7.1%)
	Europe	12 (17.1%)
	North America	51 (72.9%)
Funding type	Non-sponsored	4 (5.7%)
	Industry and public-sponsored	5 (7.1%)
	Industry-sponsored	7 (10.0%)
	Not reported	26 (37.1%)
	Public-sponsored	28 (40.0%)
Types of social media listening systems studied for drug safety surveillance	Used an available automatic information extraction system (fully developed and available for use)	8 (11.4%)
	Used a manual approach for information extraction	16 (22.9%)
	Used an experimental automatic information extraction system (at the development stage)	46 (65.7%)

5) concept normalization (e.g., converting colloquial terms to medical terms for drug names, symptoms, history, events, disease)
6) relation extraction (e.g., determining the relationship between the health product and an adverse event)

Different text processing methods were reported for each step, with varying levels of automation.

Types of social media listening systems

Most of the documents examined an experimental social media listening system that was under development (66%). Seven pre-existing social media listening systems were identified in eight documents (Additional file 1: Appendix 7): MedWatcher Social (US Food and Drug Administration), commercial systems AETracker (IMS health), Visible Intelligence (Cision), BeFree System: Bio-Entity Finder & RElation Extraction (Integrative Bioinformatics group), MeaningCloud (MeaningCloud LLC, Sngular company), Treato (Treato Ltd.), and OpenCalais (Thomson Reuters). An eighth system was identified during the environmental scan, which is known as the Web-RADR Social and is currently under development by European Union regulators. Sixteen documents studied a manual approach, whereby posts were coded manually by humans without any assistance from computers (23%).

Outcome results

Utility of social media data for pharmacovigilance

Nineteen documents provided information on the utility of social media data for pharmacovigilance; however, this was not considered to be the primary objective of the documents (Additional file 1: Appendix 8). Most of the documents focused on the detection of adverse events, while one document focused on the timing of adverse event detection [22].

Ten documents compared social media data against spontaneous reports to regulatory agencies to study the difference in the number of adverse events captured, time lag in detecting adverse events or whether the two data sources are correlated [22–31]. Specifically, 7/10 documents [25–31] compared the frequency of adverse events detected from social media source(s) versus a regulatory database, and all but one [26] reported consistent results [24–30]. In 2/10 documents, authors reported a positive correlation between adverse events reported in social media data sources and those reported by regulatory agencies [23, 31]. In one document, timing of adverse event reporting on social media was compared with the timing of the FDA's official alert or labeling revision time, and adverse events were detected on social media earlier [22].

Six documents compared adverse events reported in social media posts against published data or safety signals known by the authors, [32–38] (exact sources were not specified) and all found consistent results. One document compared weighted scores of adverse events reported in social media posts with drugs withdrawn from the market and found a positive correlation between higher weighted scores and withdrawn drugs [39]. One document compared the frequency of adverse events reported on social media with those from a large integrated healthcare system database and found that their results were generally consistent, though several less frequently reported adverse events in the medical health records were more commonly reported on social media (e.g., aspirin-induced hypoglycemia was discussed only on social media) [40]. In contrast, one document found that less than 2% of adverse events detected by AETracker (a commercially available platform) were actual events, as confirmed by pharmacovigilance experts [41].

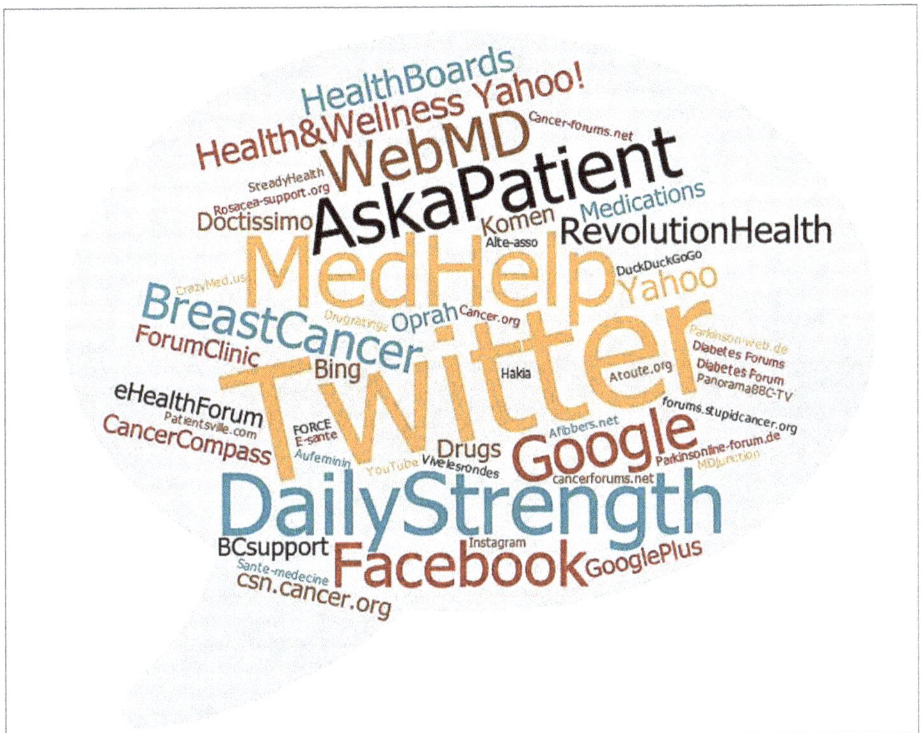

Social media source mentioned more than twice (n=70)	Count (%)
Twitter	23 (32.9%)
MedHelp	9 (12.9%)
DailyStrength	8 (11.4%)
AskaPatient	6 (8.6%)
WebMD	5 (7.1%)
Google	5 (7.1%)
Facebook	5 (7.1%)
BreastCancer.org	4 (5.7%)
RevolutionHealth	3 (4.3%)
Yahoo!	3 (4.3%)
Health & Wellness Yahoo! Groups	3 (4.3%)
HealthBoards.com	3 (4.3%)

Note: Fifty-two unique sources were reported for social media listening in 65 papers; 5 papers did not list the social media sources searched.

Fig. 2 Wordcloud of social media sources mined in the documents

Themes of utility and challenges of social media listening

Several themes emerged from the qualitative analysis of the study authors' discussions of the strengths and limitations of using social media data for pharmacovigilance. In order of prevalence, the utility of social media listening were as follows: provides supplemental data to traditional surveillance systems, captures perceptions about the effects of treatment (including adverse events), and offers an extensive source of publicly available data (Table 4). The three most common challenges were the unstructured nature of the data, complex structure of the text data, and potential lack of representativeness (i.e., posts may not be representative of all those administered health products) (Table 4). Further details can be found in Additional file 1: Appendix 17.

Validity and reliability of analytics used to process social media data

The validity and reliability measures were categorized according to the social media data processing pipeline, as follows:

Pre-processing Thirty-two documents reported methods for pre-processing (Additional file 1: Appendix 9), and provided information on the software used and accessibility of the tool (e.g., public, proprietary) [23, 26, 32, 34, 35, 42–72]. Validity or reliability of data processed in this step was not reported.

De-identification Six documents reported methods for de-identification (Additional file 1: Appendix 10), and

Table 2 Social media data characteristics

Social media data characteristics ($n = 70$)		Count (%)
Number of social media sources included by study authors	1	38 (54.3%)
	2	10 (14.3%)
	3	8 (11.4%)
	4	3 (4.3%)
	> 5	7 (10.0%)
	Not reported	4 (5.7%)
Type of social media sites	Patient-specific	35 (50.0%)
	General population	27 (38.6%)
	Both patient-specific and general population	7 (10.0%)
	Not reported	1 (1.4%)
Region of origin of the social media posts	USA	5 (7.1%)
	Spain	2 (2.9%)
	Germany	1 (1.4%)
	50+ countries	1 (1.4%)
	USA, Canada, UK, Australia, New Zealand	1 (1.4%)
	France	1 (1.4%)
	UK, North America, Australasia	1 (1.4%)
	Not reported	58 (82.9%)
Language of the social media posts	English	60 (85.7%)
	Spanish	2 (2.9%)
	French	2 (2.9%)
	German	1 (1.4%)
	Serbian	1 (1.4%)
	Multilingual	2 (2.9%)
	Not reported	2 (2.9%)
Method employed to collect social media data	Web crawling/ spidering software	19 (27.1%)
	API of the host site	14 (20.0%)
	Keyword search	7 (10.0%)
	Multiple methods	4 (5.7%)
	Other methods	13 (18.6%)
	Not Reported	13 (18.6%)
Duration (years) of social media data	Median (Q1, Q3)	1.13 (0.5, 7.13)
	Not reported	34 (48.6%)
Number of social media posts retrieved	Median (Q1, Q3)	42,594 (4608, 711,562)
	Not reported	5 (7.1%)

provided information on the software used and accessibility of the tool [31, 43, 53–56, 64, 73]. Only one study reported validity/reliability of data processed in this step, which included a precision of 67%, recall of 98%, and F-measure of 80% [43].

De-duplication Five documents reported methods for de-duplication (Additional file 1: Appendix 11), and provided information on the software used and accessibility of the tool [30, 40, 74–76]. Validity or reliability of data processed in this step was not reported.

Concept identification Forty-five documents reported on automated methods for concept identification for drugs, adverse events, and overall (i.e., drug and adverse events), which were reported using the following approaches: dictionary/lexicon-based ($n = 30$) [22, 23, 26, 30, 31, 39, 40, 43, 44, 47, 50, 51, 53–57, 59, 63–69, 72, 74, 75, 77–82],

Table 3 Health conditions, types of surveillance, and types of health products investigated

Topic ($n = 70$)		Count (%)
Health conditions studied as per ICD-10	Multiple disease system	32 (45.7%)
	Neoplasm	9 (12.9%)
	Mental illness & behavioural disorders	8 (11.4%)
	Factors influencing health status & contact with health services	6 (8.6%)
	Nervous system	6 (8.6%)
	Endocrine, nutritional & metabolic	3 (4.3%)
	Not reported	2 (2.9%)
	Circulatory system	2 (2.9%)
	Injury, poisoning and certain other consequences of external causes	1 (1.4%)
	Skin & subcutaneous tissue	1 (1.4%)
Type of surveillance studied	Any adverse event	52 (74.3%)
	Drug abuse/misuse	6 (8.6%)
	Drug-to-drug interaction	4 (5.7%)
	Specific adverse event (e.g., arthralgia, heart diseases, infertility)	7 (10.0%)
	Treatment switching	1 (1.4%)
Type of health products included	Pharmaceutical drugs (including biologics)	69 (98.6%)
	Medical devices	1 (1.4%)
	Natural health products	0 (0.0%)

supervised classifier ($n = 6$) [42, 61, 62, 71, 73, 83], mixed lexicon-based/supervised classifier ($n = 2$) [52, 58], rule-based phrase extraction ($n = 2$) [34, 35, 84], sentiment analysis ($n = 2$) [32, 46], statistical approaches ($n = 2$) [58, 70], or unspecified ($n = 1$; Additional file 1: Appendix 12) [85]. Three documents reported evaluation results for overall concept identification. In these, supervised classifier approaches were studied and their accuracy for overall concept identification ranged from 78 to 83%, precision ranged from 32 to 78%, recall ranged from 32 to 74%, and F-measure ranged from 42 to 61%. [62, 71, 73] Validity and reliability results for drug and adverse event concepts can be found in Additional file 1: Appendix 14.

Concept normalization – Drug names Nineteen documents reported on automated methods for concept normalization of drug names and all used a variation of dictionary or lexicon-based approaches ($n = 19$; Additional file 1: Appendix 13) [22, 30, 43, 47–51, 54–58, 63–66, 74, 75, 78, 79, 83, 86]. One paper also used a hybrid approach of statistical modeling using conditional random fields and dictionary-based methods [58]. Two documents reported accuracy results for dictionary/lexicon-based approaches, which ranged from 0 to 92% [58, 83]. Using a hybrid approach of statistical methods combined with dictionary-based methods, Metke-Jimenez and colleagues found accuracy results ranging from 75 to 77% [58].

Concept normalization – Medical events Thirty-four documents reported on automated methods for concept normalization of medical concepts (i.e., adverse events, symptoms, disease), of which 33 documents reported a dictionary/lexicon-based approach [22, 23, 26, 30–32, 39, 40, 43–45, 48, 50, 51, 53–59, 61, 63, 64, 66–69, 71, 72, 74, 75, 77, 81–83], and 2 documents also used statistical approaches (Additional file 1: Appendix 14) [58, 70]. Two documents reported accuracy of dictionary/lexicon approaches, which ranged from 3 to 67%. Using a hybrid approach of statistical methods combined with dictionary methods, Metke-Jimenez and colleagues found accuracy results ranging from 33 to 38%.

Relation extraction Thirty-eight documents reported on automated methods for relation extraction, which is used to establish relationships between drugs and adverse events using social media data (Additional file 1: Appendix 15). Methods were classified as rule-based or statistical association mining ($n = 16$) [22, 31, 34, 35, 40, 43, 47, 51, 60, 67–69, 75–77, 83, 85], supervised classifier ($n = 16$) [30, 39, 44, 49, 53–57, 61, 63–66, 70, 71, 73, 74, 86], dictionary/lexicon based ($n = 4$) [23, 45, 78–80] or sentiment analysis ($n = 2$) [32, 46]. Eight documents provided validity/reliability data on rule-based or statistical association mining. The precision ranged from 35 to 79%, recall ranged from 6 to 100%, F-measure ranged from 9 to 94%, and area under the curve (AUC) ranged

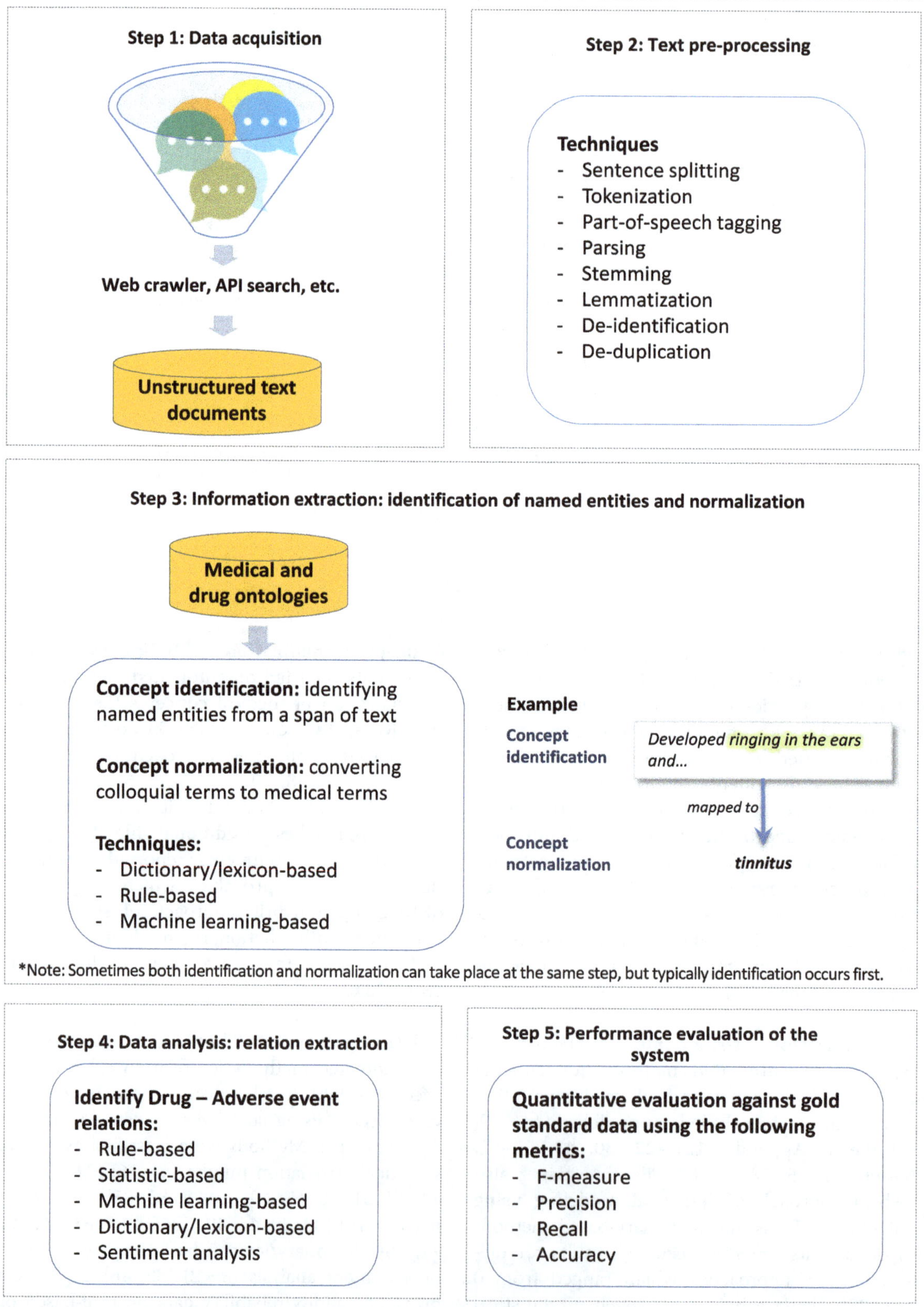

Fig. 3 Steps typically involved in social media data processing flow

Table 4 Utility and challenges of social media listening

Utility and challenges of social media listening	Count (%)
Utility of social media listening for pharmacovigilance	
Supplemental data to traditional post-marketing safety surveillance	31 (44.3%)
Captures perceptions and consequences of treatment and adverse events	14 (20.0%)
Large publicly available data source	14 (20.0%)
Able to discover undocumented or rare adverse events	11 (15.7%)
Promising early warning system	10 (14.3%)
Computationally efficient	7 (10.0%)
Captures prescription drug misuse/abuse	4 (5.7%)
Not biased towards severe adverse events	7 (10.0%)
Captures large geographical area	3 (4.3%)
Useful for risk communication	3 (4.3%)
Able to extract complex medical concepts	2 (2.9%)
Can be more accurate than spontaneous reporting systems	2 (2.9%)
Hypothesis-generating	2 (2.9%)
Able to identify undocumented drug interactions	2 (2.9%)
Findings are similar to traditional systems	1 (1.4%)
Captures information on adherence related to adverse events	1 (1.4%)
Challenges of social media listening for pharmacovigilance	
Non-standard reporting format (informal language, format used to report information, amount of information provided by each user)	30 (42.9%)
Difficult to draw complex semantic relationships from unstructured texts	14 (20.0%)
May not be a representative population	13 (18.6%)
Noise may exist in signal detection	12 (17.1%)
Inadequate information to draw causality	9 (12.9%)
Lacks comprehensive medical and demographic information	8 (11.4%)
Subjective, incomplete or misinformation	6 (8.6%)
Not a balanced coverage of all drugs and medical conditions	5 (7.1%)
Data acquisition challenges due to host site restrictions	4 (5.7%)
Duplication of data (double-counting)	4 (5.7%)
Processing multi-lingual texts	3 (4.3%)
Resource-intensive to process big data	2 (2.9%)

from 0.57 to 0.93. Fifteen documents provided validity and reliability data for the supervised classifier approach and accuracy ranged from 29 to 90%, precision from 20 to 86%, recall from 23 to 100%, F-measure from 32 to 92%, and AUC was 74%. Two documents provided data on the reliability and validity of dictionary/lexicon-based approaches, which ranged from 44 to 83% for precision, 2 to 84% for recall, and 3 to 58% for the F-measure. Validity and reliability of data for this step were not reported for sentiment analysis or semantic matching approaches.

Additional processing steps Some authors investigated additional processing steps, which included identifying the source of an adverse event report ($n = 4$; i.e,. personal experience vs. witnessed) [42, 44, 53–56], and query matching which retrieves and filters the relevant documents to answer a given user query ($n = 1$; Additional file 1: Appendix 16) [87]. Eight documents analysed user-generated texts in other languages, including Spanish [78–80], French [29, 88], German [37], Serbian [51], and multiple languages [45, 77] but only 5 reported their methods [47, 52, 62, 88–90]. One document included 53 different languages [77] and another document included English, Spanish, and French [45]. None of the papers described validity or reliability of processing non-English text.

Discussion

Most of the documents included in our scoping review dated from 2013 onwards. We identified seven pre-existing social media platforms, and another platform (Web-RADR Social) that is currently under development by European regulators. Unfortunately, no information on when this social media platform will be completed was provided. The majority of the documents primarily focused on the development of social media listening tools for pharmacovigilance (as opposed to their application), which would be useful for those interested in developing such platforms. In particular, documents authored by Freifeld et al., [74] Karimi et al., [83] and Vinod et al. [19] provide useful information on the development of such platforms.

We identified 19 documents providing some information on the utility of social media. This information was mostly abstracted from the discussion section of the documents, suggesting that the conclusions were highly speculative. Furthermore, most of the included documents only followed social media posts for a median duration of 1 year. A high-quality study that examines utility over a longer timeframe with a broader data frame may provide further useful information to the field.

According to authors' perceptions, social media can be used to supplement traditional reporting systems, to uncover adverse events less frequently reported in traditional reporting systems, to communicate risk and to generate hypotheses. However, challenges exist, such as difficulties interpreting relationships between the drugs and adverse events (e.g., there are inadequate data to draw causality), potential lack of representativeness between social media users and the general population, and the resource-intensive process of using social media data for pharmacovigilance. Evaluation studies of pharmacovigilance using social media listening are needed to substantiate these perceptions. Future studies should also consider evaluating the performance and utility of integrating social media data with other data sources, such as regulatory databases that collect spontaneous reports, as well as relevant surveillance databases.

Our results have summarized the most common elements involved in the processing of social media data for pharmacovigilance. Across the included documents, the most common steps employed were: 1) pre-processing; 2) de-identification; 3) de-duplication; 4) concept identification; 5) concept normalization; and 6) relation extraction. Validity and reliability findings varied across the different approaches that were used to mine the data, which suggests some may be more effective than others. The heterogeneous nature of the study designs and approaches reported in the documents; however, make it difficult to definitively determine which approaches are more useful than others.

As described in our protocol, we conducted this scoping review to inform members of Health Canada who are currently using our results to plan an evaluation study on utility of social media for detecting health product adverse events. They may also consider a Canadian platform to be developed in the future, depending on the results of their study.

Our results are similar to 3 other reviews on this topic. A recent review by Sarker et al. [7] described the different automatic approaches used to detect and extract adverse drug reactions from social media data for pharmacovigilance purposes in studies published in the last 10 years. Although the authors characterized existing social media listening and analytics platforms, validity and reliability of the user-generated data captured through social media and crowd-sourcing networks were not examined. Golder and colleagues [5] conducted a systematic review on adverse events data in social media. They found that although reports of adverse drug events can be identified through social media, the reliability or validity of this information has not been formally evaluated. Finally, Lardon and colleagues [6] conducted a scoping review on the use of social media for pharmacovigilance. They identified numerous ways to identify adverse drug reaction data, extract data, and verify the quality of information. However, gaps in the field were identified. For example, most studies identifying adverse drug reactions failed to verify the reliability and validity of the data and none of the studies proposed a feasible way to integrate data from social media across more than one site/information source.

The strengths of our scoping review include a comprehensive search of multiple electronic databases and sources for difficult to locate and unpublished studies (or grey literature), as well as the use of the rigorous scoping review methods manual by the Joanna Briggs Institute. In addition, we included researchers with computer science expertise (SJ, GH) to help code automated approaches. In terms of a dissemination plan, we will use a number of strategies, such as: a 1-page policy brief, two stakeholder meetings (i.e., consultation exercises), presentations at an international conference, and publications in open-access journals. Team members will also use their networks to encourage broad dissemination of results.

There are some limitations to our scoping review process. The review was limited to documents written in English to increase its feasibility, given the 5-month timeline. Additionally, due to the large number of documents identified, the data were abstracted by one reviewer and verified by a second reviewer. Lastly, although our literature search was comprehensive, there is always a chance that some social media platforms or data analytics documents were missed. Since this is a rapidly evolving and emerging field, we expect that new documents fulfilling our inclusion criteria will be released in increasing numbers [91, 92], highlighting a potential need to update our review in the near future.

Conclusion

Our results suggest that the use of social media is being investigated for drug safety surveillance from an early developmental perspective. Within this context, social media data has the potential to supplement data from regulatory agency databases, capture less frequently reported AEs, and identify AEs earlier than official alerts or regulatory changes. However, the utility, validity and implementation of information extraction systems using social media for pharmacovigilance are under-studied. Further research is required to strengthen and standardize the approaches as well as to ensure that the findings are valid, for the purpose of pharmacovigilance.

Additional file

Additional file 1: Appendix 1. Description of included and excluded interventions for drug safety surveillance. Appendix 2. Glossary of terms. Appendix 3. Medline search strategy. Appendix 4. Sources for grey literature search. Appendix 5. List of included studies. Appendix 6. Social media data processing pipeline. Appendix 7. Pre-existing social media listening platforms for drug safety surveillance. Appendix 8. Utility of social media data for drug safety surveillance. Appendix 9. Pre-processing methods and results. Appendix 10. De-identification methods and results. Appendix 11. De-duplication methods and results. Appendix 12. Concept identification methods and results. Appendix 13. Drug name normalization methods and results. Appendix 14. Medical event normalization methods and results. Appendix 15. Relation extraction methods and results. Appendix 16. Additional processing methods and results. Appendix 17. Utility and challenges with socila media listening for drug safety surveillance. (DOCX 275 kb)

Abbreviations

AE: adverse events; API: application programming interfaces; AUC: area under the curve; FDA: food and drug administration; ICD: International Statistical Classification of Diseases and Related Health Problems; PRISMA-P: Preferred Reporting Items for Systematic Reviews and Meta-analysis Protocol

Acknowledgements

We thank Dr. Elise Cogo for developing the literature search, Dr. Jessie McGowan for peer-reviewing the literature search, Ms. Alissa Epworth for performing the database and grey literature searches and all library support. We also thank Ms. Fatemeh Yazdi for helping with some screening and data extraction and Theshani De Silva for formatting the manuscript. Last but not least, we thank Jesmin Antony and Myanca Rodrigues, as well as Health Canada Products and Food Branch, in particular Dr. Laurie Chapman, for their feedback on the manuscript.

Funding

This study was funded by the Canadian Institutes of Health Research Drug Safety and Effectiveness Network (DNM–137713). ACT is funded by a Tier 2 Canada Research Chair in Knowledge Synthesis. SES is funded by a Tier 1 Canada Research Chair in Knowledge Translation.

Authors' contributions

ACT obtained funding, conceptualized the research, participated in all pilot-tests, provided methods guidance, and drafted the manuscript. WZ coordinated the study, screened citations and articles, abstracted data, cleaned data, coded open-text data, analyzed the data and helped write the manuscript. EL helped coordinate the study, screened citations, abstracted data, cleaned data, coded open-text data, and helped write the manuscript. SJ coded open-text data, verified the data and reviewed the manuscript. PK, RW, RR, and BP screened citations and articles for relevance, abstracted data, and reviewed the manuscript. GH provided content expertise, verified data categorization and reviewed the manuscript. SES obtained funding, helped conceptualize the research, and helped write the manuscript. All authors have critically reviewed the manuscript and provided substantial feedback on the content and interpretation of results, as well as provided final approval for the manuscript to be published. Each author has agreed to be accountable for all aspects of the work.

Competing interests

The authors declare that they have no competing interests. The study funder had no input into the study design; in the collection, analysis, and interpretation of data; in the writing of the report; and in the decision to submit the paper for publication.

Author details

[1]Li Ka Shing Knowledge Institute of St. Michael's Hospital, 209 Victoria Street, East Building, Toronto, ON M5B 1W8, Canada. [2]Epidemiology Division, Dalla Lana School of Public Health, University of Toronto, 6th Floor, 155 College St, Toronto, ON M5T 3M7, Canada. [3]Department of Computer Science, University of Toronto, 10 King's College Road, Toronto, ON M5S 3G4, Canada. [4]Department of Geriatric Medicine, Faculty of Medicine, University of Toronto, 27 Kings College Circle, Toronto, ON M5S 1A1, Canada.

References

1. Ross CJ, Visscher H, Sistonen J, Brunham LR, Pussegoda K, Loo TT, Rieder MJ, Koren G, Carleton BC, Hayden MR. The Canadian pharmacogenomics network for drug safety: a model for safety pharmacology. Thyroid. 2010; 20(7):681–7.
2. Lazarou J, Pomeranz BH, Corey PN. Incidence of adverse drug reactions in hospitalized patients: a meta-analysis of prospective studies. JAMA. 1998; 279(15):1200–5.
3. Environics Research Group. Adverse Reaction Reporting—Survey with Health Professionals. Ottawa: Health Canada; 2007.
4. Essential medicines and health products: Pharmacovigilance. http://www.who.int/medicines/areas/quality_safety/safety_efficacy/pharmvigi/en/. Accessed 6 June 2018.
5. Golder S, Norman G, Loke YK. Systematic review on the prevalence, frequency and comparative value of adverse events data in social media. Br J Clin Pharmacol. 2015;80(4):878–88.
6. Lardon J, Abdellaoui R, Bellet F, Asfari H, Souvignet J, Texier N, Jaulent MC, Beyens MN, Burgun A, Bousquet C. Adverse drug reaction identification and extraction in social media: a scoping review. J Med Internet Res. 2015;17(7):e171.
7. Sarker A, Ginn R, Nikfarjam A, O'Connor K, Smith K, Jayaraman S, Upadhaya T, Gonzalez G. Utilizing social media data for pharmacovigilance: a review. J Biomed Inform. 2015;54:202–12.
8. Arksey H, O'Malley L. Scoping studies: towards a methodological framework. Int J Soc Res Methodol. 2005;8(1):19–32.
9. Peters MD, Godfrey CM, Khalil H, McInerney P, Parker D, Soares CB. Guidance for conducting systematic scoping reviews. Int J Evid Based Healthc. 2015;13(3):141–6.
10. Shamseer L, Moher D, Clarke M, Ghersi D, Liberati A, Petticrew M, Shekelle P, Stewart LA, Group P-P. Preferred reporting items for systematic review and meta-analysis protocols (PRISMA-P) 2015: elaboration and explanation. BMJ. 2015;349:g7647.
11. Utility of social media and crowd-sourced data for pharmacovigilance: A scoping review protocol. https://osf.io/kv9hu/. Accessed 6 June 2018.
12. Tricco AC, Zarin W, Lillie E, Pham B, Straus SE. Utility of social media and crowd-sourced data for pharmacovigilance: a scoping review protocol. BMJ Open. 2017;7:e013474.
13. McGowan J, Sampson M, Salzwedel DM, Cogo E, Foerster V, Lefebvre C. PRESS peer review of electronic search strategies: 2015 guideline statement. J Clin Epidemiol. 2016; https://doi.org/10.1016/j.jclinepi.2016.01.021.
14. Grey Matters: a practical tool for searching health-related grey literature. https://www.cadth.ca/resources/finding-evidence/grey-matters. Accessed 6 June 2018.
15. Sinnenberg L, Buttenheim AM, Padrez K, Mancheno C, Ungar L, Merchant RM. Twitter as a tool for Health Research: a systematic review. Am J Public Health. 2016;107:e1–8.
16. Newton D. Synthesi.SR. Toronto: Knowledge Translation Program, St. Michael's Hospital; 2012.
17. Tricco AC, Lillie E, Zarin W, O'Brien K, Colquhoun H, Kastner M, Levac D, Ng C, Sharpe JP, Wilson K, et al. A scoping review on the conduct and reporting of scoping reviews. BMC Med Res Methodol. 2016;16:15.
18. Mental and behavioural disorders. In: International Statistical Classification of Diseases and Related Health Problems 10th Revision (ICD-10)-WHO Version for 2016. Geneva: World Health Organization; 2016.
19. Kumar VD, Tipney HJ. Biomedical literature mining. New York: Springer; 2014.
20. Hsieh HF, Shannon SE. Three approaches to qualitative content analysis. Qual Health Res. 2005;15(9):1277–88.
21. World Bank Country and Lending Groups. https://datahelpdesk.worldbank.org/knowledgebase/articles/906519-world-bank-country-and-lending-groups. Accessed 6 June 2018.
22. Yang CC, Yang H. Exploiting social media with tensor decomposition for pharmacovigilance. In: 2015 IEEE International Conference on Data Mining Workshop (ICDMW): 2015. Washington D.C: IEEE; 2015. p. 188–95.
23. Freifeld CC, Brownstein JS, Menone CM, Bao W, Filice R, Kass-Hout T, Dasgupta N. Digital drug safety surveillance: monitoring pharmaceutical products in twitter. Drug Saf. 2014;37(5):343–50.
24. Johnson HK. Nancy: a side effect of social media. What can twitter tell us about adverse drug reactions. In: UKMI 39th professional development seminar: 2013. 2013.
25. Kmetz J. Pharmaceutical industry special report: adverse event reporting in social media. In: Visible; 2011.
26. Leaman R, Wojtulewicz L, Sullivan R, Skariah A, Yang J, Gonzalez G. Towards internet-age pharmacovigilance: extracting adverse drug reactions from user posts to health-related social networks. In: Proceedings of the 2010 workshop on biomedical natural language processing: 2010. Upsala: Association for Computational Linguistics; 2010. p. 117–25.
27. Medawar C, Herxheimer A, Bell A, Jofre S. Paroxetine, panorama and user reporting of ADRs: consumer intelligence matters in clinical practice and post-marketing drug surveillance. Int J Risk Saf Med. 2002; 15(3, 4):161–9.
28. Discovering Drug Side Effects with Crowdsourcing. https://www.figure-eight.com/discovering-drug-side-effects-with-crowdsourcing/. Accessed 6 June 2018.

29. Pages A, Bondon-Guitton E, Montastruc JL, Bagheri H. Undesirable effects related to oral antineoplastic drugs: comparison between patients' internet narratives and a national pharmacovigilance database. Drug Saf. 2014;37(8):629–37.
30. Powell GE, Seifert HA, Reblin T, Burstein PJ, Blowers J, Menius JA, Painter JL, Thomas M, Pierce CE, Rodriguez HW. Social media listening for routine post-marketing safety surveillance. Drug Saf. 2016;39(5):443–54.
31. Yom-Tov E, Gabrilovich E. Postmarket drug surveillance without trial costs: discovery of adverse drug reactions through large-scale analysis of web search queries. J Med Internet Res. 2013;15(6):e124.
32. Akay A, Dragomir A, Erlandsson B-E. Network-based modeling and intelligent data mining of social media for improving care. IEEE J Biomed Health Inform. 2015;19(1):210–8.
33. Coloma PM, Becker B, Sturkenboom MC, van Mulligen EM, Kors JA. What can social media networks contribute to medicines safety surveillance? In: Pharmacoepidemiol drug Saf: 2015. Hoboken: Wiley; 2015. p. 467–8.
34. Liu J, Li A, Seneff S. Automatic drug side effect discovery from online patient-submitted reviews: focus on statin drugs. In: Proceedings of first international conference on advances in information mining and management (IMMM): 2011. Barcelona: IMMM; 2011. p. 23–9.
35. Li YA. Medical data mining: improving information accessibility using online patient drug reviews. Cambridge: Massachusetts Institute of Technology; 2011.
36. Mao JJ, Chung A, Benton A, Hill S, Ungar L, Leonard CE, Hennessy S, Holmes JH. Online discussion of drug side effects and discontinuation among breast cancer survivors. Pharmacoepidemiol Drug Saf. 2013;22(3):256–62.
37. Schröder S, Zöllner YF, Schaefer M. Drug related problems with antiparkinsonian agents: consumer internet reports versus published data. Pharmacoepidemiol Drug Saf. 2007;16(10):1161–6.
38. Sarrazin MSV, Cram P, Mazur A, Ward M, Reisinger HS. Patient perspectives of dabigatran: analysis of online discussion forums. Patient. 2014;7(1):47–54.
39. Chee BW, Berlin R, Schatz B. Predicting adverse drug events from personal health messages. In: AMIA Annu Symp proc. 2011. Washington DC; 2011. p. 217–26.
40. Topaz M, Lai K, Dhopeshwarkar N, Seger DL, Sa'adon R, Goss F, Rozenblum R, Zhou L. Clinicians' reports in electronic health records versus patients' concerns in social media: a pilot study of adverse drug reactions of aspirin and atorvastatin. Drug Saf. 2016;39(3):241–50.
41. Nadarajah S. Monitoring adverse events in Pharma's patient support programs: IMS Health; 2015.
42. Alvaro N, Conway M, Doan S, Lofi C, Overington J, Collier N. Crowdsourcing twitter annotations to identify first-hand experiences of prescription drug use. J Biomed Inform. 2015;58:280–7.
43. Benton A, Ungar L, Hill S, Hennessy S, Mao J, Chung A, Leonard CE, Holmes JH. Identifying potential adverse effects using the web: a new approach to medical hypothesis generation. J Biomed Inform. 2011;44(6):989–96.
44. Bian J, Topaloglu U, Yu F. Towards large-scale twitter mining for drug-related adverse events. In: Proceedings of the 2012 international workshop on smart health and wellbeing. 2012. Maui: ACM; 2012. p. 25–32.
45. Chary M, Park EH, McKenzie A, Sun J, Manini AF, Genes N. Signs & symptoms of dextromethorphan exposure from YouTube. PLoS One. 2014;9(2):e82452.
46. Chee BW, Berlin R, Schatz BR. Measuring population health using personal health messages. San Francisco: AMIA; 2009.
47. Correia RB, Li L, Rocha LM. Monitoring potential drug interactions and reactions via network analysis of instagram user timelines. In: Pacific Symposium on Biocomputing Pacific Symposium on Biocomputing. 2016. Kohala Coast: NIH Public Access; 2016. p. 492.
48. Elhadad N, Zhang S, Driscoll P, Brody S. Characterizing the sublanguage of online breast cancer forums for medications, symptoms, and emotions. In: Proc AMIA Annual Fall Symposium; Washington DC; 2014.
49. Ginn R, Pimpalkhute P, Nikfarjam A, Patki A, O'Connor K, Sarker A, Smith K, Gonzalez G. Mining twitter for adverse drug reaction mentions: a corpus and classification benchmark. In: Proceedings of the fourth workshop on building and evaluating resources for health and biomedical text processing. 2014. Reykjavik: Citeseer; 2014.
50. Gupta S, MacLean DL, Heer J, Manning CD. Induced lexico-syntactic patterns improve information extraction from online medical forums. J Am Med Inform Assoc. 2014;21(5):902–9.
51. Hadzi-Puric J, Grmusa J. Automatic drug adverse reaction discovery from parenting websites using disproportionality methods. In: Proceedings of the 2012 International Conference on Advances in Social Networks Analysis and Mining (ASONAM 2012). Istanbul: IEEE computer society; 2012. p. 792–7.
52. Jimeno-Yepes A, MacKinlay A, Han B, Chen Q. Identifying diseases, drugs, and symptoms in twitter. Stud Health Technol Inform. 2014;216:643–7.
53. Liu X, Liu J, Chen H. Identifying adverse drug events from health social media: a case study on heart disease discussion forums. In: International conference on smart health: 2014. Beijing: Springer; 2014. p. 25–36.
54. Liu X, Chen H. AZDrugMiner: an information extraction system for mining patient-reported adverse drug events in online patient forums. In: International conference on smart health: 2013. Beijing: Springer; 2013. p. 134–50.
55. Liu X, Chen H. Identifying adverse drug events from patient social media: a case study for diabetes. IEEE Intell Syst. 2015;30(3):44–51.
56. Liu X, Chen H. A research framework for pharmacovigilance in health social media: identification and evaluation of patient adverse drug event reports. J Biomed Inform. 2015;58:268–79.
57. Liu X, Chen H. Identifying adverse drug events from health social media using distant supervision. In: INFORMS Conference on Information Systens and Technology. Philadelphia: INFORMS; 2015.
58. Metke-Jimenez A, Karimi S. Concept extraction to identify adverse drug reactions in medical forums: a comparison of algorithms. Canberra: CSIRO; 2015. arXiv preprint arXiv:150406936.
59. Metke-Jimenez A, Karimi S, Paris C. Evaluation of text-processing algorithms for adverse drug event extraction from social media. In: Proceedings of the first international workshop on social media retrieval and analysis. 2014. Queensland: ACM; 2014. p. 15–20.
60. Nikfarjam A, Gonzalez GH. Pattern mining for extraction of mentions of adverse drug reactions from user comments. In. Austin: AMIA Annual Symposium proceedings; 2011. p. 1019–26.
61. Nikfarjam A, Sarker A, O'Connor K, Ginn R, Gonzalez G. Pharmacovigilance from social media: mining adverse drug reaction mentions using sequence labeling with word embedding cluster features. J Am Med Inform Assoc. 2015;22(3):671–81.
62. Patki A, Sarker A, Pimpalkhute P, Nikfarjam A, Ginn R, O'Connor K, Smith K, Gonzalez G. Mining adverse drug reaction signals from social media: going beyond extraction. Proceedings of BioLinkSig. 2014;2014:1–8.
63. Sampathkumar H, Chen X-W, Luo B. Mining adverse drug reactions from online healthcare forums using hidden Markov model. BMC Med Inform Decis Mak. 2014;14(1):1.
64. Sarker A, Gonzalez G. Portable automatic text classification for adverse drug reaction detection via multi-corpus training. J Biomed Inform. 2015;53:196–207.
65. Sarker A, O'Connor K, Ginn R, Scotch M, Smith K, Malone D, Gonzalez G. Social media mining for toxicovigilance: automatic monitoring of prescription medication abuse from twitter. Drug Saf. 2016;39(3):231–40.
66. Wu H, Fang H, Stanhope S. Exploiting online discussions to discover unrecognized drug side effects. Methods Inf Med. 2013;52(2):152–9.
67. Yang CC, Jiang L, Yang H, Tang X. Detecting signals of adverse drug reactions from health consumer contributed content in social media. In: Proceedings of ACM SIGKDD Workshop on Health Informatics: 2012. Beijing; 2012.
68. Yang CC, Yang H, Jiang L, Zhang M. Social media mining for drug safety signal detection. In: Proceedings of the 2012 international workshop on smart health and wellbeing: 2012. Maui HI: ACM; 2012. p. 33–40.
69. Yang H, Yang CC. Harnessing social media for drug-drug interactions detection. In: Healthcare Informatics (ICHI), 2013 IEEE International Conference on: 2013. Budapest: IEEE; 2013. p. 22–9.
70. Yang M, Kiang M, Shang W. Filtering big data from social media–building an early warning system for adverse drug reactions. J Biomed Inform. 2015; 54:230–40.
71. Yates A, Goharian N, Frieder O. Extracting adverse drug reactions from forum posts and linking them to drugs. In: Proceedings of the 2013 ACM SIGIR workshop on health search and discovery. 2013. Dublin; 2013.
72. Wang C, Karimi S. Differences between social media and regulatory databases in adverse drug reaction discovery. In: Proceedings of the first international workshop on social media retrieval and analysis: 2014. Queensland: ACM; 2014. p. 13–4.
73. Sarker A, Nikfarjam A, Gonzalez G. Social media mining shared task workshop. In: Proceedings of the Pacific Symposium on Biocomputing: 2016. Hawaii; 2016.
74. Freifeld CC: Digital pharmacovigilance: the medwatcher system for monitoring adverse events through automated processing of internet social media and crowdsourcing. 2014.

75. White RW, Harpaz R, Shah NH, DuMouchel W, Horvitz E. Toward enhanced pharmacovigilance using patient-generated data on the internet. Clin Pharmacol Ther. 2014;96(2):239.
76. White RW, Tatonetti NP, Shah NH, Altman RB, Horvitz E. Web-scale pharmacovigilance: listening to signals from the crowd. J Am Med Inform Assoc. 2013;20(3):404–8.
77. Carbonell P, Mayer MA, Bravo À. Exploring brand-name drug mentions on twitter for pharmacovigilance. Stud Health Technol Inform. 2015;210:55–9.
78. Segura-Bedmar I, Revert R, Martínez P. Detecting drugs and adverse events from Spanish health social media streams. In: Proceedings of the 5th International Workshop on Health Text Mining and Information Analysis (Louhi)@ EACL. Gothenburg; 2014. p. 106–15.
79. Segura-Bedmar I, De La Peña S, Martınez P. Extracting drug indications and adverse drug reactions from Spanish health social media. In: Proceedings of BioNLP: 2014; 2014. p. 98–106.
80. Segura-Bedmar I, Martínez P, Revert R, Moreno-Schneider J. Exploring Spanish health social media for detecting drug effects. BMC Med Inform Decis Mak. 2015;15(2):1.
81. Whitman CB, Reid MW, Arnold C, Patel H, Ursos L. Sa'adon R, Pourmorady J, Spiegel B: balancing opioid-induced gastrointestinal side effects with pain management: insights from the online community. J Opioid Manag. 2014; 11(5):383–91.
82. Yates A, Goharian N. ADRTrace: Detecting Expected and Unexpected Adverse Drug Reactions from User Reviews on Social Media Sites. In: Serdyukov P, Braslavski P, Kuznetsov SO, Kamps J, Rüger S, Agichtein E, Segalovich I, Yilmaz E, editors. Advances in Information Retrieval: 35th European Conference on IR Research. Berlin, Heidelberg: Springer Berlin Heidelberg; 2013. p. 816–9.
83. Karimi S, Metke-Jimenez A, Nguyen A. CADEminer: a system for mining consumer reports on adverse drug side effects. In: Proceedings of the eighth workshop on exploiting semantic annotations in information retrieval: 2015. Melbourne: ACM; 2015. p. 47–50.
84. Risson V, Saini D, Bonzani I, Huisman A, Olson M. Validation of social media analysis for outcomes research: identification of drivers of switches between oral and injectable therapies for multiple sclerosis. Value Health. 2015;18(7):A729.
85. Rizo C, Deshpande A, Ing A, Seeman N. A rapid, web-based method for obtaining patient views on effects and side-effects of antidepressants. J Affect Disord. 2011;130(1):290–3.
86. O'Connor K, Pimpalkhute P, Nikfarjam A, Ginn R, Smith KL, Gonzalez G. Pharmacovigilance on twitter? Mining tweets for adverse drug reactions. In: AMIA Annual Symposium Proceedings: 2014. Washington DC: American Medical Informatics Association; 2014:924.
87. Cameron D, Sheth AP, Jaykumar N, Thirunarayan K, Anand G, Smith GA. A hybrid approach to finding relevant social media content for complex domain specific information needs. Web Semant Sci Serv Agents World Wide Web. 2014;29:39–52.
88. Abou Taam M, Rossard C, Cantaloube L, Bouscaren N, Pochard L, Montastruc F, Montastruc J, Bagheri H. Analyze of internet narratives on patient websites before and after benfluorex withdrawal and media coverage. Fundam Clin Pharmacol. 2012;26:79–80.
89. Hanson CL, Burton SH, Giraud-Carrier C, West JH, Barnes MD, Hansen B. Tweaking and tweeting: exploring twitter for nonmedical use of a psychostimulant drug (Adderall) among college students. J Med Internet Res. 2013;15(4):e62.
90. Hughes S, Cohen D. Can online consumers contribute to drug knowledge? A mixed-methods comparison of consumer-generated and professionally controlled psychotropic medication information on the internet. J Med Internet Res. 2011;13(3):e53.
91. Pierce CE, Bouri K, Pamer C, Proestel S, Rodriguez HW, Van Le H, Freifeld CC, Brownstein JS, Walderhaug M, Edwards IR, et al. Evaluation of Facebook and twitter monitoring to detect safety signals for medical products: an analysis of recent FDA safety alerts. Drug Saf. 2017;40(4):317–31.
92. Duh MS, Cremieux P, Audenrode MV, Vekeman F, Karner P, Zhang H, Greenberg P. Can social media data lead to earlier detection of drug-related adverse events? Pharmacoepidemiol Drug Saf. 2016;25(12):1425–33.

4

An ontology-guided semantic data integration framework to support integrative data analysis of cancer survival

Hansi Zhang[1†], Yi Guo[1†], Qian Li[1], Thomas J. George[2], Elizabeth Shenkman[1], François Modave[1] and Jiang Bian[1*]

From The 2nd International Workshop on Semantics-Powered Data Analytics
Kansas City, MO, USA. 13 November 2017

Abstract

Background: Cancer is the second leading cause of death in the United States, exceeded only by heart disease. Extant cancer survival analyses have primarily focused on individual-level factors due to limited data availability from a single data source. There is a need to integrate data from different sources to simultaneously study as much risk factors as possible. Thus, we proposed an ontology-based approach to integrate heterogeneous datasets addressing key data integration challenges.

Methods: Following best practices in ontology engineering, we created the Ontology for Cancer Research Variables (OCRV) adapting existing semantic resources such as the National Cancer Institute (NCI) Thesaurus. Using the global-as-view data integration approach, we created mapping axioms to link the data elements in different sources to OCRV. Implemented upon the Ontop platform, we built a data integration pipeline to query, extract, and transform data in relational databases using semantic queries into a pooled dataset according to the downstream multi-level Integrative Data Analysis (IDA) needs.

Results: Based on our use cases in the cancer survival IDA, we created tailored ontological structures in OCRV to facilitate the data integration tasks. Specifically, we created a flexible framework addressing key integration challenges: (1) using a shared, controlled vocabulary to make data understandable to both human and computers, (2) explicitly modeling the semantic relationships makes it possible to compute and reason with the data, (3) linking patients to contextual and environmental factors through geographic variables, (4) being able to document the data manipulation and integration processes clearly in the ontologies.

Conclusions: Using an ontology-based data integration approach not only standardizes the definitions of data variables through a common, controlled vocabulary, but also makes the semantic relationships among variables from different sources explicit and clear to all users of the same datasets. Such an approach resolves the ambiguity in variable selection, extraction and integration processes and thus improve reproducibility of the IDA.

Keywords: Semantic data integration, Ontology, Semantic web, Cancer survival, Integrative data analysis

* Correspondence: bianjiang@ufl.edu
†Hansi Zhang and Yi Guo contributed equally to this work.
[1]Department of Health Outcomes and Biomedical Informatics, College of Medicine, University of Florida, Clinical and Translational Research Building Suite 3228, 2004 Mowry Road, PO Box 100219, Gainesville, FL 32610-0219, USA
Full list of author information is available at the end of the article

Background

As the second leading cause of death, cancer is responsible for one in every four deaths in the United States [1]. In 2017, there were approximately 1.68 million new cancer cases and 600 thousand cancer deaths in the US [2] estimated by the American Cancer Society. When first diagnosed with cancer, patients ask about their prognosis, whether their cancer is relatively easy or more difficult to treat, and the likelihood of survival. There is a huge variation in survival between cancer types, stages, age groups, races/ethnicities, genders, and many other factors. For example, among some of the frequently diagnosed cancers, including lung, colorectal, breast, and prostate cancers, the 5-year overall survival rates are 18.3, 64.9, 89.7, and 98.3%, respectively [3]. These rates are much worse when the cancer is metastasized, which are 4.5, 13.9, 26.9, and 29.8% for the same types of cancers, respectively [3].

To improve cancer survival rates and prognosis, one of the first steps is to improve our understanding of contributory factors associated with cancer survival. Priori research such as the National Institute on Minority Health and Health Disparities (NIMHD) Research Framework [4] and the social-ecological model [5] recognizes that individuals are embedded within the larger social system and constrained by the physical environment they lived in. Thus, the determinants of individuals' health span across different domains of influence (i.e., biological, behavioral, physical/built environment, sociocultural environment, and healthcare system) as well as different levels of influence (i.e., individual, interpersonal, community, and societal). Within these frameworks, cancer survival is influenced by multiple factors from multiple levels and multiple domains. At the individual level, cancer survival is influenced by not only cancer stage of diagnosis and treatment, demographics, and financial status, but also risky health behaviors such as smoking, alcohol drinking, and physical inactivity. For example, cigarette smoking is by far the most important risk factor for lung cancer; 80% of lung cancer deaths in the US were caused by smoking [2]. Beyond individual-level factors, occupational or environmental exposure to secondhand smoke, air pollution, radiation, and some organic chemicals are also significant risk factors. Further, at the contextual level, cancer survival is influenced by public policies that influence health care delivery which could impact patients' travel distance to the treatment facility [6].

Prior epidemiologic research on cancer survival in the US, however, has primarily focused on contributory factors from the individual level due to limited data availability. Very few studies have explored contextual factors, and certainly no study has explored all possible factors together. Most of these analyses used data from a single source, such as data from a hospital (e.g., electronic health records, EHRs), a cancer registry (e.g., the Surveillance, Epidemiology, and End Results, SEER registry) or administrative claims systems (e.g., data from Centers for Medicare and Medicaid Services, CMS) [7–10]. SEER is an extremely popular data source for studying cancer survival [8–10]. However, it is important to pool heterogeneous data sets with variables beyond the individual level for integrative data analysis (IDA) that simultaneously examine as many cancer survival predictors as possible (i.e. top down approach to the model building) so that confounding effects and interactions among predictors can be fully understood. For example, the linked SEER-Medicare data give us a more complete picture of cancer patients beyond their cancer status with other clinical characteristics such as comorbidity as well as their healthcare utilization patterns [11–14]. Nonetheless, the ability to integrate risk factors of more domains and levels from other data sources such as socioeconomic status of the community from US Census data and community smoking rate from the Behavioral Risk Factor Surveillance System (BRFSS) will further advance our understanding of the determinants of cancer survival.

Nevertheless, researchers are faced with key challenges when integrating data from different sources. Data integration is a daunting task because data from different sources can be heterogeneous in syntax (e.g., file formats, access protocols), schema (e.g., data structures), and semantics (e.g., meanings or interpretations). The effort required to connect different sources is substantial due to lack of clear definitions (i.e., data semantics) of variables, measures, and constructs. Many traditional data integration techniques have been used on large scale in biomedical research [15–17], such as rule-based links (i.e., link variables from different data sources directly base on the names and definitions), data warehouses (i.e., create a new system to store a copy of the data from difference data sources, and manage the data separately from the original data systems) and ad-hoc query optimizers (i.e., re-phrasing a user's query into multiple subqueries according to the structures of individual distributed databases) and federated middleware frameworks (i.e., link multiple applications and user interfaces to multiple data sources, act as the overarching facade across multiple applications). However, all these traditional methods did not consider the semantic knowledge, which intend to integrate information based on the meaning of the data elements. For example, how to distinguish synonyms, homonyms and related terms (e.g., different representations of the same disease using different coding standards) across different data sources. Therefore, adopting a semantic data integration approach, we propose to generate a universal conceptual representation of "information" to bridge the data heterogeneities across different sources. The "information" includes not only data elements but also their relationships, via "ontologies". An ontology is a computational representation of a domain of knowledge based upon a controlled, standardized vocabulary for describing entities and the semantic relationships between them [18–21]. The use of ontologies can facilitate data integration in many ways, including metadata representation, automatic data verification, global conceptualization, support for high-level semantic queries, and extend beyond traditional approaches of using common data elements (CDEs) and common data models (CDMs) [22–24], especially in the biomedical domain [15, 25].

Marenco et al. developed a Query Integrator System (QIS) to address robust data integration from heterogeneous data sources in the biosciences in 2004 [26]. An ontology server was used in QIS to map data sources' metadata to the concepts in standard vocabularies [26]. Cheung et al. developed a prototype web application called YeastHub based on a Resource Description Framework (RDF) database to support the integration of different types of yeast genome data in different sources in 2005 [27]. Lam et al. used the Web Ontology Language (OWL) to integrate two heterogeneous neuroscience databases [28] in 2005. In a follow-up study, Lam et al. designed AlzPharm that used RDF and its extension vocabulary, RDF Schema (RDFS), to facilitate both data representation and integration [29]. Smith et al. built the LinkHub system leveraging Semantic Web technologies (i.e., RDF and RDF queries) to facilitate cross-database queries and information retrieval in proteomics in 2007 [30]. In 2008, Shironoshita et al. introduced a query formulation method to execute semantic queries across multiple data services in the cancer Biomedical Informatics Grid (caBIG), named Semantic caBIG Data Integration (semCDI). Mercadé et al. developed an ontology-based application called Orymold for dynamic gene expression data annotation, integration and exploration in 2009. Based on the QIS [26], Luis et al. designed an automated approach for integrating federated databases using ontological metadata mappings in 2009 [31]. Chisham et al. created the Comparative Data Analysis Ontology (CDAO) and developed the CDAO-Store system to support data integration for phylogenetic analysis in 2011 [32]. Kama et al. built a Data Definition Ontology (DDO) using the D2RQ (i.e., a platform to provide RDF-based access over relational databases) for accessing heterogeneous clinical data sources [33]. Pang et al. developed BiobankedConnect to speed up the process of integrating comparable data from different biobanks to get a pooled data using ontological and lexical indexing in 2014 [34]. Ethier et al. designed the Clinical Data Integration Model (CDIM) based on the Basic Formal Ontology (BFO) [35] to support biomedical data integration in 2015 [36]. Mate et al. proposed an ontology-based approach to organize and describe the medical concepts of both source and target systems in order to integrate the data across different clinical and research systems [37]. Livingston et al. created an integrated knowledge base of biomedical data from multiple sources, called KaBOB, based on Open Biomedical Ontologies [38]. In 2016, Liang et al. proposed an ontology-oriented approach to represent the relations between genes, drugs, phenotypes, symptoms, and diseases from multiple information sources in aiding the analysis of psychiatric drug repurposing [39]. Similar to our approach, Kock-schoppenhauer et al. used the ontology-based data access (OBDA) model and the Ontop framework to access relational clinical databases with SPARQL queries [40]. However, most of these existing semantic data integration systems and frameworks have focused on 1) the harmonization and alignments of data elements using semantic resources; 2) creating tailored ad hoc resources for specific use cases that may not be generalizable; and 3) the integration of data from similar data sources (e.g., data from different electronic health record systems) and addressing the syntactic (i.e., data formats) and schematic (i.e., data models) heterogeneity. Very few studies have fully leveraged the reasoning ability provided by ontologically structured data. And none of the studies has used ontologies as a knowledge representation tool to document the data integration process.

This paper describes a case study of semantic data integration linking five data sets that cover both individual and contextual level factors for the purpose of assessing the association of predictors of interest with cancer survival. The main contribution of our work is that we applied an ontology-based data integration framework to integrate both individual and contextual level factors to facilitate integrative data analysis (i.e., pool heterogeneous data sets). The use of ontologies can facilitate data integration in many ways and extend beyond traditional data integration approaches. Unlike existing ontology-driven data integration methods, our study focused on encoding the different data integration scenarios explicitly using a formal and computational model with a shared vocabulary—the Ontology for Cancer Research Variables (OCRV). Our goal is not only to make the data integration process easier, but also to facilitate documentation and communication of the data integration processes between scientists. This is significant for research rigor, transparency, reproducibility as well as data reusability.

In our previous short paper [41], we prototyped an ontology-based data access approach to integrate three different datasets to support IDA of cancer survival. In this extended journal paper, we significantly expanded our ontology-based data integration framework.

- We used n-ary relations [42] in our ontology to represent relations among more than two individuals. For example, we created a *'ocrv:diagnosis_relation'* class to link the *'ocrv:date of diagnosis'*, the *'ocrv:-diagnosed tumor type'* and the *'ncit:patient'*.
- We adopted the Time Event Ontology (TEO) [43–45] for representing events, time, and their relationships. For example, the *'ocrv:date of diagnosis'* was represented as a *'ocrv:diagnosis_relation'* instance (event) associated with an 'teo:*timeInstance*' (time).
- We improved the reasoning ability via using OWL restrictions [46], so that we can encode certain knowledge (i.e., constrains on properties) in the ontology. For example, in our model, current smoker is defined as patients who (1) is a current everyday/someday smoker, and (2) smoked at least 100 cigarettes in the entire life. Thus, we created restrictions for the object property 'ocrv:*has_smoking_status*'.
- We leveraged the ontology to exam the consistency of the source data. For example, we used an individual's *'ocrv:date of diagnosis'* and *'ncit:birth year'* to calculate the diagnosis age and then compared with the value directly obtained from the *'ncit:age at diagnosis'* variable to check the consistency of the source data.

Methods

Our overall goal is to facilitate the data integration needs of a theory-driven multi-level IDA of cancer survival informed by the NHMID Research Framework and the socio-ecological model with an ontology-based semantic data integration approach.

Data integration use case: The multi-level integrative data analysis of Cancer survival

The goal of the multi-level IDA was to examine the predictive ability of cancer survival models under 3 common data integration scenarios that researchers often face in data analysis: (1) additional predictors, especially contextual factors such as county smoking rate become available through linking multiple datasets, (2) different predictors representing the same concept are available (e.g., different definitions of rurality based on either the rural-urban commuting area (RUCA) [47] codes or the National Center for Health Statistics (NCHS) [48] urban-rural classification scheme), and (3) different forms of the same predictor are available (e.g., different grouping strategy based on the raw 10-level RUCA classification to define metropolitan vs. non-metropolitan). To do so, we linked data from five different sources to evaluate discrimination performance of predictive models for breast, lung, and colorectal cancers.

Data sources

The multi-level IDA of cancer survival was based on data of the UF Health Cancer Center Catchment Area (CCCA) from multiple sources. The UF Health CCCA is a region in north Florida that included 20 counties: Alachua, Baker, Bradford, Citrus, Clay, Columbia, Dixie, Gilchrist, Hamilton, Jefferson, Lafayette, Leon, Levy, Madison, Marion, Putnam, Sumter, Suwannee, Taylor, and Union. The individual- and contextual-level factors were extracted from 6 data sources: (1) We collected each patient's demographic, diagnosis, treatment and survival information from the 1996–2010 Florida Cancer Data System (FCDS) [49]—a statewide cancer registry supported by the Centers for Disease Control and Prevention (CDC)—data. The FCDS followed the national data standards set forth by the American College of Surgeons, Commission on Cancer (ACoS/CoC), the North American Association of Central Registries (NAACCR) and the Surveillance, Epidemiology and End Results (SEER). (2) We obtained census tract level social vulnerability index (SVI) [50] from the Agency for Toxic Substances & Disease Registry (ATSDR). (3) We also obtained education and poverty information from the United States Census Bureau [51] (i.e., the 2000 US census). (4) We obtained county-level smoking rate, alcohol consumption rate, and health status from the Behavioral Risk Factor Surveillance System (BRFSS) [52] of the Centers for Disease Control and Prevention (CDC). Note that, each record in BRFSS is assigned with a final weight to make generalizations from the sample to the populations. BRFSS uses the raking weighting methodology, which is comprised of two parts, design weight and raking, where BRFSS final weight = Design Weight * Raking Adjustments [53]. (5) We used data from the County Health Ranking and Roadmaps [54], where we obtained county-level mental health, physical health, and primary care related information. All the raw data were in relational structures, thus, we imported and stored all of our source data in a relational database (i.e., MySQL) without any manipulations.

Adult cancer patients (18 years or older at the time of diagnosis) were identified in the FCDS data using the International Classification of Disease for Oncology 3rd edition (ICD-O-3) codes: C50.0-C50.9 for breast, C34.0-C34.3, C34.8, and C34.9 for lung, and C18.0-C18.9, and C26.0 for colorectal cancers. We obtained 50,151 unique cancer patients (18,644 breast, 21,552 lung, and 9955 colorectal). Table 1 shows a summary of the risk factors extracted from the 5 data sources. The individual-level factors were all extracted from the FCDS, reflecting individual patients' sociodemographic and clinical characteristics. The contextual-level factors such as county level average smoking rate were linked to individual patients based on their residencies. These contextual-level factors,

Table 1 Summary of the risk factors extracted from different datasets

Risk factor		Data source	Reference ontology
Individual level	Race Gender Ethnicity Marital status Smoking status Insurance payer Residency: county and census tract[a] Age at diagnosis Year of diagnosis Tumor stage Tumor type Treatment procedure	Florida Cancer Data System (FCDS)	NCIt TEO OCRV
Contextual level	Census tract SVI[b] household composition and disability Census tract SVI minority status and language Census tract SVI housing and transportation Census tract SVI socioeconomic status	Agency for Toxic Substances & Disease Registry (ATSDR)	OCRV
	Census tract high school completion rates Census tract family poverty rates[c]	United States Census Bureau	OCRV
	Census tract rurality status[d]		OCRV NCIt
	County adult mental and physical health status[e] County density of primary care physicians[f]	County Health Ranking & Roadmaps	OCRV
	County smoking rate County alcohol consumption rate	Behavioral Risk Surveillance System (BRFSS)	OCRV NCIt

[a]The residency of the individual at the county- and census tract-level (i.e., which county and census tract the individual lives in), which are the linkage variables used to connect the individuals with contextual-level risk factors

[b]Social Vulnerability Index (SVI) refers to the resilience of communities when confronted by external stresses on human health, such as when facing disasters or disease outbreaks

[c]The percentage of all families whose income in the past 12 months is below the poverty level

[d]The rurality status for each census tract is based on the RUCA code

[e]The average number of days a county's adult respondents report that their mental/physical health was not good during past 30 days

[f]The ratio of the population to total primary care physicians

contributing to individuals' cancer survivals, reflect the environmental and societal characteristics of where the individuals were embedded in. In our data analysis, these contextual-level factors were either calculated at the county level (e.g., average smoking rate from BRFSS) or the census tract level (e.g., the social vulnerability index from ATSDR), depending on the geographic resolutions of the raw data available. In addition to the risk factors, our datasets also contained variables such as survival status and cause of death (if died, and coded with the International Classification of Diseases, Ninth Revision, Clinical Modification, ICD-9-CM, codes).

Overview of a semantic data integration pipeline

Our semantic data integration workflow is based on an ontology-based data access (OBDA) framework demonstrated in Fig. 1. The first step of semantic data integration is to construct synthesized, integrated descriptions (i.e., a global ontology) of the information coming from multiple sources. An ontology—the Ontology for Cancer Research Variables (OCRV)—in our case, is a metadata representation of the data elements and their semantic relationships in a both human- and machine-understandable structure. After building the ontology, an OBDA model was created—using semantic mapping axioms—to link the source data elements to the entities in OCRV. Given a global view of available data from different sources, a user can pose data (integration) requests for the selected variables (and desired representations) against our data integration pipeline, which converts the requests to a set of SPARQL queries. Based on the semantic mapping axioms defined in the OBDA model, Ontop's Quest—a SPARQL query engine—can translate a SPARQL query over the ontology into a union of sub-queries over the data sources. The integration of the sub-query results constitutes the answer to the semantic query. The sub-queries are subject to the structure of source schemas, and often expressed in the native query languages of the sources (e.g., Structured Query Language, SQL commonly used for relational databases).

We used the Ontop platform that provides an infrastructure for querying relational databases through ontologies [55]. Within Ontop, entities (i.e., classes and properties) in the ontology are mapped to the data

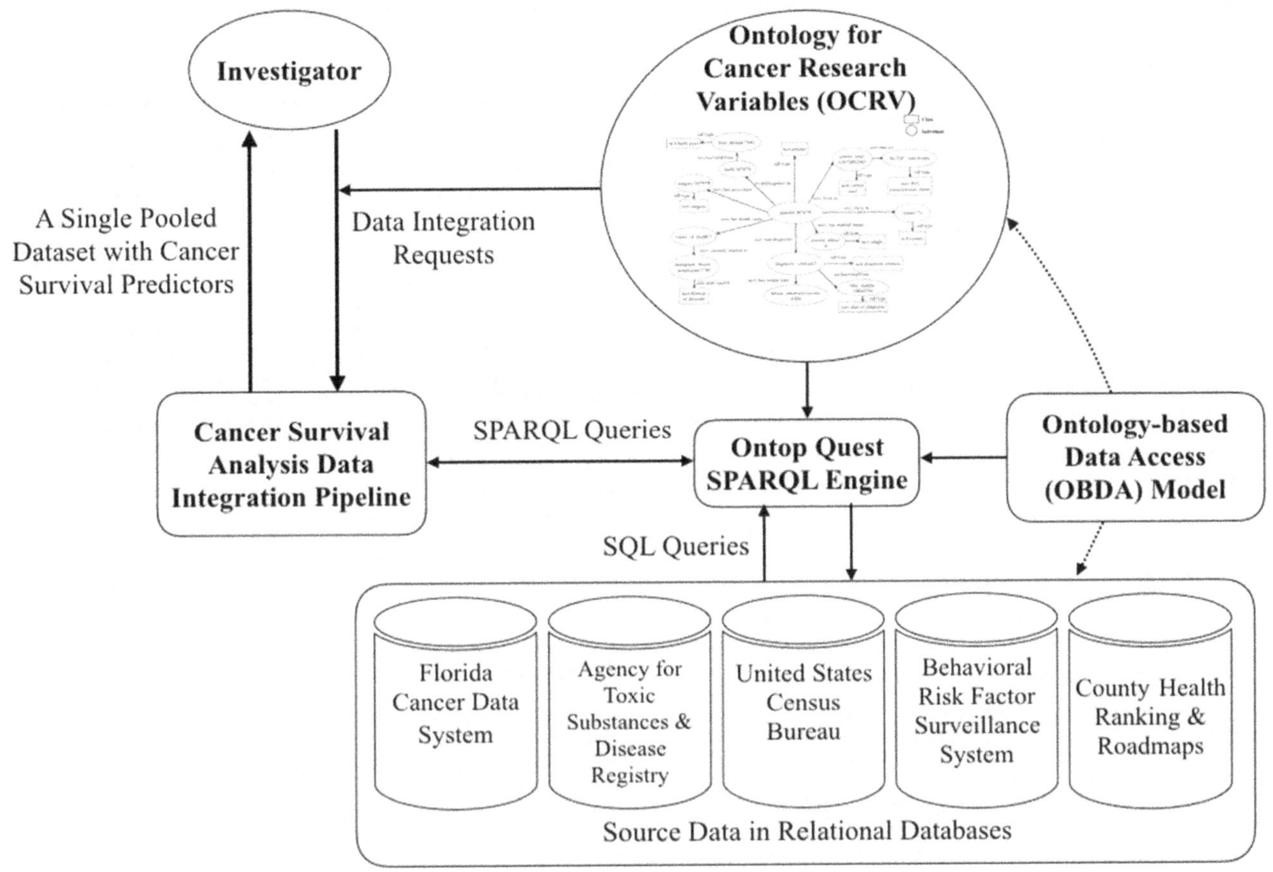

Fig. 1 The overall process of our semantic data integration approach through an ontology-based data access framework. **The user can post data integration requests according to OCRV, then the requests were converted into SPARQL queries through the data integration pipeline. The OBDA model consists of a set of semantic mappings that specify how source data are related to the entities in the ontology. The Quest is a SPARQL query engine which uses the semantic mappings in the OBDA model to translate SPARQL queries over the ontology into SQL queries over the data sources*

elements (and the relationships between the data elements) in the databases and presented as virtual Resources Description Framework (RDF) graphs. Subsequently, we can then query the virtual RDF graphs via SPQRAL queries.

Constructing an ontology for Cancer research variables (OCRV)

Scope

The OCRV was built for integrating and unifying multi-level predictors of cancer survival across heterogeneous data sources. The OCRV covered a broad range of individual- and contextual-level factors, as shown in Table 1. We used the Basic Formal Ontology (BFO) [35] as the upper-level ontology, and imported the NCI Thesaurus (NCIt) and the Time Event Ontology (TEO) as the foundation for creating the OCRV.

Approach

Using the BFO as the overarching organization, the OCRV was developed with both top-down and bottom-up strategies to catalog relevant entities. A top-down approach was followed to identify candidate entities based on the predictors (i.e., identified through a comprehensive literature review of existing predictors related to cancer survival guided by the NIMHD Research Framework and the social-ecological model) used in the cancer survival analysis. In addition, a review of existing widely accepted ontologies (using the NCBO BioPortal [56]) was conducted to find the relevant entities that can be reused in OCRV. As shown in Table 1, many of the entities that we needed are captured in the NCIt. A bottom-up approach was then used to characterize the entities that have been identified in the top-down approach. We examined the data sources that contained these risk factors, especially the metadata (i.e., the table structures of the relational database). We inspected how these risk factors were expressed in the relational source databases as well as the relationships among the raw data elements, and determined what additional entities and relations were needed to fully represent these risk factors in OCRV.

More importantly, we considered the specific data integration use cases for supporting the multi-level IDA of cancer survival. For example, in our cancer survival analysis, we only needed to model *'marital status'* as *'single'* vs. *'married'*, while the raw data has a more fine-grained categorization (e.g., *'widowed'* and *'divorced'*). Thus, we constructed our ontology to support the data analysis needs by declaring *'widowed'* and *'divorced'* as subclasses of *'single'*.

Implementation

We used Protégé 5 [57] to construct the ontology. We worked collaboratively, finalizing the list of entities based on each one's domain expertise (e.g., oncology, cancer prevention and outcomes, and cancer population science). An example of the raw data records annotated with the OCRV is shown in Fig. 2.

Designing the mapping axioms

In Ontop, the OBDA model consists of two parts: mapping axioms and data source declarations (i.e., to establish the database connections to the source databases using the Java Database Connectivity (JDBC) application program interface). The goal of the mapping axioms is to link the data elements in data sources to the entities in the OCRV. We constructed the mapping axioms using the Ontop Protégé plugin. In general, there were three types of mapping axioms (i.e., mappings for classes, mappings for object properties, and mappings for data properties). Each mapping axiom consisted of three fields: a mappingId, a source, and a target. The mappingId was used to uniquely identify a mapping axiom, the source is typically a SQL query to retrieve the necessary data from the data sources, and the target is an RDF triple template. Based on the OBDA model, Ontop was then able to realize the data in relational databases into virtual RDF graphs. Subsequently, we can use SPARQL queries to retrieve and manipulate the data stored in these virtual RDF graphs. Note that design of the mapping axioms as well as the ontology were driven by the data integration use cases, and subsequently, the required data query and manipulation needs. Based on the data integration needs, the SPARQL queries can be classified into four categories: (1) queries that extract

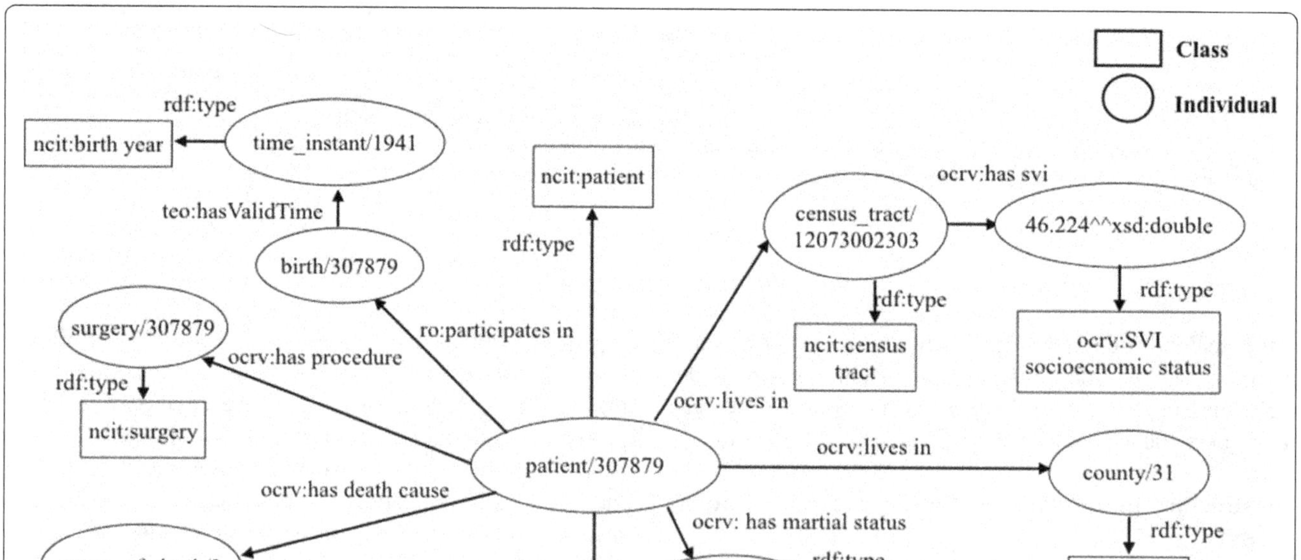

Fig. 2 An example of data records annotated with the Ontology for Cancer Research Variables (OCRV). * Square boxes are classes, and ovals are individuals

Table 2 The entities created for OCRV based on the data analysis needs

OCRV entity	Label
Classes	social vulnerability index • SVI household composition and disability • SVI housing and transportation • SVI minority status and languages • SVI socioeconomic status
	BRFSS current smoker • BRFSS current every day smoker • BRFSS current someday smoker • BRFSS smoker who smoked at least 100 cigarettes in the entire life
	BRFSS heavy drinker • male heavy drinker who reported having more than 14 drinks per week • female heavy drinker who reported having more than 7 drinks per week
	rural-urban commuting area codes • metropolitan area core • metropolitan area high commuting • metropolitan area low commuting • micropolitan area core • micropolitan high commuting • micropolitan low commuting • small town core • small town high commuting • small town low commuting • rural areas
	census tract high school completion rate
	census tract family poverty rate
	county adult mental health status
	county adult physical health status
	county density of primary care physicians
	single
	unknown marital status
Object properties	has death cause
	has diagnosis
	has marital status
	has procedure
	has smoking status
	has drinking status
	has tumor type
	has tumor stage
	has stage
	has race
	has biological sex
	has ethnicity
	has insurance payer
	has survival status
	has tumor stage
	has family poverty level
	has education level

Table 2 The entities created for OCRV based on the data analysis needs *(Continued)*

OCRV entity	Label
	has mental health condition
	has physical health condition
	has primary care physician ratio
	has svi
	lives in
Data properties	has BRFSS final weight

variables directly linked to a patient without the need for any processing; (2) queries that need to preprocess the raw data to produce the desired results; (3) queries that are used to link a patient to contextual factors through geographic variables (e.g., county, census tract); (4) queries that generate results based on the knowledge which has been encoded in ontology. We will discuss these four types of queries in detail in the RESULTS section.

Creating a data integration pipeline

The goal of our data integration tasks was to link predictors from different data sources to generate a single pooled dataset for cancer survival analysis. Thus, we created a data integration pipeline using the Ontop OWL Java application programming interface (API) [58] to translate user requests into SPARQL queries and to organize the query results into an analytic format. The OWL API [59] is a reference implementation for interacting with OWL ontologies. The Ontop OWL API extended the OWLReasoner interface in the OWL API to support SPARQL query answering against relational databases. As required by our data analysis models, the final results were organized into a data table (i.e., a matrix), where each row represented a patient's cancer diagnosis record (as one patient can have multiple cancer diagnoses in the FCDS data), and each column represented a cancer risk factor.

Results

The ontology for Cancer research variables (OCRV)

The OCRV was constructed iteratively using the Protégé tool. We used the BFO as the upper-level ontology and imported the NCIt and the TEO as the foundation for creating the OCRV. Besides reusing terms in existing

Table 3 The implementation of the OWL restrictions for *'ocrv:BRFSS current smoker'*

Class	Notation 3 (N3) code
BRFSS current smoker	@prefix: <http://www.semanticweb.org/ontologies/OCRV#> @prefix rdfs: <http://www.w3.org/2000/01/rdf-schema#> @prefix owl: <http://www.w3.org/2002/07/owl#> : BRFSS current smoker a owl:class rdfs:subClassOf ncit:smoking status.
BRFSS current every day smoker	@prefix: <http://www.semanticweb.org/ontologies/OCRV#> @prefix rdfs: <http://www.w3.org/2000/01/rdf-schema#> @prefix owl: <http://www.w3.org/2002/07/owl#> :BRFSS current every day smoker a owl:class rdfs:subClassOf [a owl:Restriction; owl:allValuesFrom: BRFSS smoker who smoked at least 100 cigarettes in the entire life; owl:onProperty:has smoking status].
BRFSS current someday smoke	@prefix: <http://www.semanticweb.org/ontologies/OCRV#> @prefix rdfs: <http://www.w3.org/2000/01/rdf-schema#> @prefix owl: <http://www.w3.org/2002/07/owl#> :BRFSS current someday smoker a owl:class rdfs:subClassOf [a owl:Restriction; owl:allValuesFrom: BRFSS smoker who smoked at least 100 cigarettes in the entire life; owl:onProperty:has smoking status].
BRFSS smoker who smoked at least 100 cigarettes in the entire live	@prefix: <http://www.semanticweb.org/ontologies/OCRV#> @prefix rdfs: <http://www.w3.org/2000/01/rdf-schema#> @prefix owl: <http://www.w3.org/2002/07/owl#> :BRFSS smoker who smoked at least 100 cigarettes in the entire life a owl:class rdfs:subClassOf ncit:smoking status.

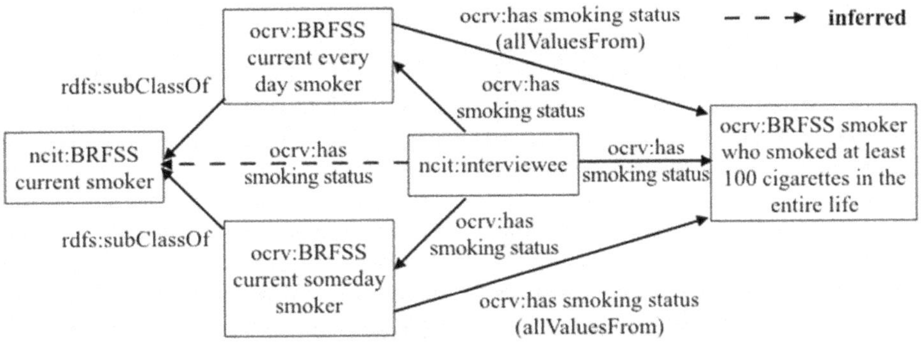

Fig. 3 The representation of the relations among *'ocrv:BRFSS current every day smoker', 'ocrv:BRFSS current someday smoker' 'ocrv:BRFSS current every day smoker'*, and *'ocrv:BRFSS smoker who smoked at least 100 cigarettes in the entire life'*

ontologies, we also created entities (i.e., classes, object properties, and datatype properties) based on the data analysis needs as shown in Table 2. Overall, we created 30 new classes, and added 23 new properties. The maximum depth of the classes is 5.

We used *owl:Restriction* and *rdfs:subClassOf* axioms to encode the knowledge of the data integration processes in OCRV, leveraging the reasoning ability. For example, to calculate the average smoking rate for a county using BRFSS, the very first step was to find the number smokers for the county in the raw BRFSS data. BRFSS is a national telephone survey that collects state data about U.S. residents regarding their health-related risk behaviors, chronic conditions, and use of preventative services. Thus, the raw BRFSS data were participants' survey responses, including answers to questions such as "Do you now smoke cigarettes every day, some days, or not at all?". According to BRFSS, a smoker was defined as a person who (1) currently smokes every day or someday, and (2) has smoked at least 100 cigarettes in the entire

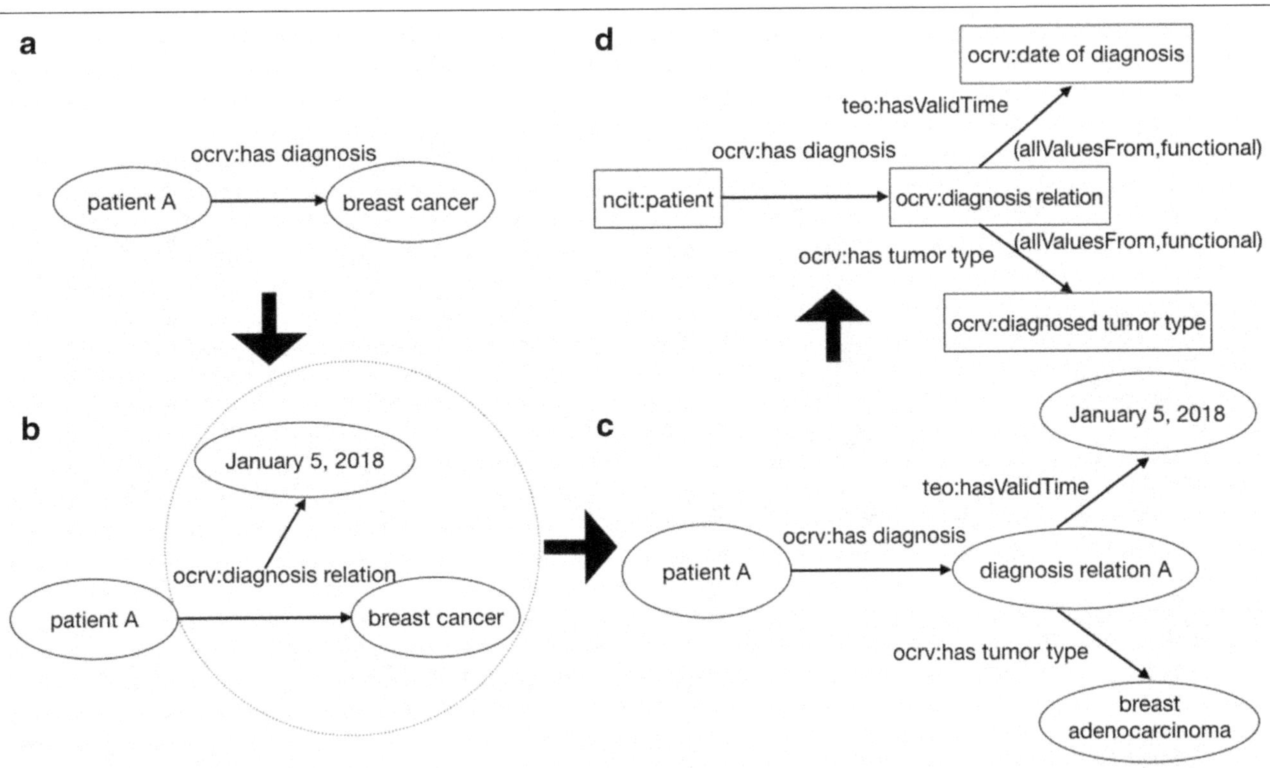

Fig. 4 The representation of the n-ary relation pattern among patient, diagnosed tumor type, and date of diagnosis, where (**a**) illustrates how a patient A links to a breast cancer diagnosis, (**b**) is a graphical representation of the diagnosis relation contains not only the diagnosis "breast cancer" but also a timestamp for the date of diagnosis, (**c**) shows on the instance level how a patient A, her diagnosis of breast adenocarcinoma, and the diagnosis date are connected, and (**d**) shows how owl:Restriction is used to implement this n-ary relation

life. The variables we used in the source data to define a smoker were: (1) SMOKDAY2 (i.e., "Do you now smoke cigarettes every day, some days, or not at all?"), and (2) SMOKE100 (i.e., "Have you smoked at least 100 cigarettes in your entire life?"). We first defined a '*ocrv:BRFSS current smoker*' class, with two subclasses as: '*ocrv:BRFSS current every day smoker*' and '*ocrv:BRFSS current someday smoker*', which were linked to a person (i.e., '*ncit:interviewee*') using the object property '*ocrv:has smoking status*'. We also created a class (i.e., '*ocrv:BRFSS smoker who smoked at least 100 cigarettes in the entire life*') to represent people who smoked at least 100 cigarettes in their entire life. To encode the BRFSS's definition of smoker, we applied OWL restrictions on the property '*ocrv:has smoking status*' for each subclass of '*ocrv:BRFSS current smoker*' as shown in Table 3 in Notation3 (N3) syntax [60], which enforces that the '*ocrv:BRFSS current every day smoker*' and '*ocrv:BRFSS current someday smoker*' need to have smoked at least 100 cigarettes in their entire life. Fig. 3 shows the relations among '*ocrv:BRFSS current every day smoker*', '*ocrv:BRFSS current someday smoker*' '*ocrv:BRFSS current every day smoker*', and '*ocrv:BRFSS smoker who smoked at least 100 cigarettes in the entire life*'.

We also followed the best practices to define n-ary [42] relations to describe relations among more than two individuals or values. In RDF and OWL, properties are binary relations, linking two individuals or an individual and a value. For example, as shown in Fig. 4a, a patient A has been diagnosed with breast cancer. However, we also want to express that the diagnosis relation happened on a specific date ('*date of diagnosis*'), as "*The patient A has been diagnosed with breast cancer on January 5, 2018.*' This is an n-ary relation, as shown in Fig. 4b, where the object property '*ocrv:diagnosis relation*' also needs to have an attribute of '*date of diagnosis*', which we cannot represent. To do so, we instead created a '*ocrv:diagnosis relation*' class; and a 'ocrv:*diagnosis relation A*' individual referring to an instance of the relation among a '*ncit:patient*', a '*ocrv:diagnosed tumor type*', and the '*ocrv:date of diagnosis*', as shown in Fig.4.c. The individual '*:diagnosis relation A*' represents a single object encapsulating both the diagnosed tumor type ('*:breast adenocarcinoma*', a specific instance of the

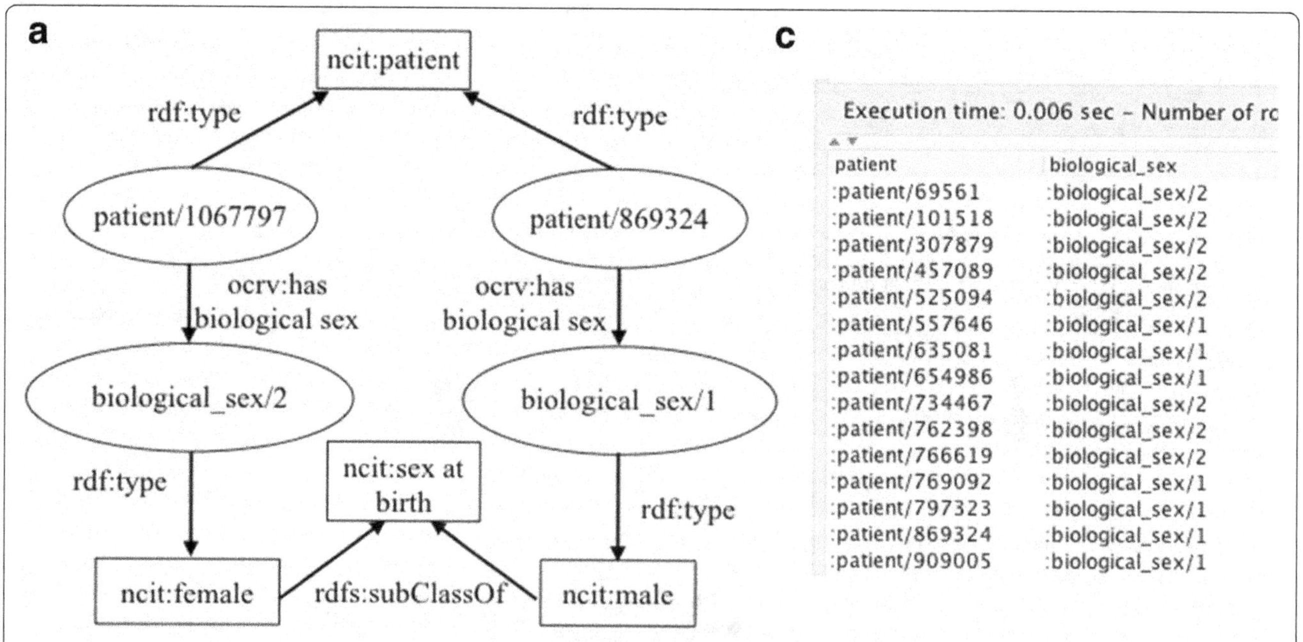

b

```
PREFIX obo: <http://purl.obolibrary.org/obo/>
PREFIX : <http://www.semanticweb.org/ontologies/OCRV#>

SELECT ?patient ?biological_sex WHERE
{?patient :has biological sex ?biological_sex.}
```

Fig. 5 A SPARQL query that extracts the sex information of all patients, where (**a**) is a graphical representation of the relationship between a '*ncit:patient*' and its '*ncit:sex at birth*', (**b**) shows the SPARQL query, and (**c**) shows the query results

tumor type) and the date of the diagnosis (*'January 5, 2018'*). Each of the 3 statements in the original n-ary relation, who was diagnosed, what the diagnosis is, and when it was diagnosed, is then a binary relationship (i.e., *'ocrv:has diagnosis', 'ocrv:has tumor type', 'teo:hasValidTime'*). The class definitions for the individuals in this pattern are shown in Fig. 4d. Both properties 'ocrv:*has tumor type*' and 'teo:*hasValidTime*" are functional properties, ensuring that each instance of *'ocrv:diagnosis relation'* class has exactly one value for *'ocrv:diagnosed tumor type'* and one value for *'ocrv:date of diagnosis'*. The OWL restrictions on these two properties restrict the values of the properties (e.g., *owl:allValuesFrom* indicates that the values of the property are all members of the class indicated by the *owl:allValuesFrom* class). We instantiated the specific *'ocrv:diagnosed tumor type'* subclasses using the ICD-O-3 codes as in the original FCDS data source (i.e., mapping axioms that linked each ICD-O-3 code to a specific tumor type as defined in the NCIt).

The four types of SPARQL queries

Type 1: Queries that extract variables directly linked to a patient without the need for any processing

Many individual-level factors such as the gender of a patient from the FCDS can be extracted with a simple SPARQL query. For example, the object property *'ocrv:has biological sex'* was used to link a *'ncit:patient'* its *'ncit:sex at birth'* as shown in Fig. 5a. Based on this relation, we can use a simple SPARQL query as shown in Fig. 5b. to retrieve all patients' sex information, where *'?patient'* represents the patients and *'?sex'* represents the patients' sex at birth information. Note that, in SPARQL, query variables are prefixed with either "?" or "$". The results of the query were shown in Fig. 5c.

Type 2: Queries that need to process the raw data to produce the desired results

In data analysis, many raw variables needed to be processed to derive new variables or converted into different formats. For example, in our cancer survival analysis, we only considered the year of diagnosis, whereas the raw data in FCDS were recorded as the date of diagnosis in 'yyyymmdd' format. In OCRV, we used *'teo:hasOrigTime'* (i.e., a data property in TEO) to link a date value to an individual of *'ocrv:date of diagnosis'*. Fig. 6 illustrates our process to convert the raw date of diagnosis to the desired year of diagnosis in a SPARQL query.

Type 3: Queries that are used to link a patient to contextual factors through geographic variables

The contextual-level factors used in our cancer survival models were linked to individual patients

a

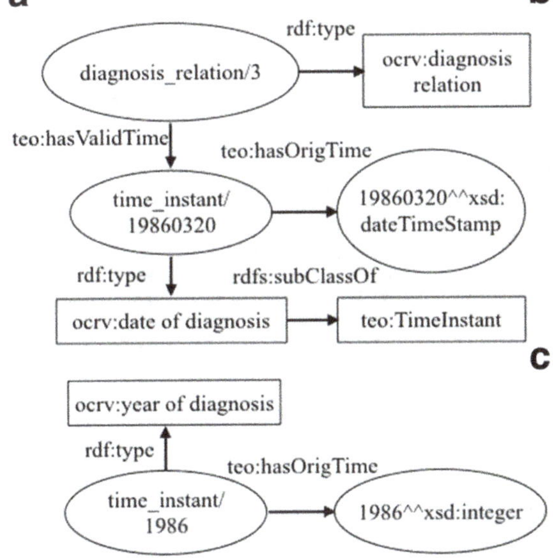

b

```
PREFIX : <http://www.semanticweb.org/ontologies/OCRV#>
PREFIX teo: <https://sbmi.uth.edu/ontology/TEO.owl#>

SELECT ?diagnosis_relation ?diagnosis_date ?diagnosis_year
WHERE
{ ?diagnosis_relation a :diagnosis relation; teo:hasValidTime ?d.
  ?d teo:hasOrigTime ?diagnosis_date.
  BIND(year(?diagnosis_date) AS ?diagnosis_year).}
```

c

Execution time: 0.018 sec - Number of rows retrieved: 15 Show: 15 All

diagnosis_realtion	diagnosis_date	diagnosis_year
:diagnosis_relation/1	"1981-09-23T00:00:00.0"^^xsd:dateTimeStamp	"1981"^^xsd:integer
:diagnosis_relation/2	"1982-05-10T00:00:00.0"^^xsd:dateTimeStamp	"1982"^^xsd:integer
:diagnosis_relation/3	"1986-03-20T00:00:00.0"^^xsd:dateTimeStamp	"1986"^^xsd:integer
:diagnosis_relation/4	"1988-09-01T00:00:00.0"^^xsd:dateTimeStamp	"1988"^^xsd:integer
:diagnosis_relation/5	"1989-09-14T00:00:00.0"^^xsd:dateTimeStamp	"1989"^^xsd:integer
:diagnosis_relation/6	"1990-02-27T00:00:00.0"^^xsd:dateTimeStamp	"1990"^^xsd:integer
:diagnosis_relation/7	"1991-03-21T00:00:00.0"^^xsd:dateTimeStamp	"1991"^^xsd:integer
:diagnosis_relation/8	"1991-06-26T00:00:00.0"^^xsd:dateTimeStamp	"1991"^^xsd:integer
:diagnosis_relation/9	"1992-06-29T00:00:00.0"^^xsd:dateTimeStamp	"1992"^^xsd:integer
:diagnosis_relation/10	"1992-11-16T00:00:00.0"^^xsd:dateTimeStamp	"1992"^^xsd:integer
:diagnosis_relation/11	"1992-12-04T00:00:00.0"^^xsd:dateTimeStamp	"1992"^^xsd:integer
:diagnosis_relation/12	"1992-10-09T00:00:00.0"^^xsd:dateTimeStamp	"1992"^^xsd:integer
:diagnosis_relation/13	"1993-04-22T00:00:00.0"^^xsd:dateTimeStamp	"1993"^^xsd:integer
:diagnosis_relation/14	"1994-10-28T00:00:00.0"^^xsd:dateTimeStamp	"1994"^^xsd:integer
:diagnosis_relation/15	"1987-01-09T00:00:00.0"^^xsd:dateTimeStamp	"1987"^^xsd:integer

Fig. 6 A SPARQL query that converts the date of diagnosis to the year of diagnosis, where (**a**) illustrates how a patient was linked to the date of diagnosis, (**b**) shows the SPARQL query, and (**c**) shows the query results

through their residencies. In FCDS, each patient's residency was mapped to both a census tract code and county code. We obtained the SVI (i.e., a census tract-level variable) from the ATSDR [61]. The SVI indicates the relative vulnerability of every U.S. census tract. The SVI ranks the tracts on 15 social factors, including unemployment and minority status, and further groups them into four themes: socioeconomic status, household composition & disability, minority status & language, and housing & transportation. Each tract receives a ranking for each factor and for each of the four themes, as well as an overall ranking. Based on the census tract codes, we can link a census tracts' SVI rankings to each patient. Fig. 7 shows an example of linking the census tract level SVI socioeconomic status to a patient.

Type 4: Queries that generate results based on the knowledge encoded in ontology

We discussed how the *'ocrv:BRFSS current smoker'* was implemented in OCRV in details above. After encoded the knowledge of what is a BRFSS current smoker, a simple SPARQL query as shown in Fig. 8b can be used to retrieve all current smokers from the source BRFSS data. The reasoner can automatically resolved the subclasses of the *'ocrv:BRFSS current smoker'* and applied the OWL restrictions to ensure that the retrieved BRFSS current smokers meet the two conditions: (1) current every day or someday smoker, and (2) has smoked at least 100 cigarettes in the entire life.

Also, according to our data analysis use cases, some of the raw categorical variables were regrouped into different subgroups—a common practice in building prediction models. To produce the desired grouping, we created new classes for the new groups and leveraged object properties to encode these grouping logics in OCRV. For example, the raw marital status had 7 categories (i.e., 'never married', 'divorced', 'widowed', 'separated', 'married', 'unknown' and 'unmarried') in FCDS. However, based on our data analysis needs, 'never married', 'divorced', 'widowed', 'separated', and 'unmarried' were considered equivalent to 'single' as shown in Fig. 9a. Thus, we created a *'ocrv:single'* class in OCRV and modeled *'ocrv:divorced', 'ocrv:widowed', 'ocrv:separated',* and *'ocrv:unmarried',* and *'ocrv:never married'* as subclasses of *'ocrv:single'*. Then, we can easily use a SPARQL query as shown in Fig. 9b to retrieve all patients whose marital statuses were single. The results of the query were showed in Fig. 9c.

a

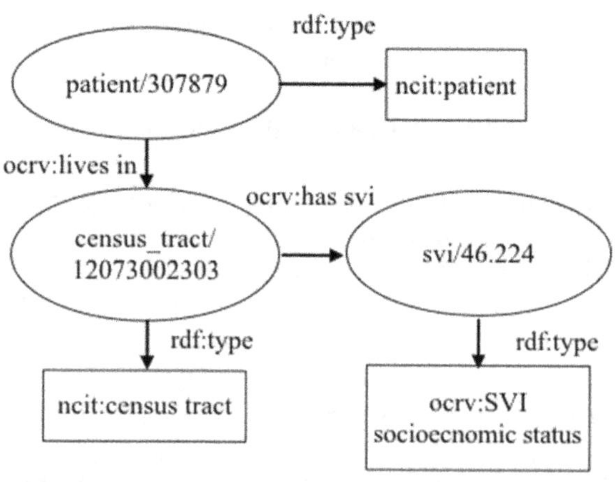

c

Execution time: 0.187 sec - Number of rows retrieved: 15

patient	censu_stract	SVI_socioeconomic_status
:patient/2407426	:census_tract/12001000500	:svi/51.744
:patient/2612697	:census_tract/12001001805	:svi/10.824
:patient/762398	:census_tract/12001001806	:svi/40.488
:patient/1029699	:census_tract/12001002219	:svi/43.68
:patient/1928938	:census_tract/12017450901	:svi/58.584
:patient/2545922	:census_tract/12017451502	:svi/91.68
:patient/1715596	:census_tract/12019030802	:svi/45.36
:patient/2644659	:census_tract/12019030904	:svi/13.104
:patient/1519626	:census_tract/12023110602	:svi/79.992
:patient/1050860	:census_tract/12031000600	:svi/91.248
:patient/1405924	:census_tract/12031000600	:svi/91.248
:patient/1409598	:census_tract/12031002300	:svi/7.008
:patient/797323	:census_tract/12031002502	:svi/35.04
:patient/2411194	:census_tract/12031002801	:svi/90.24
:patient/734467	:census_tract/12031012703	:svi/66.528

b

```
PREFIX : <http://www.semanticweb.org/ontologies/OCRV#>

SELECT ?patient ?census_tract ?SVI_socioeconomic_status
WHERE
{?patient :lives in ?census_tract.
 ?census_tract :has svi ?svi_f1.}
```

Fig. 7 A SPARQL query that links the census tract level SVI socioeconomic status to a patient, where the *'?census_tract'* query variable is the common census tract code linking the individuals of *'ocrv:SVI socioeconomic status'* and *'ocrv:patient'*. Figure (**a**) shows a graphical representation of how a patient is linked to its area-level socioeconimic status based on her residency, (**b**) is the SPARQL query, and (**c**) shows the query results

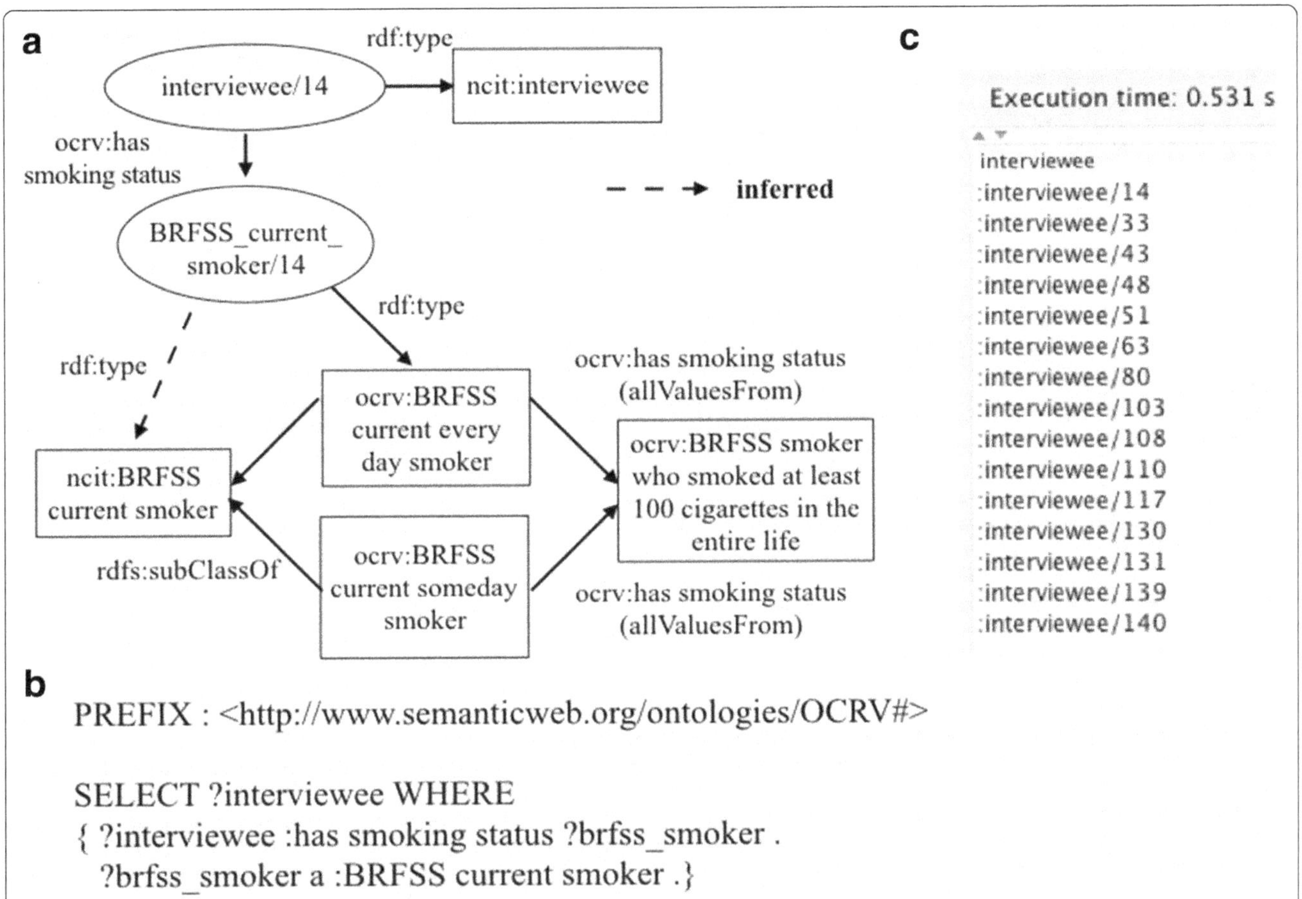

Fig. 8 A SPARQL query that lists all current smokers in BRFSS based the OWL restrictions encoded in the ontology, where (**a**) is the graphical representation, (**b**) shows the SPARQL query, and (**c**) shows the query results

The semantic data integration pipeline for Cancer survival analysis

Equipped with all the necessary SPARQL queries, our last step was to build a data integration pipeline in Java with the Ontop OWL API to produce a pooled dataset for our multi-level cancer survival analysis. The process of the data integration pipeline consists of 6 main steps: (1) set up the connections among the Ontop SPARQL query engine, reasoner, OBDA model, OCRV ontology, and underlying relational data sources; (2) load and execute a query that lists all patients (i.e., patients' unique identifiers), and use the results as the first column in the final integrated dataset; (3) load and execute the SPARQL queries corresponding to each of the risk factors that we selected, and append the results to the corresponding patients; and (4) output the final dataset in the required format (e.g., comma-separated values (CSV) format). A sample of the final integrated dataset following the process above is shown in Table 4, where each column represents a risk factor (or the outcome) and each row represents a patient record.

Discussion

Our experience in building an ontology-based data integration approach for linking heterogeneous datasets for multi-level cancer survival analysis has demonstrated the feasibility of using semantic data integration to resolve semantic, syntactic, and schematic heterogeneities across different data sources.

Benefits of an ontology-based data integration model

The use of ontologies can facilitate data integration in many ways and extend beyond traditional approaches of using common data elements (CDEs) and common data models (CDMs). First, a shared, controlled vocabulary standardizes the definitions of the data elements and makes data understandable to both human (i.e., showing the preferred names for a class, and the synonyms and properties associated with it) and computers. Second, explicitly modeling the semantic relationships among data elements makes domain and data assumptions more explicit and makes it possible to compute and reason with the data. For example, the knowledge that a current smoker in BRFSS has (1) to be a current every day or

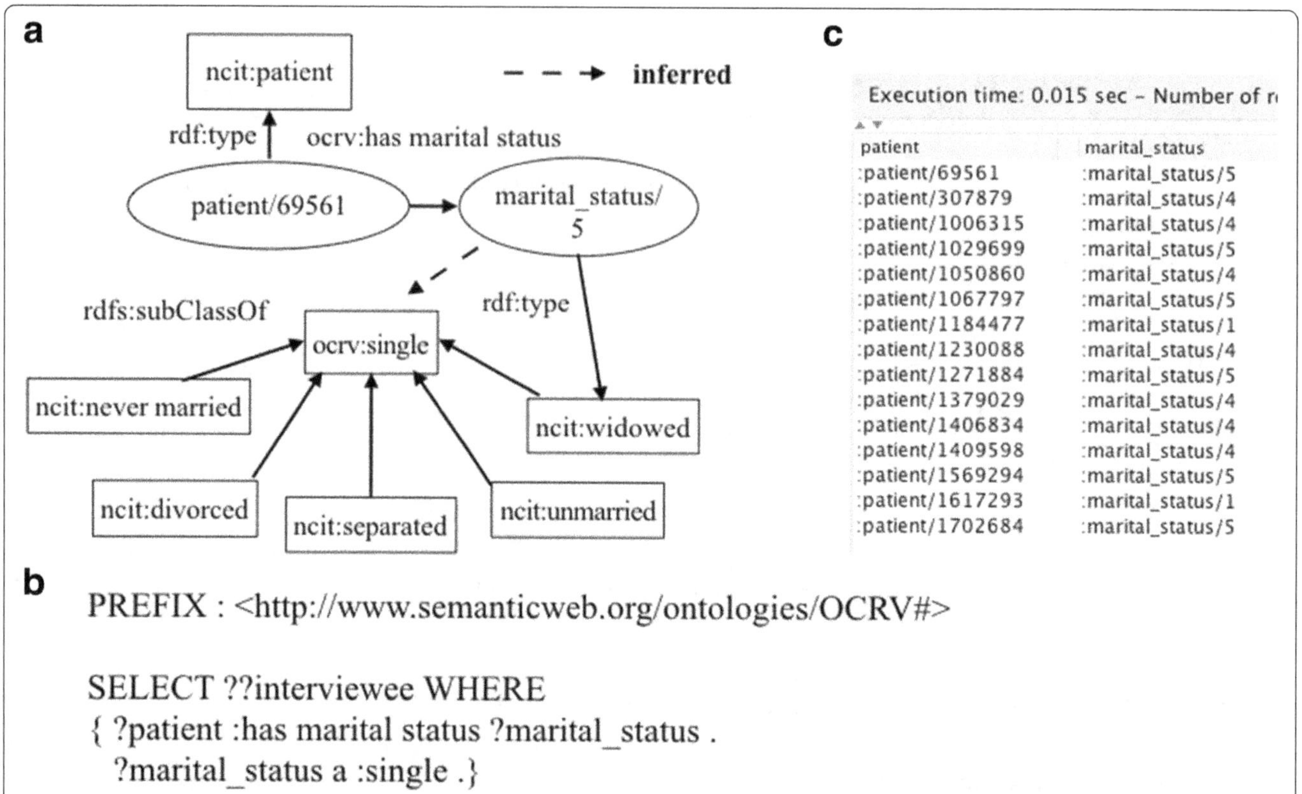

Fig. 9 A SPARQL query that lists all patients in FCDS whose marital statuses were single leveraging the grouping logics encoded in OCRV, where (**a**) is the graphical representation, (**b**) is the SPARQL query, and (**c**) shows the query results

someday smoker and (2) smoked at least 100 cigarettes in the entire life (as shown in Fig. 3), can be explicitly modeled in the ontology, which cannot be achieved with CDEs and CDMs. Third, ontologies enable modeling the constrains of data elements using a formal and machine-readable language, which facilitates automatic validation and assurance of data quality. Fourth, the need to shoehorn heterogeneous data into a CDM is replaced with a more flexible ontology-based metadata representation. Subsequently, integrating a new data source is simply connecting the entities among the different data sources without the need to modify the underlying database structures and data models. Such an approach avoids the error-prone, and labor-intensive extract, transform, load (ETL) processes when transforming the source data into a CDM. Last, ontology-based metadata representations make it possible to encode the different data integration scenarios explicitly using a formal and computational model with a shared vocabulary. This makes the data integration task easier and quicker, and more importantly, facilitates communication of the data integration processes between scientists. This is significant for research rigor, transparency, reproducibility as well as data reusability.

The ability to encode data processing and data integration knowledge in the ontology

As discussed in details above, we leveraged the OWL restrictions to properly define the *'ocrv:BRFSS current smoker'* in OCRV and used object properties to enable grouping of raw categorical variables into different subgroups based on the data analysis needs. These two examples illustrated the ability to reason with ontologically structured data to fulfill data processing and data integration needs. The same logics can indeed be achieved

Table 4 A sample result generated using the semantic data integration pipeline for cancer survival analysis

Patient ID	Biological Sex	Marital Status	Year of Diagnosis	..	SVI Socioeconomic Status	Survival
69,561	female	single	1981	…	20.256	1
…	…	...	…	…	…	…
1,785,573	male	single	2001	…	61.632	0

with having a human explicitly write out the specific queries in SQL. And, ultimately in our system, the SPARQL queries were translated into low-level SQL queries. However, the key difference is that in our case the computer was able to reason with the knowledge encoded in the ontology and generate the proper SQL queries rather than having a human to reason with the data and manually construct the SQL queries, which often time is error-prone and labor-intensive. However, not all data manipulation processes can be easily encoded in the ontology. Many of the data transformation procedures were achieved through built-in functions in the SPARQL queries. For example, the process of extracting the year of diagnosis from date of diagnosis had to be realized in SPARQL as shown in Fig. 5.

Another example of needing computing capability in addition to the logics encoded in the ontology is to calculate the average smoking rate for each Florida county using the raw data in BRFSS. The calculation is straightforward: for each county, the average smoking rate equals to the sum of the BRFSS final weights for all current smokers divided by the sum of the final weights for all BRFSS population in the county. As shown in Fig. 3, we can identify who is BRFSS defined current smoker. A county code and a BRFSS final weight were also attached to each BRFSS respondent as shown in Fig. 10. With these information, we can easily calculate the average smoking rate for each county. Nevertheless, these computations were programed in the data integration pipeline Java code.

Data quality and consistency checks of the source data using the ontology

Another advantage of using ontology as a data model is to conduct automated data quality and consistency checks of the source data, because the dependencies among and constraints of the data elements are explicitly modeled in the ontology. For example, FCDS has two related variables: *'age at diagnosis'* and *'date of diagnosis'*. As shown in Fig. 11, we explicitly modeled the relationship and constraints between these two entities, as the *'ncit:age at diagnosis'* can be calculated from the

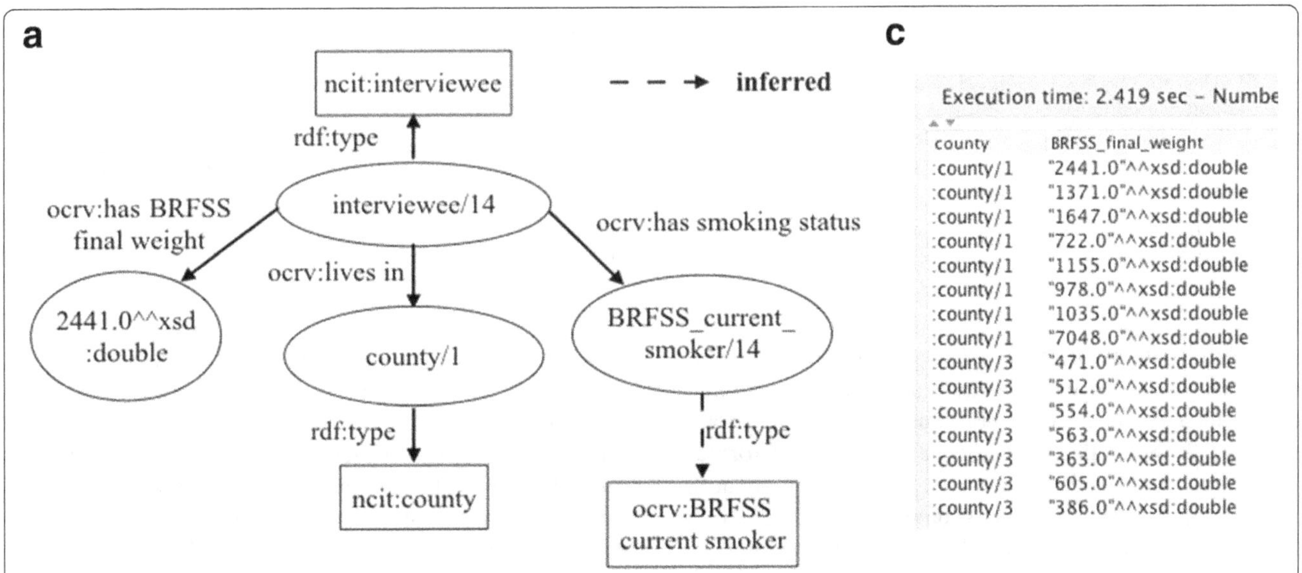

b

```
PREFIX : <http://www.semanticweb.org/ontologies/OCRV#>
PREFIX ncit: <http://purl.obolibrary.org/obo/ncit#>

SELECT ?county ?BRFSS_final_weight WHERE
{ ?interviewee :has smoking status ?brfss_smoker .
  ?brfss_smoker a :BRFSS current smoker.
  ?interviewee :lives in ?county ; :has BRFSS final weight ?BRFSS_final_weight .
  ?county a ncit:county}
```

Fig. 10 A SPARQL query that retrieves all BRFSS defined current smokers, the county codes of their residencies and BRFSS final weight, where (**a**) is the graphical representation of the relationships among these concepts, (**b**) is the SPARQL query, and (**c**) is the query results

a

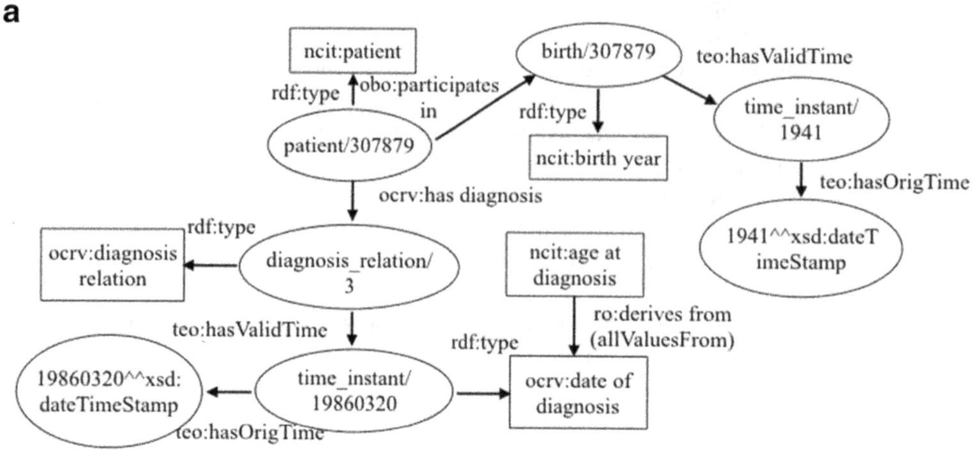

b

```
PREFIX obo: <http://purl.obolibrary.org/obo/>
PREFIX : <http://www.semanticweb.org/ontologies/OCRV#>
PREFIX teo: <https://sbmi.uth.edu/ontology/TEO.owl#>

SELECT ?patient ?birth_year ?diagnosis_year ?age_at_diangosis
WHERE
{ ?patient :has diagnosis ?diagnosis .
  ?diagnosis a :diagnosis relation; teo:hasValidTime ?d.
  ?d teo:hasOrigTime ?diagnosis_date.
  BIND(year(?diagnosis_date) AS ?diagnosis_year).
  ?patient obo:participates in ?birth.
  ?birth teo:hasValidTime ?year_of_birth.
  ?year_of_birth teo:hasOrigTime ?birth_year.}
  BIND(?diagnosis_year - ?birth_year AS ?age_at_diangosis)}
```

c

Execution time: 0.202 sec - Number of rows retrieved: 15 Show:

patient	age_of_diangosis	diagnosis_year	birth_year
:patient/69561	"76"^^xsd:integer	"1981"^^xsd:integer	"1905"^^xsd:integer
:patient/101518	"74"^^xsd:integer	"1982"^^xsd:integer	"1908"^^xsd:integer
:patient/307879	"45"^^xsd:integer	"1986"^^xsd:integer	"1941"^^xsd:integer
:patient/457089	"57"^^xsd:integer	"1988"^^xsd:integer	"1931"^^xsd:integer
:patient/525094	"59"^^xsd:integer	"1989"^^xsd:integer	"1930"^^xsd:integer
:patient/557646	"68"^^xsd:integer	"1990"^^xsd:integer	"1922"^^xsd:integer
:patient/635081	"81"^^xsd:integer	"1991"^^xsd:integer	"1910"^^xsd:integer
:patient/654986	"69"^^xsd:integer	"1991"^^xsd:integer	"1922"^^xsd:integer
:patient/734467	"64"^^xsd:integer	"1992"^^xsd:integer	"1928"^^xsd:integer
:patient/762398	"68"^^xsd:integer	"1992"^^xsd:integer	"1924"^^xsd:integer
:patient/766619	"28"^^xsd:integer	"1992"^^xsd:integer	"1964"^^xsd:integer
:patient/769092	"87"^^xsd:integer	"1992"^^xsd:integer	"1905"^^xsd:integer
:patient/797323	"72"^^xsd:integer	"1993"^^xsd:integer	"1921"^^xsd:integer
:patient/869324	"64"^^xsd:integer	"1994"^^xsd:integer	"1930"^^xsd:integer
:patient/909005	"78"^^xsd:integer	"1987"^^xsd:integer	"1909"^^xsd:integer

Fig. 11 An example of using a SPARQL query to calculate the *'age at diagnosis'* from the *'date of diagnosis'* and *'birth year'* for data consistency checks, where (**a**) shows a graphical representation, (**b**) is the SPARQL query, and (**c**) shows the query results

'*ocrv:date of diagnosis*' and '*ncit:birth year*'. We can then compare the raw *'age of diagnosis'* and the computed age of diagnosis to exam data consistency. Further, we also used OWL restrictions to enforce the required formats and ranges of the data elements. Equipped with automated data consistency checks, data analysts shall follow best practices in dealing with data quality issues [62].

Limitations and future work

The current OCRV stemmed from our particular IDA for cancer survival use case does not cover all possible modeling needs in cancer research. More use cases need to be considered to expand our ontology. In addition, we instantiated classes '*ncit:disease or disorder*' and '*ocrv:diagnosed tumor type*' ICD-9-CM code and the International Classification of Diseases for Oncology 3rd Edition(ICD-O-3), respectively, through Ontop's mapping axioms. Currently, the knowledge of linking a specific disease to the corresponding ICD-9-CM/ICD-O-3 codes is manually expressed in the SQL queries when creating the mapping axioms. In the future work, we will import the disease ontology, where the corresponding ICD codes have already been encoded in the classes as annotation properties. Nevertheless, we will need to extract and convert these annotation properties to data properties (i.e., create individual mapping axioms linking the individuals of diseases to individuals of ICD codes). Consequently, the reasoner can leverage these mapping axioms to infer the knowledge of how to connect a set of ICD codes to corresponding diseases automatically.

Conclusions

We have presented an ontology-based semantic data integration approach for multi-level integrative data analysis of cancer survival. Our approach solves key data integration challenges: (1) not only provide clear definitions of the data elements using standardized common vocabulary, but also explicitly expressed the relationships among the variables, (2) be able to clearly document data processing and integration procedures, (3) leverage ontologically structured data to infer and derive the required data elements and formats automatically, (4) provide a convenient mechanism for documenting data quality and consistency checks, and most importantly (5) allows scientists to clearly document and communicate their data manipulation processes, which is significant for research rigor, transparency, reproducibility as well as data reusability.

Abbreviations

ACoS/CoC: American College of Surgeons, Commission on Cancer; API: Application Programming Interface; ATSDR: Agency for Toxic Substances & Disease Registry; BRFSS: Behavioral Risk Factor Surveillance System; caBIG: cancer Biomedical Informatics Grid; CCCA: Cancer Center Catchment Area; CDC: Centers for Disease Control and Prevention; CDE: Common Data Element; CDIM: Clinical Data Integration Model; CMD: Common Data Model; CMS: Centers for Medicare and Medicaid Services; CSV: Comma-Separated Values; DDO: Data Definition Ontology; EHR: Electronic Health Record; ETL: Extract, Transform, Load; FCDS: Florida Cancer Data System; ICD-9-CM: International Classification of Diseases, Ninth Revision, Clinical Modification; ICD-O-3: International Classification of Diseases for Oncology 3rd Edition; IDA: Integrative Data Analysis; JDBC: Java Database Connectivity; N3: Notation 3; NAACCR: North American Association of Central Registries; NCHS: National Center for Health Statistics; NCI: National Cancer Institute; NIMHD: National Institute on Minority Health and Health Disparities; OBDA: Ontology-Based Data Access; OCRV: Ontology for Cancer Research Variables; OWL: Web Ontology Language; QIS: Query Integrator System; RDF: Resource Description Framework; RDFS: Resource Description Framework Schema; RUCA: Rural-Urban Commuting Area; SEER: Surveillance, Epidemiology, and End Results; semCDI: Semantic caBIG Data Integration; SVI: Social Vulnerability Index; TEO: Time Event Ontology

Funding

This work was supported in part by NIH grants UL1TR001427, the OneFlorida Cancer Control Alliance (funded by James and Esther King Biomedical Research Program, Florida Department of Health Grant Number 4 KB16), the OneFlorida Clinical Research Consortium (CDRN-1501- 26692) funded by the Patient Centered Outcomes Research Institute (PCORI). The content is solely the responsibility of the authors and does not necessarily represent the official views of the NIH or PCORI.

Authors' contributions

The work presented here was carried out in collaboration among all authors. YG and JB designed the study. YG, QL and HZ were involved in acquisition of the data. HZ and BJ carried out the experiments. HZ, YG, and QL analyzed the data. HZ wrote the initial draft of the manuscript with substantial support from YG and JB. TG, ES, FM, YG, and JB provided expert opinion during the ontology curation process, and guided the design of the ontology. All authors provided critical feedback on the study design, reviewed and edited the manuscript. All of the authors have read and approved the final manuscript.

Competing interests

The authors declare that they have no competing interests.

Author details

[1]Department of Health Outcomes and Biomedical Informatics, College of Medicine, University of Florida, Clinical and Translational Research Building Suite 3228, 2004 Mowry Road, PO Box 100219, Gainesville, FL 32610-0219, USA. [2]Division of Hematology and Oncology, Department of Medicine, College of Medicine, University of Florida, Gainesville, Florida, USA.

References

1. CDC. Statistics for Different Kinds of Cancer 2017. https://www.cdc.gov/cancer/dcpc/data/types.htm. Accessed 30 Jan 2018.
2. Siegel RL, Miller KD, Jemal A. Cancer statistics, 2017. CA Cancer J Clin. 2017;67:7–30.
3. Howlader N, Noone A, Krapcho M, Miller D, Bishop K, Kosary C, et al. SEER Cancer Statistics Review, 1975–2014, National Cancer Institute. Bethesda, MD, https://seer.cancer.gov/csr/1975_2014/, based on November 2016 SEER data submission, posted to the SEER web site, April 2017.
4. NIMHD. NIMHD Research Framework https://www.nimhd.nih.gov/about/overview/research-framework.html. Accessed 31 Jan 2018.
5. Golden SD, Earp JAL. Social ecological approaches to individuals and their contexts: twenty years of health education & behavior health promotion interventions. Health Educ Behav Off Publ Soc Public Health Educ. 2012;39:364–72.
6. Vetterlein MW, Löppenberg B, Karabon P, Dalela D, Jindal T, Sood A, et al. Impact of travel distance to the treatment facility on overall mortality in US patients with prostate cancer. Cancer. 2017;123:3241–52.
7. Shao S, Gill AA, Zahm SH, Jatoi I, Shriver CD, McGlynn KA, et al. Diabetes and overall survival among breast Cancer patients in the U.S. military health system. Cancer Epidemiol Biomark Prev. 2018;27:50–7.
8. Iqbal J, Ginsburg O, Rochon PA, Sun P, Narod SA. Differences in breast Cancer stage at diagnosis and Cancer-specific survival by race and ethnicity in the United States. JAMA. 2015;313:165.
9. Eng LG, Dawood S, Sopik V, Haaland B, Tan PS, Bhoo-Pathy N, et al. Ten-year survival in women with primary stage IV breast cancer. Breast Cancer Res Treat. 2016;160:145–52.
10. Smith CB, Bonomi M, Packer S, Wisnivesky JP. Disparities in lung cancer stage, treatment and survival among American Indians and Alaskan natives. Lung Cancer. 2011;72:160–4.
11. Nipp R, Tramontano AC, Kong CY, Pandharipande P, Dowling EC, Schrag D, et al. Disparities in cancer outcomes across age, sex, and race/ethnicity among patients with pancreatic cancer. Cancer Med. 2018; https://doi.org/10.1002/cam4.1277.
12. Gourin CG, Herbert RJ, Fakhry C, Quon H, Kang H, Kiess AP, et al. Quality indicators of oropharyngeal cancer care in the elderly: quality of oropharynx Cancer care in the elderly. Laryngoscope. 2017; https://doi.org/10.1002/lary.27050.
13. Khan SA, Pruitt SL, Xuan L, Makris U, Gerber DE. How does autoimmune disease impact treatment and outcomes among patients with lung cancer? A national SEER-Medicare analysis. Lung Cancer. 2018;115:97–102.
14. Lichtensztajn DY, Giddings B, Morris C, Parikh-Patel A, Kizer K. Comorbidity index in central cancer registries: the value of hospital discharge data. Clin Epidemiol 2017;Volume 9:601–9.
15. Gardner SP. Ontologies and semantic data integration. Drug Discov Today. 2005;10:1001–7.
16. Goble C, Stevens R. State of the nation in data integration for bioinformatics. J Biomed Inform. 2008;41:687–93.
17. Lapatas V, Stefanidakis M, Jimenez RC, Via A, Schneider MV. Data integration in biological research: an overview. J Biol Res Thessalon Greece. 2015;22:9.
18. Gruber TR, Olsen GR. An ontology for engineering mathematics. Proc of KR. 1994;1994:258–69.
19. Gruber TR. A translation approach to portable ontology specifications. Knowl Acquis. 1993;5:199–220.
20. David D. Tim V den B. Towards a Flexible Semantic Framework for Clinical Trial Eligibility using Topic Maps. 2012;
21. Guarino N. Formal ontology in information systems: proceedings of the 1st international conference June 6–8, 1998, Trento, Italy. 1st edition. Amsterdam, the Netherlands. The Netherlands: IOS Press; 1998.
22. Wache H, Vögele T, Visser U, Stuckenschmidt H, Schuster G, Neumann H, et al. Ontology-based integration of information - a survey of existing approaches. In: In IJCAI'01 workshop. On ontologies and information sharing; 2001.
23. Xiao H. Query processing for heterogeneous data integration using ontologies: University of Illinois at Chicago; 2006.
24. Noy NF. Semantic integration: a survey of ontology-based approaches. ACM SIGMOD Rec. 2004;33:65.
25. Dhombres F, Charlet J. Knowledge representation and management, It's time to integrate! Yearb Med Inform. 2017;26:148–51.
26. Marenco L, Wang T-Y, Shepherd G, Miller PL, Nadkarni P. QIS: a framework for biomedical database federation. J Am Med Inform Assoc. 2004;11:523–34.

27. Cheung K-H, Yip KY, Smith A, deKnikker R, Masiar A, Gerstein M. YeastHub: a semantic web use case for integrating data in the life sciences domain. Bioinformatics. 2005;21(Suppl 1):i85–96.
28. Lam HYK, Marenco L, Shepherd GM, Miller PL, Cheung K-H. Using web ontology language to integrate heterogeneous databases in the neurosciences. AMIA Annu Symp Proc AMIA Symp. 2006:464–8.
29. Lam HY, Marenco L, Clark T, Gao Y, Kinoshita J, Shepherd G, et al. AlzPharm: integration of neurodegeneration data using RDF. BMC Bioinformatics. 2007; 8(Suppl 3):S4.
30. Smith AK, Cheung K-H, Yip KY, Schultz M, Gerstein MB. LinkHub: a semantic web system that facilitates cross-database queries and information retrieval in proteomics. BMC Bioinformatics. 2007;8(Suppl 3):S5.
31. Marenco L, Wang R, Nadkarni P. Automated database mediation using ontological metadata mappings. J Am Med Inform Assoc. 2009;16:723–37.
32. Chisham B, Wright B, Le T, Son T, Pontelli E. CDAO-store: ontology-driven data integration for phylogenetic analysis. BMC Bioinformatics. 2011;12:98.
33. Ariane AK, Audi P, Rémy C, Douglas T, Frank E, Catherine D, et al. Data Definition Ontology for clinical data integration and querying. Stud Health Technol Inform. 2012;:38–42.
34. Pang C, Hendriksen D, Dijkstra M, van der Velde KJ, Kuiper J, Hillege HL, et al. BiobankConnect: software to rapidly connect data elements for pooled analysis across biobanks using ontological and lexical indexing. J Am Med Inform Assoc. 2015;22:65–75.
35. Arp R, Smith B, Spear AD. Building ontologies with basic formal ontology: The MIT Press; 2015. https://doi.org/10.7551/mitpress/9780262527811.001.0001.
36. Ethier J-F, Curcin V, Barton A, McGilchrist MM, Bastiaens H, Andreasson A, et al. Clinical data integration model: Core interoperability ontology for research using primary care data. Methods Inf Med. 2014;54:16–23.
37. Mate S, Köpcke F, Toddenroth D, Martin M, Prokosch H-U, Bürkle T, et al. Ontology-based data integration between clinical and research systems. PLoS One. 2015;10:e0116656.
38. Livingston KM, Bada M, Baumgartner WA, Hunter LE. KaBOB: ontology-based semantic integration of biomedical databases. BMC Bioinformatics. 2015;16 https://doi.org/10.1186/s12859-015-0559-3.
39. Liang C, Sun J, Tao C. Semantic web ontology and data integration: a case study in aiding psychiatric drug repurposing. Stud Health Technol Inform. 2015;216:1051.
40. Kock-Schoppenhauer A-K, Kamann C, Ulrich H, Duhm-Harbeck P, Ingenerf J. Linked data applications through ontology based data access in clinical research. Stud Health Technol Inform. 2017;235:131–5.
41. Zhang H, Guo Y, Li Q, George TJ, Shenkman EA, Bian J. Data integration through ontology-based data access to support integrative data analysis: a case study of cancer survival. IEEE. 2017:1300–3. https://doi.org/10.1109/BIBM.2017.8217849.
42. Noy N, Rector A. Defining N-ary relations on the. Semantic Web. 2006; https://www.w3.org/TR/swbp-n-aryRelations/. Accessed 31 Jan 2018
43. Tao C. Time event ontology. 2012. https://bioportal.bioontology.org/ontologies/TEO. Accessed 31 Jan 2018.
44. Tao C, Wei WQ, Solbrig HR, Savova G, Chute CG. CNTRO: a semantic web ontology for temporal relation Inferencing in clinical narratives. AMIA Annu Symp Proc AMIA Symp. 2010;2010:787–91.
45. Tao C, Solbrig HR, Chute CG. CNTRO 2.0: A Harmonized Semantic Web ontology for temporal relation Inferencing in clinical narratives. AMIA Jt summits Transl Sci Proc AMIA Jt summits Transl Sci 2011;2011:64–68.
46. McGuinness DL, van Harmelen FOWL. Web ontology. Language. 2004; https://www.w3.org/TR/owl-features/. Accessed 31 Jan 2018
47. United States Department of Agriculture. USDA ERS - Rural-Urban Commuting Area Codes. 2017. https://www.ers.usda.gov/data-products/rural-urban-commuting-area-codes/. Accessed 31 Jan 2018.
48. United States Department of Agriculture. Data Access - Urban Rural Classification Scheme for Counties. 2016. https://www.ers.usda.gov/data-products/rural-urban-commuting-area-codes.aspx. Accessed 31 Jan 2018.
49. CDC. Florida Cancer Data System. https://fcds.med.miami.edu/inc/welcome.shtml. Accessed 31 Jan 2018.
50. Agency for Toxic Substances and Disease Registry. The Social Vulnerability Index (SVI). 2013. https://svi.cdc.gov/. Accessed 31 Jan 2018.
51. U.S. Department of commerce. United states census bureau. 2016. https://www.census.gov/. Accessed 31 Jan 2018.
52. CDC. Behavioral Risk Factor Surveillance System. https://www.cdc.gov/brfss/index.html. Accessed 8 Oct 2017.
53. Iachan R, Pierannunzi C, Healey K, Greenlund KJ, Town M. National weighting of data from the behavioral risk factor surveillance system (BRFSS). BMC Med Res Methodol. 2016;16:155.
54. University of Wisconsin Population Health Institute, Robert Wood Johnson Foundation. County Health Rankings & Roadmaps. 2017. http://www.countyhealthrankings.org/. Accessed 31 Jan 2018.
55. Calvanese D, Cogrel B, Komla-Ebri S, Kontchakov R, Lanti D, Rezk M, et al. Ontop: answering SPARQL queries over relational databases. Semantic Web. 2017;8:471–87.
56. Whetzel PL, Noy NF, Shah NH, Alexander PR, Nyulas C, Tudorache T, et al. BioPortal: enhanced functionality via new web services from the National Center for biomedical ontology to access and use ontologies in software applications. Nucleic Acids Res 2011;39 Web Server issue:W541–W545.
57. Musen MA. The protégé project: a look back and a look forward. AI Matters. 2015;1:4–12.
58. Horridge M, Bechhofer S. The OWL API: A Java API for Working with OWL 2 Ontologies.
59. Palmisano I. The OWL API. 2017. https://github.com/owlcs/owlapi. Accessed 3 Feb 2018.
60. Tim B-L, Dan C. Notation3 (N3): a readable RDF. Syntax. 2011; https://www.w3.org/TeamSubmission/n3/. Accessed 11 Feb 2018
61. U.S. Department of health and human services. Agency for Toxic Substances & disease registry (ATSDR). 2018. https://www.atsdr.cdc.gov/. Accessed 11 Feb 2018.
62. Visochek A. Practical Data Wrangling: Expert techniques for transforming your raw data into a valuable source for analytics. Packt Publishing; 2017.

5

Smart medical beds in patient-care environments of the twenty-first century

Ignacio Ghersi[1,2*], Mario Mariño[1] and Mónica Teresita Miralles[1,2]

Abstract

Background: Recent scientific achievements and technological advances have brought forward a massive display of new or updated medical devices, enabled with highly-developed embedded-control functions and interactivity. From the final decade of the twentieth century, medical beds have particularly been affected by this surge, taking on new forms and functions, while accommodating to established properties that have become well-known for these devices. The past fifteen years have also brought forward changes to conceptual frameworks, concerning the product design and manufacturing processes (standards), as well as the patient (perspectives on patient-care environments and accessibility). This work presents a state-of-art survey on electric medical beds, representing what is defined as the time of "smart beds", as part of an increasingly comprehensive patient-care environment.

Methods: A survey and assessment of market trends, research efforts and standards related to smart medical beds was performed, covering a wide range of public records of intellectual property, models and related healthcare solutions, as well as relevant research efforts in the field between 2000 and 2016. Contextual topics, necessary for the understanding of this subject, on novel technologies, disability and the reach of healthcare systems, were also researched and interpreted.

Results: The new generation of electric medical beds is defined, with the final stage of the proposed timeline for these devices being covered. Functional, aesthetic and interactive features are presented, and the current global market for medical beds and related standards are also assessed. Finally, discussions concerning rising challenges and opportunities for these systems are explored, with the potential for adding further monitoring and assistive implementations into medical devices and environments being highlighted.

Conclusions: Smart medical beds are integrated solutions for patient care, assistance and monitoring, based on a comprehensive, multidisciplinary design approach. Research in this field is critical in a context of global ageing, and powered by a surge in opportunities for accessibility solutions. Smart beds, seamlessly integrated into the healthcare system, have a unique opportunity in enabling more efficient efforts for caregivers, and more responsive environments for patients.

Keywords: Electric bed, Smart medical bed, Patient-centered, Technology, Accessibility

* Correspondence: igghersi@gmail.com
[1]Centro de Investigación en Diseño Industrial de Productos Complejos (CIDI-FADU-UBA), Facultad de Arquitectura, Diseño y Urbanismo, Universidad de Buenos Aires, 2160 Intendente Güiraldes Ave, Buenos Aires, Argentina
[2]Laboratorio de Biomecánica e Ingeniería para la Salud (LaBIS-FI-UCA), Facultad de Ingeniería y Ciencias Agrarias, Pontificia Universidad Católica Argentina, 1600 Alicia Moreau de Justo Ave, Buenos Aires, Argentina

Background

Electric medical beds have accumulated almost one hundred years of history. An essential part of the healthcare environment, the medical bed is also used as a measure of its *reach* [1], its *efficiency* (for occupancy and bed-management strategisation [2]), *development* (representing funding and investment in healthcare systems, see [3]) and *diversity*. For the case of automated, electric devices such as these, technological and contextual factors have resulted in significant changes to their appearance and their expected functionality over this period, while retaining original features that have guided the first exponents of this medical device. It is, however, in the twenty-first century, that an unprecedented, innovative stage in the development of these devices has peaked, taking advantage of all technological means at the disposal of developers, and resulting in new vectors of added value for these products: this stage can be referred to as the time of *smart medical beds*.

Previous work [4] has detailed the evolution of medical beds form initial, push-button models, to the year 2000, dividing such period into two stages: *electric beds* (1940's to 1980's) and *mechatronic*[1] *beds (1990's)*. Highlights from this diachronic study over a sixty-year period were:

a) Spreading of these devices outside the hospital environment from the 60's, towards institutional or residential facilities.
b) Development of particular regulatory frameworks
c) Growing invention and commercialization of dedicated accessories
d) Incipient incorporation of new technologies into the devices (second stage)

Mechatronic beds became a reality in the 90's, when inventions, commercial products (i.e. Hill-Rom TotalCare -1998), and dedicated research work [5] accumulated ergonomics, functions and accessories (alternative actuators, pressure mattresses, weighing scales), incorporating informatics and communications into these devices.

In the past decades, the medical-bed market has further changed, responding to also-changing structural, functional, and social-economic demands concerning the performance of medical beds. From the year 2000 to the present, these highly elaborate mechatronic devices have consolidated into what can be called the segment of smart mechatronic beds or *smart beds*, a term that describes a comprehensive *synthesis* between new materials, design and higher functionality and autonomy for these systems, all under advanced user interfaces. Smart beds implement new technologies (graphical interfaces, novel environment-aware sensors and actuating solutions, etc.), to provide a higher level of service and function, like real-time monitoring, caregiver and patient assistance, automated functions and positions (chair, assisted bed exit), and data logging, as well as more advanced means of communication.

This work presents a survey on medical beds in the healthcare environments between the years 2000 and 2016, leading to an analysis on their current product and research state-of-art, as well as on their potential for development and market perspectives. Focused on the final stage of the product timeline, it proposes a study of wide scope on the many factors affecting medical beds over this reduced time range, through a deeper assessment of current technologies, challenges and views that are set to shape the healthcare environment and delivery methods in the near future.

Methods

This work presents the results of a survey on electric medical beds from the year 2000, and up to 2016. Three different topics were assessed:

a) Trends and changes found in medical beds over this period (section "Twenty-first century medical beds: Trends and changes (2000–2016)").
b) Current market-reach and features of smart beds (section "Twenty-first century medical beds: Current market-reach and features").
c) Research efforts with an impact on the experience or capabilities of the medical bed, as part of more comprehensive healthcare environments (section "Research shaping the future of smart healthcare environments").

As a characterization of the current state of a specific medical device, sources for this article have been the result of a thorough literature survey on its core subject (medical, long-term care beds, patients and operators). In order to form a comprehensive view on the matter and its perspectives, however, other relevant sources representing economic, social/political and cultural implications to such a relevant medical device were also involved in this study:

- Current models of medical beds (significant brands, models of medical beds, and products found through dedicated catalogs [6]).
- Relevant research findings and publications (*IEEExplore, JSTOR, PubMed, SpringerLink, EBSCOhost, ScienceDirect*), concerning mechatronics, patient/bed monitoring, advances in user interfaces, accessibility and sensors. Terms (with combinations): *Hospital Bed/s, Control, Bedridden, Stretcher, MEMS, Face* (for face control in accessibility*), BCI, Ergonomics, Motor Impairment,*

South America (for local research and product state-of-art), *Trends, Long term, Technology, Cost Nursing Beds, Design.*
- Public records of intellectual property (hospital/electric bed control interfaces, accessibility-enabled beds, networking and communication): United States Patent and Trademark Office, German Patent and Trademark Office, The Lens database, INPI (Argentina).
- Standards relevant to the implementation of new technologies into these devices, based on reports from regulatory agencies and certifications declared by medical-bed models.
- Commercial solutions and technological news at a global scale on these topics (*IEEE Spectrum, Scientific American, Wired Magazine, Popular Mechanics).* Terms: *BCI, Bedridden, Hospital, Bed, Control, Face Control, MEMS.*

Inclusion criteria restricted models between 2000 and 2016, and to those designed for medium to long-term care scenarios, for which patient/caregiver/environment interactions become most relevant. Scientific publications included research on novel sensors and assistive technologies, implemented or believed to be compatible with the use or improvement of the experience of the medical bed (motion sensors, brain-computer interfaces, image processing, speech recognition, and adapted push-buttons). Changes to regulations covering medical beds in this period were also assessed. Unlike commercial models of medical beds, patents were not restricted to the period 2000–2016 because the priority or issue date may not be indicative of when the invention is actually implemented or distributed. Criteria for the evaluation of innovations and changes to medical beds in this period were a) user interfaces, b) accessories, c) aesthetic-morphological properties, and d) embedded functions.

Results

A total 85 distributors and manufacturers of medical beds from America, Europe and Asia were found and evaluated. A wide range of beds covering home-care, institutional-care, emergency, surgical and therapeutic beds (bariatric, elderly, long-term) have been detected. Given the inclusion criteria of this work, emergency, psychiatric, obstetric and surgical beds were not assessed. Nine companies were found to be distributors from other brands. Out of the rest, two manufacturers were discarded for lack of data concerning the specifics of the manufactured beds, resulting in a group of 74 manufacturers of medical beds.

Figure 1 is an illustration of a smart medical bed summarizing the changes that were found to be most significant to these medical devices in the twenty-first century: innovative interfaces, increased functionality and dedicated accessories, with customization and finishing options.

Integration of features like those in Fig. 1 into medical beds has been a result of technological advances of the past decades. Table 1 is a list of records of intellectual property, found to be associated to smart features compatible with medical beds and patient-care environments of this period (see Section "Smart features"). Accessibility, networking and environmental control from the bed, as well as improved function and design features are exemplified in these patents, with many of these concepts or variations currently available in smart beds.

Table 2 lists 20 models from 13 manufacturers that have been selected as representative of the different criteria that were chosen for the evaluation of smart beds (user-interfaces, accessories, aesthetics/design, functions). Highlights of these models are further explored in sections "Twenty-first century medical beds: Trends and changes (2000–2016), Twenty-first century medical beds: Current market-reach and features and Research shaping the future of smart healthcare environments", with each

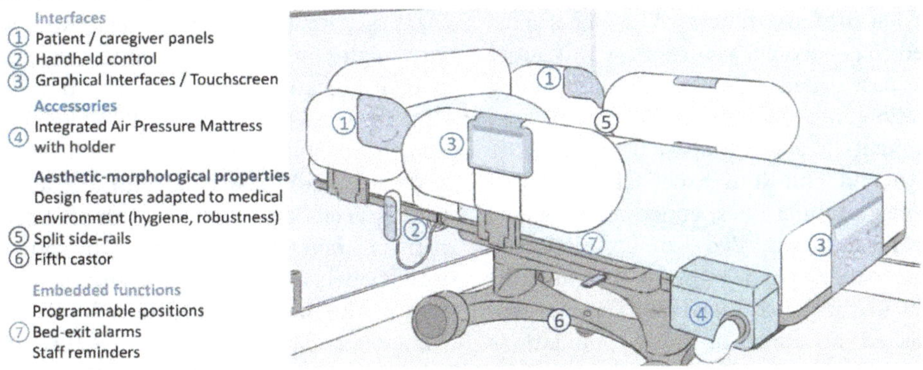

Fig. 1 Illustration of a smart medical bed for clinical use: directed at multiple settings, smart medical beds integrate an array of innovative interfaces, functions and accessories, with distinct design features and customizations

Table 1 Selected records of intellectual property concerning smart functions, design features and connected patient-care environments

Priority Year	Ref	Patent	Title	Highlight
1991	[35]	US5335313A	Voice-actuated (...) control system for hospital bed	Speech Recognition
1992	[17]	US6481688	Hospital bed communication and control device	Accessibility Accessory for Beds
1994	[48]	US5831221A	Caster mounted weighing system	Integrated Scale
	[49]	US5454126A	Foot egress chair bed	Chair Position
1995	[50]	US5542138	Bedside control unit for a hospital bed	Environmental Control through bed Adjustable interface
	[51]	US7017208B2	Hospital Bed	Graphical Interface
1998	[52]	US6781517B2	Communication and Bed Function Control Apparatus	Multiple Integrated Controls
2001	[53]	US8334779	Touch Screen Control of a Hospital Bed	Touchscreen
2004	[8]	US7852208B2	Wireless Bed Connectivity	Networking Functionality
2005	[10]	US20080172789A1	Patient Support with Improved Control	Integrated Front Panel, Side-rail Controls (patient and caregiver). Touchscreen, Graphical Interface. Environmental Control
2007	[54]	EP2027844A1	Proximity Activation of Voice Operation of Hospital Bed	Different Operation for Caregiver and Patient, Voice control
2010	[11]	US20110214234A1	Multifunctional Display for Hospital Bed	Touchscreen for Patient and Caregiver. Environmental control
2010	[55]	EP2438897A2	Hospital bed with graphical user interface having advanced functionality	Graphical User Interface, Networking, Communication
2010	[56]	EP2460503A2	Biometric Bed Configuration	Biometrics, Conditional Control

section detailing findings on the three areas of interest that were listed in section "Methods".

Twenty-first century medical beds: Trends and changes (2000–2016)

Market expansion and technological availability

In accordance with the aforementioned results, a growing number and variety of medical beds has been found in this period, with increased mechanical and autonomous functions, reaching up to novel devices, like a continuous-use bed that turns into a wheelchair for disabled patients [7], and models with embedded networking, communication, monitoring and integrated alarms [8] (i.e. Stryker iBed Awareness). The global market for medical beds has become, as a result, vastly more competitive in the past decades [9], and the continuing trend of specialization into different sub-groups of patients and environments is evident: apart from *bariatric* (i.e. Joerns Bari10A and Hill-Rom Excel Care ES) and *domiciliary* beds, new product lines, aimed at the aid of the *elderly* (Japan's Paramount Bed Co. Ltd. Rakusho Series) or *pediatric* patients appear more prominently, while other models (for instance Merivaara Carena) display features directed at many of these populations under a single model.

Following the trend of all medical devices, the integration of more-developed technologies into electric medical beds became the most significant in this period, resulting in examples with multi-language speech synthesis for patient-caregiver communication (Stryker InTouch), and recommending [10], and even implementing speech-recognition functions for their control (Vallitech-2015). With significant embedded capabilities and autonomy, user interfaces (detailed in section "User interfaces") continue to stand out as relevant weighting factors in the evaluation of these products. A patent of 2005 shows multiple potential configurations for side-rail integrated controls [10], and a subsequent patent of 2010 updates these alternatives with touchscreen functions, for both patient and caregiver use [11]. In 2004, a patent displaying a bed with wireless connectivity, high-complexity user interfaces, and incorporating patient-blocking functions, foot pedals, and automated functions was presented [8]. The TotalCare SpO_2RT bed, from Hill-Rom, as well as Stryker's InTouch Care bed and SizeWise's Navigator models, show integrated touchscreens and dedicated graphical user interfaces as part of their developments. Upgraded, comprehensive front panels and alternate controls continued to proliferate in this period, and the redundancy of controls became a standard feature (for instance, visible in Haelvoet Olympia Hospital and Linet Eleganza Smart models). Improved ergonomics and risk-reducing articulations have also been included into new devices, modifying the

Table 2 Smart medical beds: models exhibiting state-of-art functional, design and interactive features

Brand	Model	Year (where available)
ArjoHuntleigh	Enterprise 9000	2010
Haelvoet	Olympia Hospital	2013
Hill-Rom	TotalCare SpO_2RT	2004
	TotalCare Bariatric	2007
	Excel Care ES	2013
Joerns	Bari10A	2012
	UltraCare XT	2013
Linet	Eleganza Smart	2009
	Eleganza 3XC	2013
Merivaara	Carena	2012
Paramount Bed Co. Ltd.	Rakusho Series	–
	METIS VIP Series	–
	KA6600 Series	–
Pro Bed	Freedom Bed	–
Rotec	Versatech 600	2013
SizeWise	Navigator	2013
Stryker	InTouch II	2008/2011
	S3 Med/Surg Bed	2015
Vallitech	VLT-931	2015
Völker	LTC Beds	2016

hip-section articulation when the backrest is lifted (TotalCare SpO_2RT model), and/or compensating the position of the patient in its environment (Stryker S3 Med/Surg Bed).

Changing (and keeping) the face of the medical bed

Over the past years, trends and most relevant innovations to medical beds have been notably related to design aspects, referred to materials (more hygienic and resistant), population-specific models, ergonomic manual commands, and morphological changes associated to updated mobility-options (elevation, front-back and lateral inclination, etc.), updated side-rails, patient-support structures, castors (fifth castor for enhanced transport), while embedded with the aforementioned new technologies.

In the competitive scenario presented in previous sections, aesthetic and comprehensive design features stand out as a differentiating factor between products. These features, prominently represented by the side-rails and panels, also serve in adapting the beds to different environments and populations. An analysis of these products, and their means of diffusion, allowed inferring a set of values and responses that this new generation of smart beds aims to provoke:

- They are highly and increasingly user-oriented (institutions, operators and patients), which is expressed in their form, function, interactivity and ergonomics.
- They strongly express the ideas of hygiene, safety, durability, comfort, ease of use (both for patients and caregivers), reliance on technology and caregivers, with panels and side-rails as main differentiating factors (full/split rails, integrated controls).
- They emphasize embedded functions and high-end technologies, displaying the power embedded into these products, and in line with a growing technological awareness. However, they also allude to the invisibility of this elaborate technology with simple, intuitive controls.

In sum, the following trends, exemplified in Fig. 2, have been associated to the design of smart beds:

- While these devices highlight their advanced functionality, they maintain simplified control interfaces, relying on known structures and signals, to ease their use by patients or caregivers.
- For *residential* or *residential-inspired beds*, they assimilate into these daily environments (Haelvoet Olympia Hospital, Völker LTC Beds, Paramount Bed Co. Ltd. METIS VIP).
- Oppositely, *critical-care beds* highlight robustness, embedded technologies, and their reliability for medical use through their design (Stryker InTouch, Hill-Rom TotalCare Bariatric, Linet Eleganza 3XC, Paramount Bed Co. Ltd. KA6600 series). Other models can be customized for both scenarios (i.e. Rotec Versatech 600).

Regulatory consolidation

Regulatory frameworks have an impact on the design-process and requisites expected of different families of devices in order to reach their potential users. In the sector of medical beds, there have been advances in this field between 2000 and 2016. After the development of particular standards for electric medical beds in the late 90's [4], the first decades of the twenty-first century have seen the convergence of these standards into a unified reference. ISO/IEC standard 60,601–2-52:2009 (basic safety and essential performance of medical beds) [12] was issued in 2009 as a combination of previous standards IEC 60601–2-38:1996 (requirements for the safety of electrically operated hospital beds) [13], and EN 1970:2000 (adjustable beds for disabled persons: requirements and test methods). This document, which covers issues like safe working loads, mechanical and electrical safety, ergonomic requisites and

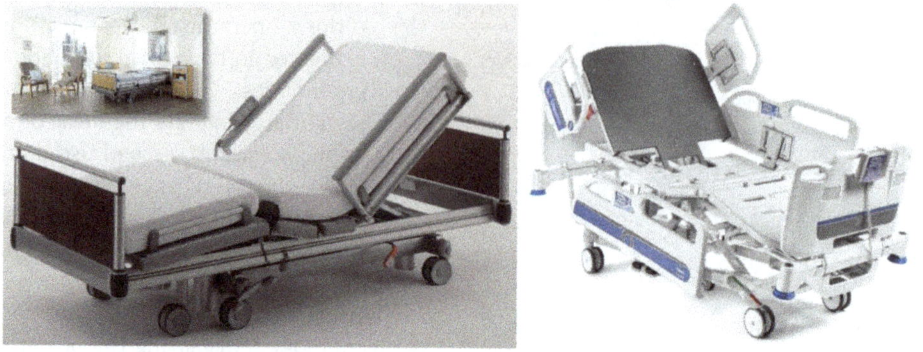

Fig. 2 Aesthetic and design customizations stand out in state-of-art medical beds, serving a purpose of adaptation to different environments. Left: residential-inspired, long-term care (Völker LTC Vis-à-vis bed) [43]; Right: cardiac and progressive-care for hospital ward (Malvestio Sigma PCU Electric Bed Scale System) [44]. Permission for use of images granted by Völker and Malvestio

risk-management strategies as a consolidated reference among five scenarios for medical beds (from hospital to nursing and home environments) [12], was first amended in 2015 [14], and falls within the updated scope of IEC 60601 [15].

Twenty-first century medical beds: Current market-reach and features

Current market reach

The current number of developers and manufacturers of medical beds, their associated products and accessories, as well as healthcare-management technologies, falls easily within the hundreds. Significant market actors, as described by medical-bed market surveys [9, 16], include Hill-Rom, Linet, ArjoHuntleigh, Stryker, Paramount Bed Co. Ltd. and Invacare.

The global market of electric and smart medical beds, both for healthcare facilities and residential use, reaches its highest degree of development in the United States and Europe, with the Asian market showing great potential for growth in the following years, and within this market, pressure-relief surfaces and beds are among the most prominent sub-groups [9]. Figure 3 shows the global distribution of the reviewed companies (accessed 04/2018).

Smart features

Table 3 shows a set of stand-out curent medical-bed properties found on the reviewed systems, ranging from

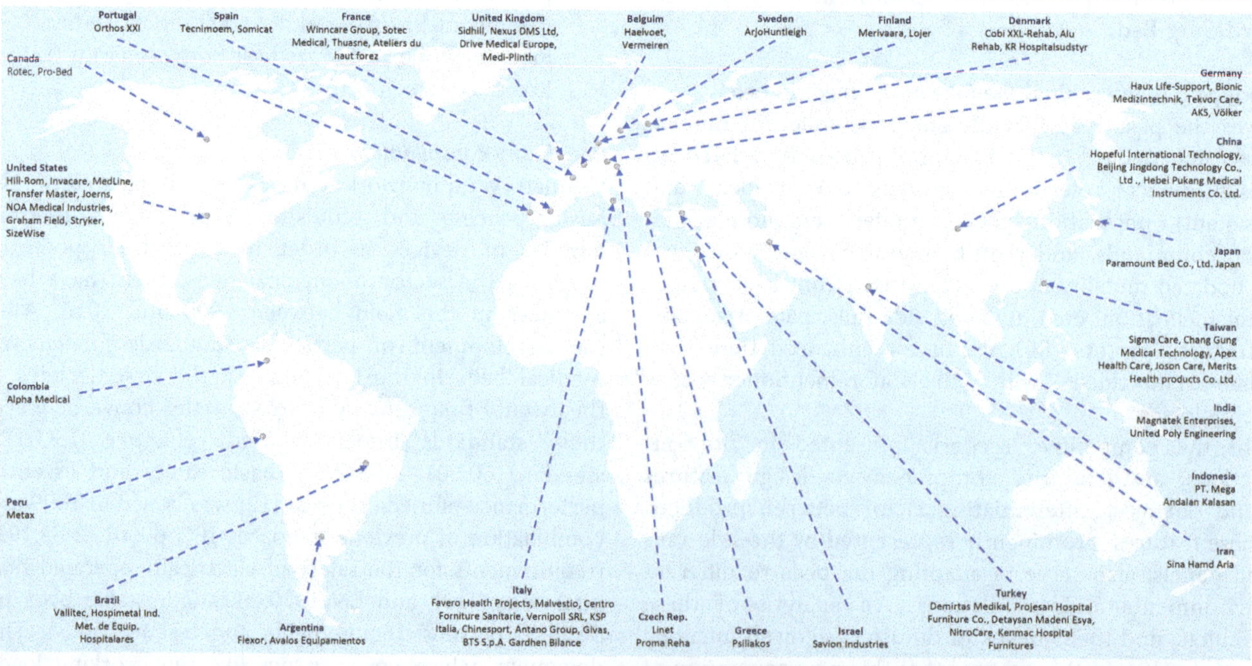

Fig. 3 Global distribution of the reviewed electric and smart-bed manufacturers. World map adapted from [45]

Table 3 Standout features of current medical beds

	Related to the device	Related to the patient/caregiver	Related to the environment
Description	• Ergonomic • Low: controllable frame height, significantly lowering the frame to mitigate consequences of bed falls	• Universal • Bariatric • Critical • Acute • Early Mobility	• Hospital • Intensive Care • Long-Term • Residential • Medical-Surgical • Multiple
Aesthetic/design features	• 5th castor for eased bed transportation • Robustness, removable panels for hygiene • Controllable height (including low-frame models) • Side-rail shock absorbers • Advanced mechanics	• Frame extension (length-width) • Ergonomics for patient, caregiver • Movable, adaptable side-rail controls • Autoregression: the back section is moved towards the headboard when lifted, reducing applied pressure to the lower back	• Optional panels, side-rails, colors and materials for environmental adaptation • Under-Bed Lighting • Chair position • Concealable controls • Customizable for medical or residential scenarios
Standout functions	• Backup power • Accessory support • Mechanical/Digital head of bed angle indicators • Predefined, programmable positions (cardiac chair, Trendelenburg, etc.) • Usage History (positions, etc.) • Integrated accessories (i.e. active mattress) • Motion Programs	• Lit Controls • Integrated scale • Braden Scale Calculation • Nursing staff reminders • Patient blocking functions • Translation for basic questions • Monitoring (i.e. bed-exit) • Eased CPR control • Motion Support • Treatment/Preventive therapies/systems	• Patient exit alarm • Remote-local alarms • Obstacle detection • Communication functions

homecare to intensive-care solutions, detailing *aesthetic-morphological properties* (section "Changing (and keeping) the face of the medical bed") and *special functions* that are available in these devices, stemming from the integration of multiple technological solutions into one device (section "Market expansion and technological availability"). As a group, these devices directly highlight the different *specific purposes* that medical beds can be intended for (see "description"), as well as the increased level of technology embedded into them over time. These features are divided in the table, according to their relation to the *device* itself, the *user* (caregiver or patient), or the *healthcare environment*.

Features mentioned in the table (i.e. bed-exit alarms, obstacle detection, advanced motion options, therapy routines, patient and bed history logging, integrated scale, head-of-bed angle monitoring and measurements, patient-blocking, local and remote information on patient conditions, integrated accessory-controls), are all relevant in their own right, but most impactful when controlled under a single patient-care interface. Most of these features are shared among models, and not only isolated cases, representing the increased expectations that their users have developed.

As indicated in section "Changing (and keeping) the face of the medical bed", design highlights, including patient and caregiver ergonomics and environmental adaptations for clinical and/or residential settings, are most significant and prominently present across the growing family of smart beds. Similarly, access to pre-programmed positions, dedicated accessories and optional features are also largely visible. For instance, 85% of the models highlighted in Table 2 include positions like cardiac chair and automatic CPR (cardiopulmonary resuscitation), and 95% have dedicated accessories like specialty mattresses, IV-holders and options for a fifth castor. From the perspective of robustness and safety, battery backup and eased CPR release, mentioned in Table 3, provide for fast responses to emergencies under power-failure conditions, another functionality mentioned in the current standard.

Supplementing design features, customization of finishings, materials, colors and side-rail styles for a single model are also distinct, but present to a lesser extent (corresponding to a 60% of the models in Table 2), while proving a meaningful addition to the design of dedicated, more patient-conscious environments. Finally, adjustable bed sections (frame width and length), particularly useful for bariatric patients, have become a widespread feature, found in the form of integrated mechanics, or as optional additions, across all models from Table 2.

User interfaces

As a result of this analysis, it has become evident how user interfaces in medical beds have progressively diversified in this period. Starting with wired hand-held controls (which persist in most models, for instance Joerns UltraCare XT), interfaces have advanced up to solutions with redundant side-rail integrated controls (exterior and interior, i.e. ArjoHuntleigh Enterprise 9000), remote controls, foot-pedals, integrated numeric displays and touchscreens (mostly directed to caregiver control), and variants like hanging controls reachable by the patient (see Linet Eleganza Smart and Haelvoet Olympia). Figure 4 shows examples of these alternatives, supplementing handheld and side-rail controls, which are also visible in Fig. 2. Additionally, current inventions contemplate new integrations between these technologies for future devices [10, 17].

Smart medical-bed interfaces count on the aforementioned, now-standard features like patient blocking, nurse-call functions, networking and interaction with other devices and accessories (i.e. air-pressure mattresses), and redundancy through multiple controls is available for most options, favoring robust and reliable operation. Based on years of interdisciplinary experience, currently-enforced standards have regulated requisites for these interfaces (indicators, size, means of operation) [12]. The addition of advanced graphical means and touchscreens with dedicated user interfaces is currently present in a select number of beds, however (20% of the highlighted cases in this article), while it provides eased access to features like alarm setup and monitoring, and is essential to the control of a growing number of states and functions in smart beds, like bed-history functions. For this reason, their presence is expected to increase in the future.

Research shaping the future of smart healthcare environments

Monitoring and assistive solutions

Available as integrated functions for commercial beds and research proposals, patient monitoring is the most extended group among comprehensive proposals for the care of high-risk or long-term patients. Varied systems for fall [18] and agitation detection, around the bed, can be valuable additions to the medical bed, allowing for patient-aware care environments and active sensor-networks [19]. Similarly, pressure-distribution matrices over the support surface of the bed allow a comprehensive analysis on patient position, and may reduce the risk of developing pressure ulcers [20]. Based on acquired data concerning the state of the patient or device, these monitoring proposals can either show the detected state [21], emit alarms [18], or act autonomously against detected hazards [22, 23]. Patient-motion sensors, in contact with the subject, can perform similar tasks concerning the detection and alert of lack of mobility (Leaf Healthcare Inc. developed one such device), as isolated additions.

Integrated, non-invasive vital-sign acquisition from the bed has also been a matter of research over the past years. A consumer-ready device [24] can be placed under the mattress, and acquire heart and breathing rates, as well as estimate patient motion and register caregiver-response time. Outside the medical bed, entertainment systems with infrared sensors have been valued and are being studied for non-invasive heart rate detection [25].

Head-of-bed angle indication and logging is important for the prevention of secondary conditions associated to immobility, and requisites concerning its state vary depending on the condition of the patient (prevention of pressure ulcers requires low angles, and risk of aspiration in intubated patients requires head-rest angles of over 30 degrees, according to the experience of nursing and medical staff) [26]. While incorporated into high-end current devices, the addition of this functionality to manual devices through MEMS [27] sensors is a low-cost addition with great positive potential [28]. Many current technologies are, likewise, sufficiently developed to allow for low-cost derived solutions, integrating these into less-developed healthcare environments.

Finally, patient-motion assistance is another field of research that is valued for the care of the older and disabled patients, with research solutions [29], as well as consumer-ready devices incorporating such features, so that the device supports patient motion, instead of replacing it.

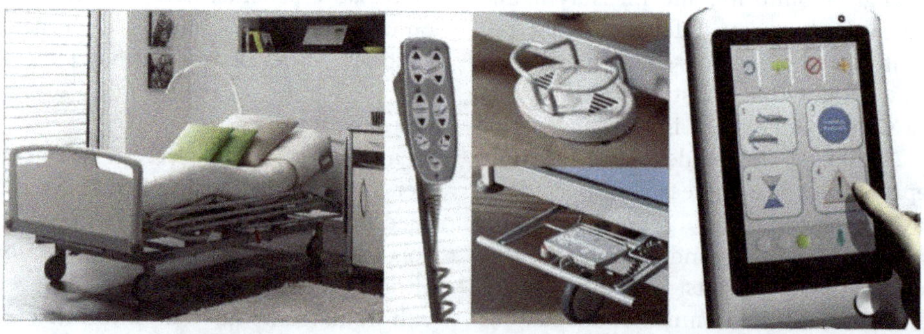

Fig. 4 User interfaces in smart beds are multiple, robust and dedicated to the patient and/or caregiver. Integration of new technologies, ergonomics and graphical interfaces allows for improved control over a broader range of functions. Left: Olympia Hospital bed, developed and manufactured by Haelvoet [46]. Right: example of a graphical-user interface designed for the control of a new generation of medical beds [47]. Permission for use of images granted by Haelvoet

Accessibility interfaces for smart beds

Directed to the treatment of subjects with temporary or permanently-restricted mobility, medical beds benefit from past and current accessibility inventions and developments, both in terms of their actuation-means, as well as in terms of their user-interfaces.

Among these solutions, environmental control units (ECU, see [30] for a review on incipient models of the late 90's) currently stand out as available additions to the medical bed environment, controlling some medical beds. These systems are among the most used accessibility-technologies by patients with spinal cord injury [31]. Basic inputs to ECUs include accessibility switches, sip-puff controls and pressure sensors (see [32]), and their impact on the quality of life of patients is a matter of research [33]. Over the past decades, this concept has been considered by research solutions for healthcare facilities, with inventions aiming at supplementing bed control [17]. Speech control, for instance, is considered and implemented on a limited number of cases, as an accessory ECU (as the one developed for the Pro Bed Medical Technologies Freedom Bed) or incorporated into some devices [34]. The promise of speech control for these devices is not new, with a patent from 1991 describing an ECU for a hospital bed and its environment [35]. The effectiveness of speech recognition, however, was more limited at that time, as compared to current models and consumer-ready systems.

Another example is the development of Brain-Computer Interfaces [36], powerful technologies for the aid of critically impaired patients, which are seen as possible inputs for ECUs and medical beds with basic actuating functions. This promising technology, however, presents specific difficulties [37] and is under development, limiting its current reach.

Technology-assisted healthcare environments

Surrounding the medical bed, the integration of information-technologies into the patient-care environment has changed the way patient-information and treatments are handled. Updated user interfaces, dedicated to patients and caregivers, have emerged over the past decade, both as consumer-ready solutions [38] and research projects [34], covering the management of patient records, and control over the near environment (like TV, lights, etc.). As medical beds become smarter, interaction with these smart environments becomes a possibility [8].

A growing trend looks to change the experience of the healthcare environment for patients, providing new means of communication and entertainment at their reach, particularly aimed at patients with restricted mobility (acute, recovering, and long-term patients). These proposals integrate connectivity and a higher control over the environment, while including informative resources (tutorials [38], etc.) concerning different conditions. Even when not including control over the bed itself, these "Interactive Patient-Care Systems" [39] may integrate a touchscreen through adjustable stands (e.g. Siemens HiMed Cockpit, visible in Fig. 5).

The development of personalized healthcare and medical devices for injuries and chronic diseases has been deemed as one of the most impactful and feasible challenges to be tackled by biomedical engineers in the near future [40], and the evolution of medical beds and devices in the immediate surroundings of the patient is instrumental to these advances. The core of these projects stems from a thorough vision concerning the patient's experience of this environment, valuing the possibility of *empowering patients* on their own care, through a more fluid interaction with their surroundings.

Discussion

Medical beds have changed, in the past decades, from technological, aesthetic, and functional perspectives. Smart medical beds are a comprehensive synthesis of these three: integrated solutions for patient care, assistance and monitoring. Powered by a surge in user technological-awareness, the acceptance of new technologies into smart beds and accessories will likely continue to grow in developed regions, reaching more complex, upgraded, and even bold iterations in the near future.

The future of medical beds will be shaped by the continued, conscious supplement of technologies into the healthcare environment. A prospective analysis on the evolution of healthcare systems will be necessary for the definition of proper strategies, in order to provide better, adapted services (expectations concerning number of beds and resources needed [41]). As for patients and environments, research is heading in the way of providing even further functionality and integration with the medical bed. Embedded monitoring, autonomous responses and accessibility-enabled systems can take full advantage of the potential of these devices, while also posing future challenges in the development of reliable solutions for the severely-disabled.

Technologies implemented into smart medical beds may, at this point, result in derived, low-cost upgrades to other devices, like manually-operated beds, which less-developed regions can benefit from.

While features like autonomy and embedded functionality may hint at an apparent detachment form the work of health specialists at this point in time, the need for multidisciplinary insight will, actually, become more urgent in the development of successful healthcare solutions. Research and study on healthcare-environment related solutions is of great need in a context of a globally-ageing population [42], where disability will have

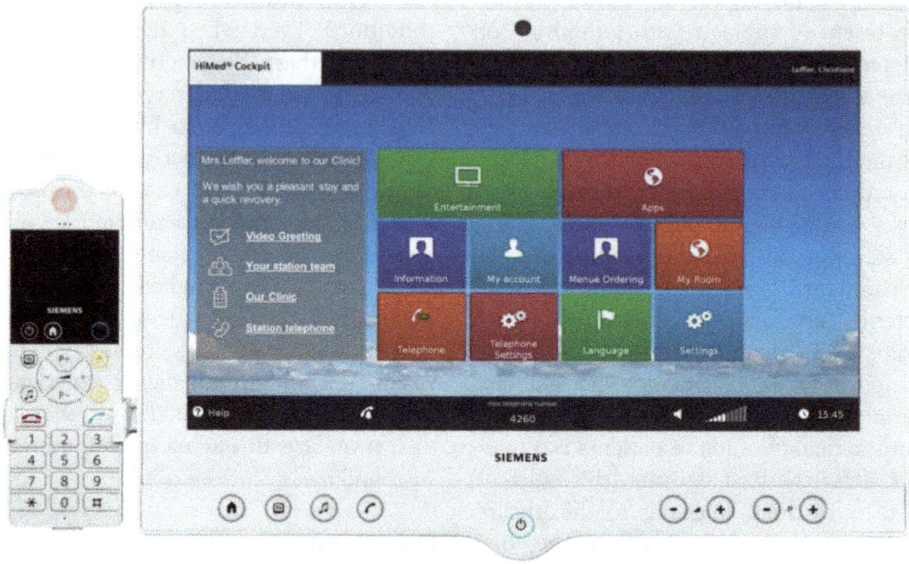

Fig. 5 Interactive patient-care systems integrate technology, information and communications into the healthcare environment [38]. Permission for use of images granted by Siemens

an even greater impact. Accessibility-enabled smart medical beds have the potential of becoming the center of new, comprehensive and patient-conscious healthcare environments.

Conclusions

Smart medical beds have emerged in the past decades as integrated solutions for patient care, assistance and monitoring, based on a comprehensive, multidisciplinary design process. The global market of medical beds is currently broad, competitive, and still has potential to spread. Dedicated devices for different demographics are developed, and high-end functionality under customizable solutions have become common features, expected of these devices. Research is also continuously promoting novel or updated integrations of technology into this family of devices. It is expected that these changes will continue to spread into further automation and design adaptations, with the smart bed becoming the heart of the smart patient-care environment of the future. The full potential of smart beds will not only be achieved with isolated technological or morphological advances, but when they are seamlessly integrated into the healthcare system, enabling more efficient efforts for caregivers, and more responsive environments for patients.

Endnotes

[1]*Mechatronics* refers to a multi-disciplinary field, combining knowledge from mechanics, electronics, informatics and communications engineering, as well as control theory, into the design of a broad range of products [57], among which are medical devices.

Abbreviations

CPR: Cardiopulmonary Resuscitation; ECU: Environmental Control Units; IEC: International Electrotechnical Commission; ISO: International Organization for Standardization; MEMS: Micro-ElectroMechanical System

Funding

This work was supported in part by Universidad de Buenos Aires, Programación Científica 2013–2016, Proyecto Interdisciplinario PIUBAMAS 20621201000011BA: "Evaluación del riesgo de caídas en adultos mayores y en pacientes geriátricos".
This work was supported in part by Facultad de Ingeniería y Ciencias Agrarias, Pontificia Universidad Católica Argentina: "Modelos biomecánicos y desarrollos de dispositivos para la cuantificación del movimiento humano en individuos normales y/o disfuncionales".

Authors' contributions

IG, MM and MTM contributed to the design of the research and to the analysis of its results. MM and MTM directed the project. IG took the lead in writing the manuscript with input from all authors. All authors read and approved the manuscript, provided critical feedback and helped shape the state-of-art survey, analysis and figures.

Author's information

IG: PhD in Design (UBA). Eng. in Electronics and Communications (UCA). Researcher in Biomechanics and Health Engineering at LaBIS-UCA. PhD work on updated mechatronics and interfaces for a novel medical bed design (CIDI-UBA & LaBIS-UCA).
MM: Emeritus Professor (FADU-UBA). PhD in Industrial Design (UBA). Founding member of the Center for Research in Industrial Design CIDI-FADU-UBA, with patented work and extensive research on mechatronic beds and products.
MTM: PhD in Physics (UBA). Academic, researcher, and director of the Biomechanics and Health Engineering Laboratory LaBIS-UCA. Member of CIDI-FADU-UBA, with research on biomechanics, medical technology and human balance.

Competing interests

The authors declare that they have no competing interests.

References

1. World Health Organization (2014) World Health Statistics Italy. ISBN 978 92 4 156471 7.
2. de Bruin AM, Bekker R et Al GM (2010) Dimensioning hospital wards using the Erlang loss model. Ann Oper Res 178(1): 23–43 doi:https://doi.org/10.1007/s10479-009-0647-8.
3. World Health Organization (2015) Chapter 3. In: Service Availability and Readiness Assessment - Reference Manual, Version 2.2 (online) http://www.who.int/healthinfo/systems/sara_reference_manual/en/. Accessed 2016.
4. Ghersi I, Mariño M, Miralles M (2016) From modern push-button hospital-beds to 20th century mechatronic beds: a review. J Phys Conf Ser 705(2016), Conference 1, 012054. doi:https://doi.org/10.1088/1742-6596/705/1/012054
5. Goldschwartz M (1995) Mario Mariño, el primer Doctor La Prensa (online) http://www.cidi.bime.com.ar/publicaciones2.php?id=8. Accessed 2018.
6. MedicalExpo catalog. http://www.medicalexpo.com/. Accessed 2018.
7. Panasonic (2014) Care Serv Robot is First in the World to Obtain ISO 13482 (online) http://news.panasonic.com/global/topics/2014/26411.html. Accessed 2016.
8. Collins WF, Allen JM, Huster KA et al. (2007) Patent: Wireless bed connectivity.
9. Norville L (2012) Market Analysis: Hospital Beds (online) http://medicaldealer.com/market-analysis-hospital-beds/. Accessed 2016.
10. Elliott D, Moreno DM et al. (2013) Patent: Patient support with improved control.
11. Herman FJ (2014) Patent: Multifunctional display for hospital bed.
12. IEC/ISO (2009) IEC 60601–2-52:2009 Medical electrical equipment - Part 2–52. (online) https://www.iso.org/. https://webstore.iec.ch/. Accessed 2016.
13. IEC (1996) IEC 60601–2-38:1996 (online) https://webstore.iec.ch/
14. IEC/ISO (2015) IEC 60601–2-52: Amd 1 (online) https://webstore.iec.ch/. Accessed 2016.
15. IEC (2012) Preview IEC 60601–1 (online) https://webstore.iec.ch/
16. Kalorama Information (2013) Abstract: The World Market for Medical Beds (online) http://www.kaloramainformation.com/Medical-Beds-7888742/. Accessed 2016.
17. Welling JR, Poehner ME (2003) Patent: Hospital bed communication and control device.
18. Banerjee T, Enayati M, Keller JM, Skubic M, et al. Monitoring patients in hospital beds using unobtrusive depth sensors. In: EMBC 36th annual international conference of the IEEE, 26–30 Aug, vol. 201; 2014. p. 5904–7. https://doi.org/10.1109/EMBC.2014.6944972.
19. Acampora G, Cook DJ, Rashidi P, Vasilakos AV. A survey on ambient intelligence in healthcare. IEEE Proc. 2013;101:2470–94. https://doi.org/10.1109/JPROC.2013.2262913.
20. Gunningberg L and Carli C (2014) Reduced pressure for fewer pressure ulcers: can real-time feedback of interface pressure optimise repositioning in bed? Int wound J. Sept 16, 2014. doi:https://doi.org/10.1111/iwj.12374.
21. Scott RG, Thurman KM. Visual feedback of continuous bedside pressure mapping to optimize effective patient repositioning. Advances in wound care. 2014;3:376–82. https://doi.org/10.1089/wound.2013.0519.
22. Yousefi R, Ostadabbas S, Faezipour M, Nourani M, et al. A smart bed platform for monitoring & ulcer prevention. In: BMEI 2011 4th international conference, 15–17 Oct, vol. 2011; 2011. p. 1362–6. https://doi.org/10.1109/BMEI.2011.6098589.
23. Stepowska J, Sharkey K. In bed with robots: the future of patient transportation. 2014. UTS Newsroom (online) http://newsroom.uts.edu.au/news/2014/11/bed-robots-future-patient-transportation.
24. Klap T, Shinar Z. Using piezoelectric sensor for continuous-contact-free monitoring of heart and respiration rates in real-life hospital settings. In: Computing in cardiology conference (CinC), 22–25 Sept, vol. 2013; 2013. p. 671–4.
25. Zeng W, Zhang Q, Zhou Y, Xu G et al. (2015) Infrared video based non-invasive heart rate measurement. In: 2015 IEEE International Conference on Robotics and Biomimetics (ROBIO), 6–9 Dec 2015. pp 1041–1046. doi: https://doi.org/10.1109/ROBIO.2015.7418909.
26. Bachman T. Patient positioning: more than just "turn every 2h". BNI. 2006;22:3.
27. Crone WC. A brief introduction to MEMS and NEMS, Chapter 9. In: Springer handbook of experimental solid mechanics. USA: Springer-Verlag; 2008. p. 203–6. ISBN: 978–0-387-26883-5.
28. Staub M. Senior design team helps hospital staff regulate bed angle. 2013. Department of Mechanical Science and Enginering, University of Illinois at Urbana-Champaign. (online) https://mechanical.illinois.edu/news/senior-design-team-helps-hospital-staff-regulate-bed-angle. Accessed 2016.
29. Seo KH, Choi TY, Oh C. Development of a robotic system for the bed-ridden. Mechatronics. 2011;21:227–38. https://doi.org/10.1016/j.mechatronics.2010.10.011.
30. Wellings DJ, Unsworth J. Fortnightly review: environmental control systems for people with disability: an update. BMJ. 1997;315(7105):409–12.
31. World Health Organization and International Spinal Cord Society. International Perspectives on Spinal Cord Injury. 2013. World Health Organization (online) http://apps.who.int/iris/bitstream/handle/10665/94190/9789241564663_eng.pdf?sequence=1. Accessed 2018.
32. AbleNet Switch Selection Guide (online) https://www.ablenetinc.com/. Accessed 2016.
33. Verdonck M, Steggles E, Chard G. The meaning of living with or without environmental control Systems for People with tetraplegia: an Irish focus group study. In: assistive technology from adapted equipment to inclusive environments. Amsterdam, Netherlands: IOS press; 2009. ISBN 978–1607500421.
34. Servicio de Información y Noticias Científicas. 2012. Una pantalla lleva la historia clínica electrónica a pie de cama del hospital (online) https://www.agenciasinc.es/Noticias/Una-pantalla-lleva-la-historia-clinica-electronica-a-pie-de-cama-del-hospital. Accessed 2016.
35. Douglas TL (1994) Patent: Voice-actuated, speaker-dependent control system for hospital bed.
36. van Gerven M, Farquhar J, Schaefer R, et al. The brain–computer interface cycle. J Neural Eng. 2009;6:041001. 10pp
37. Westly E. Fixing the Brain-Computer Interface (online). 2011. https://spectrum.ieee.org/biomedical/bionics/fixing-the-brain-computer-interface/. Accessed 2016.
38. Siemens. HiMed – The intelligent answer to the challenges of everyday clinical life (online) https://w3.siemens.com/mcms/topics/en/himed/Pages/default.aspx. Accessed 2018.
39. U.S. Dept. of Veteran Affairs. New System Is More Than Just Great TV (online). 2013. https://www.tampa.va.gov/features/New_System_Is_More_Than_Just_Great_TV.asp. Accessed 2016.
40. College of Fellows, American Institute for Medical and Biological Engineering. Medical and biological engineering in the next 20 years: the promise and the challenges. IEEE Trans Biomed Eng. 2013;60(7):1767–75.
41. Oberlin P, Mouquet MC (2008) Number of hospital beds in 2030: projection with national French case-mix data, BMC Health Serv Res 2008, 8 (Suppl 1): A6 doi:10.1186/1472-6963-8-S1-A6.
42. United Nations DoEaSA (2013) World population ageing. New York. ST/ESA/SER.A/348.
43. Völker. Völker LTC Vis-a-Vis (online) http://www.voelker.de/cms/en/products-healthcare/products-healthcare-beds/vis-a-vis.html. Accessed 2018.
44. Malvestio. *Sigma PCU Electric Bed Scale System* (online) https://malvestio.it/en/prodotti/ward/sigma-cardiac-and-progressive-care-unit/sigma-pcu-electric-bed-346950be/33. Accessed 2018.
45. World Map Without Antarctica (online) https://commons.wikimedia.org/wiki/File:BlankMap-World-noborders.png. Accessed 2018.
46. Haelvoet. *Olympia Hospital by Haelvoet (online)* https://www.haelvoet.be/uploads/documents/pdf/201705/HAE-OLYMPIA-HOSPITAL-EN1.pdf. Accessed 2018. Haelvoet nv, Leon Bekaertstraat 8, 8770 Ingelmunster, Belgium.
47. Ghersi I (2016) Comprehensive electronic Interface for the control of a new generation of mechatronic beds, doctorate thesis in Facultad de Arquitectura, Diseño y Urbanismo Universidad de Buenos Aires Advisors: Mariño M and Miralles MT In press (Digital Repository - Universidad de Buenos Aires) http://repositoriouba.sisbi.uba.ar/gsdl/cgi-bin/library.cgi. 245 pp.
48. Geringer ER, Goldberg J (1998) Patent: Caster mounted weighing system.
49. Foster LD, Ruehl JW, Vogel, JD (1996) Patent: Foot egress chair bed. Hill-Rom Services Inc.
50. Williams TN, Parrish GR (1996) Patent: Bedside control unit for a hospital bed.
51. Weismiller MW, Kummer JA, Kramer KL, Schulte SR, Palermo PD, Dlugos DF (1995) Patent: Hospital Bed. Hill-Rom Services Inc.
52. Moster J, Zerhusen R, Hamilton M et al. (2005) Patent: Communication and bed function control apparatus.
53. Reeder RA Zerhusen RM, Vogel JD, Cerimele ME, Riley CW and Wildman TD (2012) Patent: Touch Screen Control of a Hospital Bed.
54. Dixon SA (2009) Patent: Proximity Activation of Voice Operation of Hospital Bed.
55. Huster KA, Tallent DR et al. (2012) Patent: Hospital bed with graphical user interface having advanced functionality.
56. Andrienko K (2012) Patent: Biometric Bed Configuration.
57. Bishop RH. What is mechatronics? In: Mechatronics, an Introduction. United States: Taylor & Francis Group LLC; 2005. ISBN 978-0849363580.

6

Traditional Chinese medicine pharmacovigilance in signal detection: decision tree-based data classification

Jian-Xiang Wei[1*], Jing Wang[2], Yun-Xia Zhu[2], Jun Sun[3], Hou-Ming Xu[3] and Ming Li[3]

Abstract

Background: Traditional Chinese Medicine (TCM) is a style of traditional medicine informed by modern medicine but built on a foundation of more than 2500 years of Chinese medical practice. According to statistics, TCM accounts for approximately 14% of total adverse drug reaction (ADR) spontaneous reporting data in China. Because of the complexity of the components in TCM formula, which makes it essentially different from Western medicine, it is critical to determine whether ADR reports of TCM should be analyzed independently.

Methods: Reports in the Chinese spontaneous reporting database between 2010 and 2011 were selected. The dataset was processed and divided into the total sample (all data) and the subsample (including TCM data only). Four different ADR signal detection methods-PRR, ROR, MHRA and IC- currently widely used in China, were applied for signal detection on the two samples. By comparison of experimental results, three of them—PRR, MHRA and IC—were chosen to do the experiment. We designed several indicators for performance evaluation such as *R* (recall ratio), *P* (precision ratio), and *D* (discrepancy ratio) based on the reference database and then constructed a decision tree for data classification based on such indicators.

Results: For PRR: R_1-R_2 = 0.72%, P_1-P_2 = 0.16% and D = 0.92%; For MHRA: R_1-R_2 = 0.97%, P_1-P_2 = 0.20% and D = 1.18%; For IC: R_1-R_2 = 1.44%, P_2-P_1 = 4.06% and D = 4.72%. The threshold of *R*,*P*and *D*is set as 2%, 2% and 3% respectively. Based on the decision tree, the results are "separation" for PRR, MHRA and IC.

Conclusions: In order to improve the efficiency and accuracy of signal detection, we suggest that TCM data should be separated from the total sample when conducting analyses.

Keywords: Adverse drug reaction, Signal detection, Data classification, Decision tree

Background

The World Health Organization (WHO) defines adverse drug reactions (ADRs) as harmful and unintended reactions, which occur from the standard use of medicinal dosages for prophylaxis, diagnosis or treatment of diseases, or for the modification of physiological functions. ADRs include side effects, toxic effects, residual effects, idiosyncratic reactions, multiple infections arising from anti-infectives, drug dependence, and carcinogenic and mutagenic actions [1]. It is very difficult to identify the potential drug risks in clinical tests due to a range of issues, such as small sample size, limited observation time and scope. Subsequently, unintended adverse reactions may occur during medication use posing further threats to health and causing a financial burden on the patients. To strengthen monitoring of ADRs, China has established the ADR Monitoring Center and carried out appropriate endeavors since 1989. China established a national network system for ADR monitoring in 2003. By the end of 2016, the number of spontaneous reports submitted through the network has reached nearly 10,750,000 and has been drastically increasing at a rate of 1 million per year.

Currently, the methods used in signal detection in China mainly include Proportional Reporting Ratio (PRR), Reporting Odds Ratio (ROR), Medicines and

* Correspondence: jxwei@njupt.edu.cn
[1]School of Internet of Things, Nanjing University of Posts and Telecommunications, Nanjing 210003, China
Full list of author information is available at the end of the article

Healthcare products Regulatory Agency (MHRA) and Information Component (IC) [2–9]. These methods calculate signal scores, i.e., the values for PRR, ROR and IC, to assess whether a drug is significantly associated with an adverse event. These calculations or algorithms, so-called the disproportionality analyses or measures, however, differ from one another in that the PRR, MHRA and ROR are frequentist (non-Bayesian), whereas the IC is Bayesian [10]. Many scholars of China have applied these methods on Chinese ADR data, but consistency in the detection results is poor [11–13]. So, no signal detection method that conforms to ADR data quality in China has been established. The co-existence of multiple detection methods causes challenge in signal detection. Moreover, the Chinese ADR database includes all drugs such as TCM, Western medicine, and biological products, but signal detection is not categorized by drug types. Owing to the large volume of data (about ten million), the variety of methods and the complexity of data processing, the China National Center for ADR Monitoring requires approximately two weeks to perform signal detection for all data, and the large amount of selected signals still need to be manually analyzed by experts. Thus, the efficiency of signal discovery is very low. Presently, there is no research on whether ADR data can be categorized by drug type before signal detection.

Combining TCM pharmacology with modern technologies, more drug types and preparations have entered Chinese market increasingly. The data system of the China Food and Drug Administration (CFDA) has shown 60,029 authorized TCMs as of October 17, 2013 [14]. Because of increased usage, the lack of knowledge about TCM and misuse, there is a surge in the amount of TCM ADR reports and the types of drugs involved. In the past few years, the CFDA has warned about the severe adverse reactions of Xiangdan, Shengmai, Xiyanping, Mailuoning, and Honghua (*Safflower*) injections, the safety issues of Lei Gong Teng (*Tripterygium wilfordii*) preparation, and the digestive reactions of the compound Qingdai pill. For example, Shengmai injection is a traditional Chinese medicine injection composed of Red Ginseng, *Ophiopogon japonicus* and Schisandra Chinensis. The adverse reactions of Shengmai injection in severe cases are as follows: body as a whole-general disorders accounted for about 53.2%, respiratory system disorders accounted for 20.7% and cardiovascular disorders accounted for about 11.4%. A total of 179 cases of Shengmai injection were reported, including anaphylactic shock (90) and severe anaphylactoid reaction (89), accounting for about 35.2% of all severe cases [15].

TCMs can be relatively crude preparations usually prepared as formula of numerous herbal and other natural-source ingredients, and as patent medicines i.e. manufactured, formulated products also containing numerous ingredients (sometimes they include conventional drug ingredients). TCMs have a botanical name, prescription name, trade name and pharmaceutical name. Usually, their names include Chinese names, Pin Yin names and Latin names. In China, generic drug names refer to China Approved Drug Names (CADN), which are the legal names of drugs formulated by the Pharmacopoeia Committee in accordance with the principle of CADN and submitted to the Ministry of public health for the record. All drugs composed of the same ingredients or the same formula have generic drug names are mandatory and binding. Generic drug names must be used on the label, instruction or package of listed drugs. So, each TCM in the spontaneous reporting data owns a unique generic drug name, named by Chinese characters (includes Pin Yin). ADR signal detection is based on generic drug names. In contrast with conventional medicines, TCMs are chemically rich complex mixtures comprising several hundreds of constituents, often more [16]. Owing to the inherent characteristics of TCM, the factors influencing its ADRs are more complicated than Western medicine. An understanding of the evaluation criteria on TCM ADR has always been vague. There is a lack of scientific, objective, and unbiased methods to evaluate TCM ADR [17, 18]. Some experts have pointed out that because of the special nature of TCM, its ADR data are quite different from those of Western medicine; thus, its ADR signal detection should be performed separately [16, 19]. The purpose of this paper is to solve the problem whether TCM should be separated for signal detection.

Methods

Data resource

A total of 1,823,144 ADR reports from 2010 and 2011 were obtained from the CFDA. Of these, 608,710 (33.4%) reports had one drug linked to multiple ADRs. The reports were further split into one drug to one ADR relationship. Reports with "unknown" drug name or ADRs were excluded. Following data processing, a total of 2,221,942 records were obtained. There are 317,417 records of TCM accounting for 14.29%; 1,874,904 records of "Western medicine" accounting for 84.38%; and 29,621 records of "biological products" accounting for 1.33%. The overall data were aggregated based on generic drug names of drugs and names of ADRs; as such, 139,281 drug-ADR pairs with their corresponding frequencies were obtained: this data set is `Data1`. This data set included 6174 drugs and 2458 ADRs.

In order to determine the effectiveness of classifying data for signal detection, a reference database of known ADRs needed to be established for comparison. The reference database was obtained from the CFDA and it was extracted from drug product labeling manually. The

ADRs in the drug product labeling were collected primarily from pre-market clinical trials. In addition, side effects detected by the ADR monitoring system and verified by the experts would also be added to the drug product labeling during post-marketing. The drug name and ADR name of the reference database were mapped to the spontaneous reporting data. It includes 53,774 drug-ADR pairs and involves 2401 different drugs and 2460 different ADRs. The reference database will be noted as `Data2`.

Based on the two datasets, we make the further data processing as follows:

1. For `Data1`, because usually a minimum occurrence of 3 is accepted in signal detection, ADR data with an occurrence of less than 3 were removed from `Data1`. Further, for consistency in the reference database, drugs that were present in `Data1` but absent in `Data2` were removed from `Data1`. This resulted in a dataset with 39,782 records, involving 1692 different drugs and 877 ADRs. This dataset is referred to as `the total sample`.
2. TCM data were extracted from `the total sample`, generating a TCM dataset. The dataset included 4697 records, involving 326 drugs and 283 ADRs. This dataset is referred to as `the subsample`, and it is a proper subset of `the total sample`.
3. Fields in the two datasets include "type of drug", "generic drug name", "name of ADR", "occurrence frequency", "known or not", etc. The `Data2` is used to annotate the field "known or not" in `the total sample` and `the subsample`: if the drug-ADR pair that appeared in the reference database, it was annotated as "1," otherwise it was annotated as "0."

Selection of signal detection methods

Currently, ADR signal detection methods in China utilize such four mainstream methods as: PRR, ROR, MHRA, and IC, and the calculations of measures of disproportionality are primarily based upon a two-by-two contingency table (Table 1) [20].

The four methods are applied to `the subsample` respectively. The signal detection of `the subsample` was done at the TCM product level. The results of positive signals are listed in Table 2.

Table 1 Two-by-two contingency table

	Target ADRs	Other ADRs	Total
Target drugs	a	b	$a+b$
Other drugs	c	d	$c+d$
Total	$a+c$	$b+d$	$a+b+c+d$

Table 2 The number of positive signals in the two samples, detected by the four methods

Signal detection methods	The number of positive signals in the total sample	The number of positive signals in the subsample
PRR+	18,780	2209
ROR+	18,568	2145
MHRA+	15,952	1820
IC+	7196	660

As shown in Table 2, the numbers of positive signals generated by PRR, ROR, MHRA and IC showed a decreasing relationship. Using "1" to indicate positive signal and "0" to indicate non-positive signal, the correlation coefficients of the detection results of the four methods are shown in Table 3 and Table 4.

We knew from Tables 3 and 4 that the correlation coefficient of PRR and ROR was close to 1(0.9887 and 0.9721), that is, the outcomes of the two methods are basically identical. At the same time, the two approaches are based on the theory of disproportionality. Therefore, it's necessary to use both PRR and POR. We chose PRR, MHRA, and IC as the three methods for signal detection in this study. All the methods of signal detection were implemented with Visual FoxPro database software 6.0.

Decision-making process

To judge the superiority and inferiority of the signal detection outcomes in the two samples before and after data separation, the following issues needed to be addressed: How to evaluate the difference of results of signal detection methods applied to the two samples before and after data separation? What indicators were needed to be set for discrimination? What was the decision- making process? Flowchart on decision-making process is presented as follows (Fig. 1).

Detecting signals in `the total sample` and `the subsample` respectively. Then, two results were obtained. Some indicators of evaluation method were constructed and used to evaluate the superiority and inferiority of the two results. The decision-making was conducted based on the reference database and the evaluation results.

Table 3 Correlation coefficients of four methods in the total sample

	PRR	ROR	MHRA	IC
PRR	1			
ROR	0.9887	1		
MHRA	0.8670	0.8613	1	
IC	0.5009	0.5055	0.5069	1

Table 4 Correlation coefficients of four methods in the subsample

	PRR	ROR	MHRA	IC
PRR	1			
ROR	0.9721	1		
MHRA	0.8441	0.8219	1	
IC	0.4205	0.4275	0.4241	1

Fourfold table design based on the reference database

The reference database provided an objective evidence for classification decisions. Signal detection of the two samples was performed and compared with the reference database, which could be structured into a fourfold table as follows (Table 5).

In Table 5, a represents the number of ADR pairs with positive signals in both `the total sample` and `the subsample`, a_1 represents the number of ADR pairs that are present in `the total sample`, `the subsample`, and the reference database, a_0 represents the number of ADR pairs that are present in `the total sample` and `the subsample` but are absent in the reference database, and $a = a_1 + a_0$. The other symbols such as $b(b_1, b_0)$, $c(c_1, c_0)$ and $d(d_1, d_0)$ are analogous to $a(a_1, a_0)$. The ADR pairs in b_1 and c_1 are distinct signals between two samples, and thus can be used as a basis for classification decision.

Evaluation method

1) Indicator *R - Recall ratio*

The recall ratio, a measure of the coverage of known signals, represents the ratio of the signals detected from the reference database. Using recall ratio R_1 to describe the ability to detect known signals in `the total sample`, as represented by formula (1):

$$R_1 = \frac{a_1 + b_1}{a_1 + b_1 + c_1 + d_1} \tag{1}$$

From Table 5, we can see that $a_1 + b_1 + c_1 + d_1$ is the total number of known signals and $a_1 + b_1$ is the number of known signals detected in `the total sample`. Similarly, using recall ratio R_2 to describe the ability to detect known signals in `the subsample`, as represented by formula (2):

$$R_2 = \frac{a_1 + c_1}{a_1 + b_1 + c_1 + d_1} \tag{2}$$

By comparing the recall ratios between the two samples, the differences in the ability to detect known signals can be distinguished, which also reflect the differences in signal detection sensitivities between these two samples based on the reference database. Therefore, the recall ratio is a key indicator that should be used as the primary basis for classification decisions.

2) Indicator *P - Precision ratio*

The drawback of formula (1) and (2) lies in the fact that when a_1 is much greater than b_1 and c_1, there is no significant difference between b_1 and c_1 even though they have markedly distinct values. Therefore, if the difference between R_1 and R_2 is slight, it is necessary to define the precision ratio. The precision ratio, a measure of the accuracy of detecting known signals, is the proportion of the known signals detected based on a certain sample. We use precision ratio P_1 to describe the ability to detect known signals in `the total sample`, which is represented by formula (3).

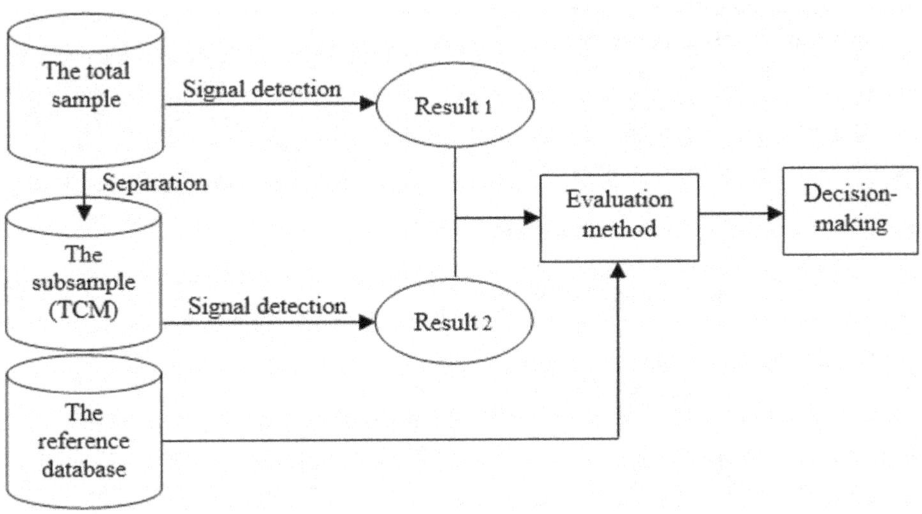

Fig. 1 Decision-making process flowchart

Table 5 Two-by-two contingency table of the two samples

	The subsample +	The subsample -
The total sample +	$a(a_1, a_0)$	$b(b_1, b_0)$
The total sample -	$c(c_1, c_0)$	$d(d_1, d_0)$

$$P_1 = \frac{a_1 + b_1}{a + b} \tag{3}$$

From Table 5, we can see that $a + b$ is the total number of signals detected in `the total sample` and $a_1 + b_1$ is the number of known signal detected in `the total sample`. Similarly, using precision ratio P_2 to describe the ability to detect known signals in `the subsample`, as represented by formula (4).

$$P_2 = \frac{a_1 + c_1}{a + c} \tag{4}$$

3) Indicator D - *discrepancy ratio*

Discrepancy ratio represents the diversity measurement of the detection outcomes in the two samples, represented by formula (5).

$$D = \left| \frac{b_1 - c_1}{b + c} \right| \tag{5}$$

In formula (5), $b + c$ represent the total number of different detection outcomes in the two samples.

Decision tree

Using the indicators of R, P and D in `the total sample` and `the subsample` to decide whether to classify TCM data, the process is as follows.

1) The primary basis is to consider the coverage percentage of known signals based on the detected outcomes in the two samples. Specifically, the indicator R of the two samples is considered (See formula 1 and 2). Sample with high recall ratio is chosen. If $R_1 - R_2 > R_t$, it is recommended to not perform classified detection of TCM data; if $R_2 - R_1 > R_t$, it is recommended to perform classified detection of TCM data; if the recall ratio difference is slight, further decision is needed (R_t represents the threshold of R).
2) When there is little difference in recall ratios of the two samples, the indicator P of the signal detection needs to be considered, which is the precision ratio of the two samples (See formula 3 and 4). If $P_1 - P_2 > P_t$, it is recommended to not perform classified detection of TCM data; if $P_2 - P_1 > P_t$, it is recommended to perform classified detection of TCM data; if the precision ratio difference is slight, further decision is needed (P_t represents the threshold of P).
3) When there is little difference in both recall ratio and precision ratio of the two samples, then indicator D is compared. If the discrepancy ratio exceeds the prescribed threshold ($D > D_t$), the decision outcome is "non-separation", otherwise is "separation" (D_t represents the threshold of D).

Based on the above analysis, the decision tree for determining whether to perform classified detection of data is constructed as Fig. 2.

Results

The statistical results of the two samples are shown in Table 6 and Table 7.

The PRR, MHRA, and IC methods are used to perform experiments with `the total sample` and `the subsample` and the results are shown in Table 8.

A decision-making table (Table 9) is established using data from Table 8 and the classification decision tree. The thresholds of three indicators are set based on the mean of the differences of R, P and D across three signal detection methods. For R, the difference of PRR, MHRA and IC is 0.72%, 0.97% and 1.44%, so the mean of three differences about equal to 1.04%. Thus, the threshold of R is set to 2%, an integer slightly larger than the mean. Similarly, for P, the mean of the differences is $(0.16\% + 0.20\% + 4.06\%)/3 \approx 1.47\%$, so the threshold of P is set to 2%. For D, the mean of the differences is $(0.92\% + 1.18\% + 4.72\%)\ /3 \approx 2.73\%$, so the threshold of D is set to 3%. In brief, we set R_t to 2%, P_t to 2% and D_t to 3% in the following decision process. Based on the decision tree (see Fig. 2), the decision-making process is as follows:

1) PRR: because R_1-R_2 = 0.72% < 2%, P_1-P_2 = 0.16% < 2% and D = 0.92% < 3%, the conclusion is "Separation".
2) MHRA: because R_1-R_2 = 0.97% < 2%, P_1-P_2 = 0.20% < 2% and D = 1.18% < 3%, the conclusion is "Separation".
3) IC: because R_1-R_2 = 1.44% < 2%, P_2-P_1 = 4.06% > 2%, the conclusion is "Separation".

Thus, the conclusion of "Separation" is reached by using all three methods.

Discussion

Comparative analysis of two samples

The statistical results of two samples are shown in Table 6.

`The total sample` includes 1,972,008 ADR reports, involving 1692 drugs, 39,782 drug-ADR pairs, and 877 ADRs. The average number of ADRs is 1165.49 for each

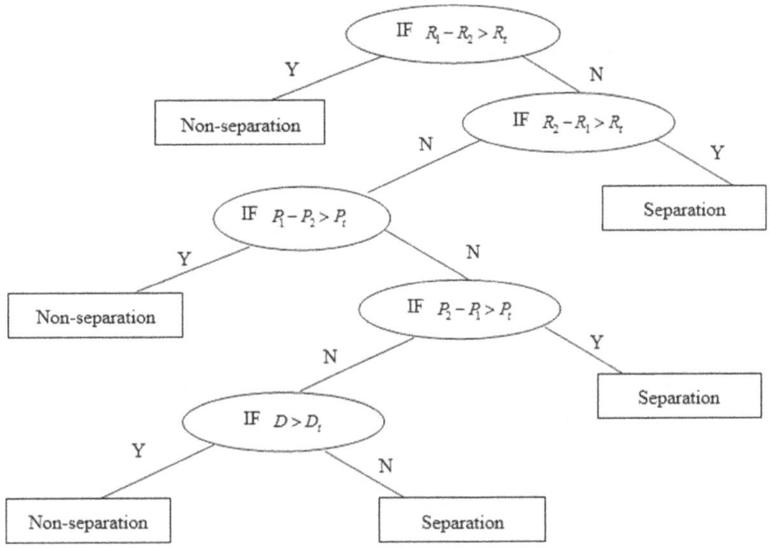

Fig. 2 Decision tree for determining whether to classify data. Note: R_1 and R_2 represent the recall ratios of the total sample and the subsample. P_1 and P_2 are the precision ratios of two samples. D is the discrepancy ratio of two samples. R_t, P_t and D_t represent the threshold of each indicator respectively

drug and 49.57 for each drug-ADR pair, whereas each ADR has an average frequency of 2248.58.

The subsample is a collection of all reports of TCM removed from the total sample. It contains 199,115 ADR reports of TCM, accounting for 10.1% of the total sample, in which 326 drugs, 4697 drug-ADR pairs, and 283 ADRs are involved. The average number of ADRs is 610.78 for each drug and 42.39 for each drug-ADR pair, whereas each ADR has an average frequency of 703.59. Compared with the total sample, the average frequency of the subsample is respectively reduced by 554.7, 7.18 and 1545.

Compared with the reference database, the total sample contains 13,555 known drug-ADR pairs, and the proportion is 34.07%; the subsample contains 830 known drug-ADR pairs, and the proportion is 17.67%, 16.4% less than that in the total sample. Specifically, known drug-ADR pairs in the TCM database are far less than those in the total sample.

The total sample contains 88,083 serious reports, accounting for 4.47%. The subsample contains 10,007 serious reports, accounting for 5.03%. Therefore, the subsample has relatively higher serious report proportion than the total sample.

Table 6 Statistical results of the two samples

Type	The total sample	The subsample
ADR reports	1,972,008	199,115
Drugs involved	1692	326
ADRs involved	877	283
Drug-ADR pairs (known drug-ADR pairs)	39,782 (13,555)	4697 (830)
Serious ADR reports	88,083	10,007

Table 7 shows the top ten ADRs with highest frequency in two samples. For each sample, the sum of their frequency is close to 60%. Seven of the top ten adverse reactions are the same between the two samples. The obvious difference between the two samples is that "headache" (2.87%), "abdominal pain" (2.65%) and "diarrhea" (2.53%) in the total sample, and "palpitation" (4.38%), "chest tightness" (3.14%) and "fever" (2.94%) in the subsample. The top three adverse reactions in both samples are "rash" (14.27% vs 16.15%), "nausea" (11.48% vs 7.20%) and "pruritus" (8.78% vs 11.42%), but the proportion of "nausea" is 4.28% higher in the total sample than that in the subsample, while "pruritus" is 2.64% lower than that in the subsample.

Discussion of methods

This paper presents a decision method by comparing signal detection results before and after separating TCM data from the total sample. The method employs two important formulas of information retrieval theory: recall ratio and precision ratio. Recall ratio is an indicator of success which represents the proportion of known ADRs retrieved from all known TCM ADRs. Precision ratio refers to the proportion of known ADR in all retrieved signals, and is an indicator of signal-noise ratio. In the design of decision-making tree, we first consider the recall ratio, which is about whether more known signals can be detected with independent signal detection in TCM sample. If there is no difference in recall ratio, further consideration should be given to the precision

Table 7 Top ten ADRs with highest frequency in two samples

Adverse reaction	Frequency of ADRs in the total sample (proportion)	ADR	Frequency of ADRs in the subsample (proportion)
Rash	281,399 (14.27%)	Rash	32,161 (16.15%)
Nausea	226,368 (11.48%)	Pruritus	22,736 (11.42%)
Pruritus	173,111 (8.78%)	Nausea	14,339 (7.20%)
Vomiting	141,098 (7.16%)	Dizziness	9577 (4.81%)
Dizziness	83,278 (4.22%)	Shivering	9206 (4.62%)
Headache	56,507 (2.87%)	Palpitation	8728 (4.38%)
Abdominal pain	52,291 (2.65%)	Vomiting	8661 (4.35%)
Diarrhea	49,839 (2.53%)	Anaphylactoid reaction	7182 (3.61%)
Anaphylactoid reaction	49,261 (2.50%)	Chest tightness	6251 (3.14%)
Shivering	39,066 (1.98%)	Fever	5847 (2.94%)
Total	1,152,218 (58.44%)		124,688 (62.62%)

ratio. In addition, the discrepancy ratio is added for decision-making when the above two indicators cannot work well. The decision method is based on the reference database and the proportion of known ADRs of TCM in it is very low (17.67%), this could result in uncertainty of the decision outcome. At the same time, according to the previous data analysis, there have been some differences in the two samples. Thus, according to the TCM data characteristics, the decision result is biased towards "separation" when the corresponding values of the three indicators are relatively close before and after data separation.

Discussion of results

Table 8 shows the experiment results with the three detection methods. For PRR, the total number of signals detected in `the total sample` is 2209, `the subsample` is 2218, and the number of common signals is 1888. For MHRA, the number of signals detected in `the total sample` is 1820, `the subsample` is 1836, and the number of common signals is 1488, which is 389, 382, and 400 less than that of the PRR method. For IC, the total number of signals detected in `the total sample` is 660, `the subsample` is 752, and the number of common signals is 579. Obviously, among the three methods, IC detects the lowest number of signals.

Table 9 gives the values of all indicators of the three methods. Since the PRR method detects the most signals, it contains the largest number of known ADR, resulting in the highest recall ratio of 72.41%. The recall ratios of MHRA and IC are 61.69% and 38.19% respectively. But the precision ratio is opposite. Although the total amount of signals detected by IC is the smallest, its precision ratio is the highest, 42.15%, while the precision ratios of PRR and MHRA are 27.10% and 27.89% respectively.

For PRR and MHRA, decision-making paths are consistent and the results are all "Separation" because all the values of three indicators fall within the according thresholds. For IC, however, decision-making path is deferent from PRR and MHRA. The recall ratio of the two samples is very similar, but `the subsample` has a significantly high precision ratio than `the total sample`. So, the conclusion is "Separation" for IC.

The dataset of this research is fixed, that is to say, `the total sample` and `the subsample` are fixed, so the values of three indicators calculated based on two samples are constant, and they will not change with the different threshold. Thus, it is impossible to determine the optimum threshold in traditional ways such as Precision Recall curve, Receiver Operating Characteristic

Table 8 Experiment results through the three detection methods

Detection method		The subsample +	The subsample -
PRR	The total sample +	$a = 1888$ ($a_1 = 561$, $a_0 = 1327$)	$b = 330$ ($b_1 = 40$, $b_0 = 290$)
	The total sample -	$c = 321$ ($c_1 = 34$, $c_0 = 287$)	$d = 2158$ ($d_1 = 195$, $d_0 = 1963$)
MHRA	The total sample +	$a = 1488$ ($a_1 = 456$, $a_0 = 1032$)	$b = 348$ ($b_1 = 56$, $b_0 = 292$)
	The total sample -	$c = 332$ ($c_1 = 48$, $c_0 = 284$)	$d = 2529$ ($d_1 = 270$, $d_0 = 2259$)
IC	The total sample +	$a = 579$ ($a_1 = 274$, $a_0 = 305$)	$b = 173$ ($b_1 = 43$, $b_0 = 130$)
	The total sample -	$c = 81$ ($c_1 = 31$, $c_0 = 50$)	$d = 3864$ ($d_1 = 482$, $d_0 = 3382$)

Table 9 Decision-making table

Detection method	Indicators	The total sample	The subsample	Difference
PRR	Recall ratio (%)	$R_1 = 72.41\%$	$R_2 = 71.69\%$	0.72%
	Precision ratio (%)	$P_1 = 27.10\%$	$P_2 = 26.94\%$	0.16%
	Discrepancy ratio (%)	$D = 0.92\%$		
MHRA	Recall ratio (%)	$R_1 = 61.69\%$	$R_2 = 60.72\%$	0.97%
	Precision ratio (%)	$P_1 = 27.89\%$	$P_2 = 27.69\%$	0.20%
	Discrepancy ratio (%)	$D = 1.18\%$		
IC	Recall ratio (%)	$R_1 = 38.19\%$	$R_2 = 36.75\%$	1.44%
	Precision ratio (%)	$P_1 = 42.15\%$	$P_2 = 46.21\%$	−4.06%
	Discrepancy ratio (%)	$D = 4.72\%$		

Curve or Mean Average Precision. In this paper, the choice of the threshold is mainly based on the mean value of the difference between the same indicator across all methods before and after data separation. If the ADR data of more years can be obtained, we can group data by increasing year by year to observe change trends of the difference value of the three indicators. It will help to determine the thresholds more accurately. This will be the further work we need to do.

Limitations

Our research has a few limitations. First, the low quality of the ADR report data and the co-existence of multiple signal detection methods may bring uncertainty to the results. Second, this study is based on the data provided by the CFDA during 2010–2011. The limited amount of data (approximately 2.2 million) may not be representative of the total data of the CFDA (approximately 10 million). Third, another limitation of the study is the use of only the ADRs extracted from drug product labeling manually. In China, there is a requirement that all ADRs observed in clinical studies should be submitted as spontaneous reports and those verified by the experts should be added to the drug product labeling. But the reference database might not include the kinds of signals which are novel and unexpected associations that appear once a drug is used by a broader group of individuals.

Conclusion

Whether TCM should be independent signal detection or not has become an important issue of pharmacovigilance in China. In order to address this problem, we propose a method based on decision tree in this study. We first analyze the results of applying four mainstream ADR signal detection methods that have been used widely in China and select three of these four methods. We set three indicators used for performance evaluation such as R, P and D based on the reference database, and then construct a decision tree for data classification. Finally, we conduct experiment on `the total sample` and `the subsample` (TCM). Experiment results show that the conclusions are all "Separation" for PRR, MHRA and IC. Thus, we suggest that TCM data should be separated from the total data when conducting analyses.

Abbreviations

ADR: Adverse drug reaction; CADN: China approved drug names; CFDA: China food and drug administration; IC: Information component; MHRA: Medicines and healthcare products regulatory agency; PRR: Proportional reporting ratio; ROR: Reporting odds ratio; TCM: Traditional Chinese medicine

Acknowledgements

Thanks to the CFDA for providing data necessary for this research.

Funding

This study was funded by National Social Science Foundation (14BTQ036).

Authors' contributions

JXW conceived of the study. JW and YXZ participated in data processing. JXW participated in data analysis, and drafting of the manuscript. JS, HMX and ML were involved in critically revising the manuscript and reviewing experiment results. All authors gave final approval of the submitted manuscript, and agreed to be accountable in all aspects for the submitted manuscript.

Competing interests

The authors declare that they have no competing interests.

Author details

[1]School of Internet of Things, Nanjing University of Posts and Telecommunications, Nanjing 210003, China. [2]School of Computer Science and Technology, School of Software, Nanjing University of Posts and Telecommunications, Nanjing 210023, China. [3]Jiangsu Center for ADR Monitoring, Nanjing 210002, China.

References

1. Edwards IR, Aronson JK. Adverse drug reactions: definitions, diagnosis, and management. Lancet. 2000;356(9237):1255–9.

2. Evans SJW, Waller PC, Davis S. Use of proportional reporting ratios (PRRs) for signal generation from spontaneous adverse drug reaction reports. Pharmacoepidemiol Drug Saf. 2001;10:483–6.
3. Wilson AM, Thabane L, Holbrook A. Application of data mining techniques in pharmacovigilance. J Clin Pharmacol. 2003;57(2):127–34.
4. Van Puijenbroek EP, Diemont WL, Grootheest K. Application of quantitative signal detection in the Dutch spontaneous reporting system for adverse drug reactions. Drug Saf. 2003;26(5):293–301.
5. Hauben M, Zhou XF. Quantitative methods in pharmacovigilance: focus on signal detection. Drug Saf. 2003;26(3):159–86.
6. Bate A. Bayesian confidence propagation neural network. Drug Saf. 2007;30(7):623–5.
7. Bate A, Lindquist M, Edwards IR, Orre R. A data mining approach for signal detection and analysis. Drug Saf. 2002;25(6):393–7.
8. Bate A, Lindquist M, Edwards IR, Olsson S, Orre R, Lansner A, De Freitas RM. A Bayesian neural network method for adverse drug reaction signal generation. Eur J Clin Pharmacol. 1998;54:315–21.
9. DuMouchel W. Bayesian data mining in large frequency tables, with an application to the FDA spontaneous reporting system. Am Stat. 1999;53:177–90.
10. Sakaeda T, Tamon A, Kadoyama K, et al. Data mining of the public version of the FDA adverse event reporting system. Int J Med Sci. 2013;10(7):796–803.
11. Li C, Xia J, Deng J, et al. A comparison of measures of disproportionality for signal detection on adverse drug reaction spontaneous reporting database of Guangdong province in China. Pharmacoepidemiol Drug Saf. 2008;17(6): 593-600.
12. Jing J, Yongfang H, Xiujuan L, Jingtian R, Shaohong J. Application of different signal detection methods in ADR self-reporting systems in China. Chinese Journal of Pharmacovigilance. 2010;3:154–5.
13. Jingtian R, Wang S, Yongfang H, Xiaoxi D, Liming L. Comparative research of common ADR signal detection methods. Chinese Journal of Pharmacovigilance. 2011;6:356–9.
14. Wu J, Lin X, Lijun J, et al. Developmental status and case study of traditional Chinese medicine ADR monitoring. Pharmaceutical Analysis. 2014;1:22–5.
15. Information on adverse drug reactions (No.44): a severe anaphylactic reaction to Shengmai injection. http://114.255.93.201/xxtb_255/ypblfyxxtb/201201/t20120111_4856.html. Accessed 6 Sep 2016.
16. Barnes J. Pharmacovigilance of herbal medicines : a UK perspective. Drug Saf. 2003;26(12):829–51.
17. Tian YJ, Jiao B, Xie JZ, et al. The programming and application of analysis system for adverse drug reactions of traditional chinese medicine. Chin J Pharmacovigilance. 2007;4(4):217-21.
18. Zhang L, Yan J, Liu X, et al. Pharmacovigilance practice and risk control of traditional Chinese medicine drugs in China: current status and future perspective. J Ethnopharmacol. 2012;140(3):519–25.
19. Bate A, Ericsson J, Farah M. International data mining for signals of herbal ADRs. Drug Saf. 2006;29(4):353.
20. Puijenbroek EPV, Bate A, Leufkens HGM, et al. A comparison of measures of disproportionality for signal detection in spontaneous reporting systems for adverse drug reactions. Pharmacoepidemiology & Drug Safety. 2002;11(1):3–10.

SNOMED CT standard ontology based on the ontology for general medical science

Shaker El-Sappagh[1,3], Francesco Franda[2], Farman Ali[3] and Kyung-Sup Kwak[3*]

Abstract

Background: Systematized Nomenclature of Medicine—Clinical Terms (SNOMED CT, hereafter abbreviated SCT) is a comprehensive medical terminology used for standardizing the storage, retrieval, and exchange of electronic health data. Some efforts have been made to capture the contents of SCT as Web Ontology Language (OWL), but these efforts have been hampered by the size and complexity of SCT.

Method: Our proposal here is to develop an upper-level ontology and to use it as the basis for defining the terms in SCT in a way that will support quality assurance of SCT, for example, by allowing consistency checks of definitions and the identification and elimination of redundancies in the SCT vocabulary. Our proposed upper-level SCT ontology (SCTO) is based on the Ontology for General Medical Science (OGMS).

Results: The SCTO is implemented in OWL 2, to support automatic inference and consistency checking. The approach will allow integration of SCT data with data annotated using Open Biomedical Ontologies (OBO) Foundry ontologies, since the use of OGMS will ensure consistency with the Basic Formal Ontology, which is the top-level ontology of the OBO Foundry. Currently, the SCTO contains 304 classes, 28 properties, 2400 axioms, and 1555 annotations. It is publicly available through the bioportal at *http://bioportal.bioontology.org/ontologies/SCTO/*.

Conclusion: The resulting ontology can enhance the semantics of clinical decision support systems and semantic interoperability among distributed electronic health records. In addition, the populated ontology can be used for the automation of mobile health applications.

Keywords: SNOMED CT, Ontology, Clinical terminology, Electronic health records, Description logic

Background

Clinical terminology is "a representational artifact containing a list of lexical entities, complete with definitions, used in some domain and formulated in a natural language" [1]. The goal of standardized clinical terminology such as Systematized Nomenclature of Medicine—Clinical Terms (SNOMED CT, hereafter abbreviated SCT) is to create a taxonomy of terms referring to entities in a given medical environment [2–8] and a framework of rules guaranteeing that each term is used with exactly one meaning; each meaning salient in the environment is expressed using exactly one term [9]. Each term in this taxonomy is in one or more parent–child relationships to some other terms in the taxonomy. For a full definition and examples of clinical terminologies, readers are guided to Ivanovic and Budimac [10]. SCT is not compliant with any formal upper-level ontology, and it allows for multiple inheritances, which causes a messy situation in the classification of entities [11]. SCT has been implemented in a variety of operational systems, including electronic health record (EHR) semantic queries, cross mapping, and clinical decision support systems (CDSSs) [2]. However, SCT is still normally distributed as pipe ("|")-separated text files [3]. These files are used to encode and retrieve medical data using text-based matching. The structure and the expressiveness of the SCT underlying formalism has not changed significantly since the mid-1990s. On the other hand, there have been significant developments in both logic-based formalisms and ontology design since then.

* Correspondence: kskwak@inha.ac.kr
[3]Department of Information and Communication Engineering, Inha University, Incheon, South Korea
Full list of author information is available at the end of the article

SNOMED CT and the ontology

An ontology can solve many challenges in the SCT structure and semantics [12]. It is a formal and explicit representation of a shared conceptualization [13]. More formally, an ontology (O) is defined as: $O = TBOX + ABOX$. In this expression, $TBOX=(C, \leq_C, R, \sigma_R, \leq_R, A, \sigma_A, T)$ is the ontology terminology, where *C*, *R*, *A*, and *T* represent disjoint sets of concepts, relations, attributes, and data types; $\leq_C$ is the taxonomy or concept hierarchy; $\leq_R$ is the relations' hierarchy; $\sigma_R : R \longrightarrow C^+$ represents the relations' signatures, which define what concepts are involved in one specific relation of the set *R*; and $\sigma_A : A \longrightarrow C \times T$ is the signature of an attribute of a certain concept, *C*, which takes values of a certain data type T. And *ABOX* is the ontology instantiation in the form $C(I_1)$, with $R(I_1, I_2)$ for I_j as the ontology instances. From this definition, the terminology can be considered a lightweight ontology with low semantics. Ivanovic and Budimac [10] defined medical terminologies and vocabularies, and compared them with ontology semantics.

he large size of SCT makes defining new terms and maintaining the existing collection a challenging task [14]. According to Zhang et al. [15], SCT data released to third parties do not have integrity constraints between relationships in the release data, in the database sense of the term. In other words, there are no optionality/mandatory constraints, and cardinality is always many-to-many, creating a completely unconstrained model; any system implementation will have to create its own integrity maintenance.

Bodenreider et al. [16] evaluated the consistency of SCT with seven ontology principles, such as subsumption and a hierarchical structure according to a description logic (DL) perspective, and their study shows that the current form of SCT has many limitations. For example, many classes have only a single child, such as {*Multiple polyps*, child: *Multiple adenomatous polyps*} (*morphologic abnormality*), whereas some other classes have an unusually large number of children, such as *Oxidoreductase (substance) (571 children)*. Children must be different from their parents. It is common to find properties or relationships specific to the parent class not being inherited by the children, as for example in the case of the parent class *Subjective visual disturbance*, which is described as having possible clinical courses of *sudden onset* or *gradual onset*; but the child *sudden visual loss* has *sudden* as its only valid *onset*. Given that each term in this taxonomy is in one or more parent–child relationships to some other terms in the taxonomy, another problem related to the hierarchical structure of SCT is multiple inheritances, which causes confusion in classification of the entities [11].

In addition, SCT exploits its taxonomy structure for classifying concepts, but it has an uncontrolled use of IS_A to signify a variety of different types of relations (such as PART_OF, IS_A_INSTANCE_OF, and so on), which results in IS_A overload and incorrect subsumption. Dentler and Cornet [17] discovered that 35,010 concepts (12%) contained redundant elements in their definitions in the July 2012 version of SCT. Other issues detected with SCT are false synonymies, failure in the use-mention distinction, and "incoherent ontological commitment" [18]. According to Bodenreider et al. [16], compliance with sound ontological principles would guarantee the accuracy of reasoning based on SCT.

SNOMED CT and the database

Many efforts have been made to enhance the SCT structure and semantics by using a database technology [15, 19]. But Campbell et al. [20] asserted that SCT databases have limitations, including reduction of data richness, limitations on the query capability, and increased systems overhead. A database converts the SCT main text-based data files (i.e. concepts, descriptions, and relationships) into three interrelated database tables based on CONCEPT_IDs [19]. As a result, the SCT knowledge base is $\Sigma = (T, A)$, where T is the schema, and A represents the instances. Structured Query Language (SQL) queries on Σ can be used to fetch specific concepts, descriptions, or relationships that are used for medical data encoding, natural language processing, and building a user interface in EHR ecosystems [21]. Regarding intelligence and inference capabilities, databases are weak in making inferences, because databases support queries only based on explicitly stated data instances, and they are based on a closed-world assumption (CWA) [22, 23]. CWA assumes that Σ contains complete data. Based on Σ, if a SQL query asking for fact C did not find it explicitly stated, then a clear result will be returned (0 or NULL). This concept is known as negation as failure (NaF) or (NOT TRUE = FALSE), or $\Sigma \nvDash C$. The resulting database models for SCT cannot be utilized to answer semantic queries, and no reasoner has been used to make inferences from databases. Some studies, such as the one by Schadow et al. [24], implemented the logical model of SCT in relational database format by transitive closure Table (TC), which represents only subsumptive relationships in the form < Ancestor, Descendant>. However, this limited table requires extensive recursive calculations. For example, the TC table for the 2014 SCT exceeds five million rows [20]. In its application programming interface (API) called Snofyre [25], National Health Services proposed an SCT object model where SCT contents are implemented as Java classes, but this object model still lacks inference capabilities.

An ontology has more advantages than a database, because it is based on a formal description logic and open-world assumption (OWA) [22, 23]. The ontology knowledge base is $\Sigma = (T, A)$, where T = TBOX, and A = ABOX. Based on the formal DL, reasoners infer hidden knowledge and add it to Σ. OWA assumes that the Σ contains incomplete knowledge, so no existing knowledge means "NOT KNOWN." For example, if Σ does not include knowledge about a patient's allergy, it is not correct to say that the patient does not suffer from an allergy (i.e. NOT TRUE = UNKNOWN). Additional information is required to confirm or refute this hypothesis. A negative answer (i.e. NaF) is returned if the query contradicts other axioms in Σ. There are many reasoners and tools in the literature to support ontology engineering and semantic reasoning [26]. As a result, thanks to formal ontology principles, converting this terminology into an ontology enhances the formal logic–based inference (e.g. subsumption and equivalence) capabilities, redundancy checking, semantic consistency checking, and the definition of formal logic–based semantics for defining concepts. Campbell et al. [20] asserted that access to the full logical model of SCT is necessary. Souvignet et al. [27] and Schulz et al. [28] asserted that although SCT was not developed using OWL DL standard language, its general structure and formalism could be converted into an ontological representation by using EL++ DL[1,2] [29].

SNOMED CT and top-level ontologies

The ontological foundations of the large clinical terminology in SCT have substantially evolved; the International Health Terminology Standards Development Organization (IHTSDO) [3] and Gao and Khazai [30] showed how SCT conforms to the OWL standards. However, there are no upper-level ontologies to describe the SCT concept model (SCM) [31], i.e. formal or semiformal systems of categories, relationships, and axioms. Héja et al. [32] and Lopez-Garcia and Schulz [33] asserted that the SCT ontology (SCTO) is error prone without alignment with highly constrained and formal upper-level ontologies, such as BFO, Descriptive Ontology for Linguistic and Cognitive Engineering (DOLCE), or BioTopLite [1, 31, 34]. Rodrigues et al. [35] asserted that to build a common ontology, you have to agree on a common model of meaning. Although SCT is published twice a year (January and July) in Release Format 2 (RF2), the 19 top-level concepts are not changed between these releases; new releases mainly try to fix redundancies, inconsistencies, errors, and shortages [6, 36]. For each new release, IHTSDO provides textual release notes and delta files to determine the atomic additions and removals of concepts and relationships [7]. However, SCT top-level concepts or categories, which are formally modeled by the SCM, are stable. The Open Biomedical Ontologies (OBO) Foundry advocates the use of an upper-level ontology [37]. Using a common upper-level ontology for building the SCTO has several advantages, such as

(1) forced categorization of domain entities into well-defined upper-level categories;
(2) standardized ways in which entities are related to each other through a well-defined canon of relations;
(3) better interoperability with other heterogeneous semantic resources and biomedical ontologies in the future; and
(4) support for coordination between the structure of the terminology and medical records, which is one of the requirements that Cimino [38] and Rector [39] mentioned.

There are many existing biomedical top-level ontologies, such as the Ontology for General Medical Science (OGMS), BioTop, BioTopLite, the Basic Formal Ontology (BFO), etc. [34, 40, 41]. OGMS extends BFO [42]. Most of the OBO Foundry ontologies are aligned with BFO, which makes BFO the best choice for building the SCT upper-level ontology [31, 41]. One of the main advantages of BFO is its *realism-based* approach, namely, the view that our thoughts, representations, beliefs, and knowledge are about reality [1]. Thus, an ontology is a *representational artifact* about the world itself and not concepts [43]. The problem arising from concept-based ontologies is that the term *concept* is often ambiguous [44]. Taking, for example, SCT itself, we know that *concept* can refer to 1) the clinical idea (for instance, the concept of kidney disease), 2) the ConceptId (a string, for example, "90,708,001"), and 3) the entity itself in the real world (the instances of kidney disease we actually find in patients' bodies) [42]. Thus, the ambiguity often neglects the use-mention distinction. Resorting to the ontologically realistic perspective of BFO, the ambiguity is resolved: the terms in ontologies refer to universals, which are not concepts or strings, but mind-independent and repeatable features of reality where existence depends on the particulars (the concrete entities) by which they are instantiated [1, 16]. So, when we talk about *kidney disease*, we are sure we are talking about something in reality (namely, all the instances in the world of the kinds of kidney disease). Thus, we avoid use-mention mistakes, and we avoid incorrect conclusions (for example, that kidney diseases are concepts instead of real things in people's bodies).

In order to build the SCT ontology, the SCT international release comes with a Perl transform script that converts the RF2 files into OWL format. This converter translates the concept hierarchy into an OWL taxonomy hierarchy by using the lightweight OWL EL description logic based on the *owl:subClassOf* property [3, 31]. To achieve balance between expressiveness of the used DL and its computation time, EL++ DL is commonly used in medical informatics [27–29] because it offers sufficient expressiveness and is computable within a reasonable time. According to the World Wide Web Consortium (W3C) guide for OWL 2, EL formalism *"is particularly suitable for applications employing ontologies that define very large numbers of classes and/or properties, captures the expressive power used by many such ontologies, and for which ontology consistency, class expression subsumption, and instance checking can be decided in polynomial time."* EL++ DL will be discussed in Section "Discussion"; for more knowledge about it, see Dentler et al. [45] and Penaloza and Sertkaya [29].

Using EL++ DL supports its reasoners (e.g. CEL[3]) to compute the subclass hierarchy of a given ontology in polynomial time; however, the resulting OWL ontology is of such a big size (> 140 MB) that it runs into memory problems when loaded into most of the popular ontology tools [46]. Many projects on BioPortal are based on SCT, such as nursing, etc. [40]. We studied all of these ontologies and discovered that none of them have object and data properties, or axioms for post-coordination expressions. They are all lightweight taxonomies based on the *116,680,003|is a|* relationship. Recently, Schulz and Martínez-Costa [31] proposed a method for harmonizing SCT with BioTopLite [34]. However, this study has a critical limitation: it implemented the SCT relationships as object properties without preserving the hierarchical relationships between them. The semantics of the resulting ontology is not suitable for creating SCT post-coordinated expressions, because OWL does not support the creation of properties for object properties. Moreover, they used different terminologies to map SCT relationships to BioTopLite object properties, such as "has condition" to model a relationship between *clinical finding* and *procedure*.

The ultimate goal of this paper is to develop the SCTO upper level to manage and enforce the logical consistency of SCT concepts, descriptions, and relationships. This ontology is not populated with the SCT concepts, but that process is straightforward and will be handled in future research. The ontology designed here allows researchers to logically check the consistency and content coverage of SCT. Moreover, the proposed ontology can be used in EHR environments to provide data entry, information retrieval, and decision support capabilities in a more intelligent way based on the logical semantics of ontologies. The proposed ontology is built based on BFO as its top-level ontology [42, 44]. The SCTO is general enough so that it can be used as an overarching ontology for other domain-specific ontologies derived from SCT. OGMS is, in turn, based on BFO 2[4] as the overarching top-level ontology [41, 42]. This binding process is critical in order to accomplish the following.

(1) Identify a standard understanding of the SCT concepts' semantic meanings. It forces the categorization of domain entities into well-defined upper-level categories connected with canonical relations. For instance, *allergy* can be a disposition or a process; *fracture* can be a damaged anatomical entity (the fractured bone) or a fracturing event. Ontology reasoners can detect inconsistencies and redundancies in the resulting ontology. This is helpful for SCT versioning, EHR coding, and terminology mapping [5, 11].
(2) Build up logically coherent hierarchies. Using unified semantics for top-level classes prevents ambiguities. In addition, BFO and OGMS support only single inheritance, which can solve many inconsistencies that currently exist in SCT [1].
(3) Solve the problem of the dynamic nature of post-coordinated concept definitions. The same complex concept can be represented with different post-coordinated concepts. Using unified OWL 2 axioms can define complex post-coordinated expressions in a unified and accurate way [3].
(4) Facilitate the creation of CDSS systems using rule formats, such as Semantic Web Rule Language (SWRL), and rule engines such as Pellet, the Java Expert System Shell (JESS), or fuzzy JESS. SCTO's TBOX and ABOX form a knowledge base. In addition, OWL 2 format supports the addition of IF-THEN rule axioms using SWRL. These rules can be utilized to build CDSSs for specific purposes based on all SCT semantics [47, 48]. In addition, semantic interoperability between distributed CDSSs and EHR systems is achieved.
(5) Facilitate integration, harmonization, interoperability, data exchange, and mapping with other ontologies, like Gene Ontology (GO), International Classification of Disease, etc., because mapping is based on intelligent semantic similarity between classes, and not just lexical matching between the terms' text [2, 5, 11, 19, 31, 49]. For a full list of supported mappings between SCT and other terminologies, readers can refer to Cardillo [50].

It is our hope that this study will provide a way for other researchers to use SCT for significant knowledge-engineering tasks. Our work is based on the 31/07/2015 release of SCT [3, 4, 30, 51].

Methods

SCT to OGMS mapping process

The mapping process is manually done for the 19 SCT top-level concepts according to the SCM [3]. First, we map each of the SCT top-level concepts to a specific class in OGMS [42]. Secondly, we use subClassOf and equivalentTo properties to build axioms to restrict the semantic meaning of each of these top-level universals. The mapping decision is made by analyzing the meaning of the candidate classes and relations, considering formal axioms as well as text definitions and hierarchical contexts of both OGMS and SCT classes. The mapping is iteratively checked by using some DL reasoners in the Protégé environment, such as Pellet. For identified inconsistent classes or axioms, we found a solution. In order to implement the SCTO, we used the Protégé 5 knowledge engineering tool,[5] together with HermiT, Pellet, and FaCT++ ontology reasoners.

Modeling pre-coordinated expressions

SCT expressions are defined as a structured combination of one or more concept identifiers used to express an instance of a clinical idea [3]. The expression consists of one or more focus concepts and optional refinements. To improve readability, SCT terms will be printed in italics rather than placed in single quotes. Clinical expressions in SCT concepts can be of two types: pre-coordinated expressions, which use a single SCT concept identifier, and post-coordinated expressions, which contain more than one SCT identifier. In pre-coordinated expressions, the clinical meaning of the expression matches the meaning of the unique listed concept, e.g. *73,211,009 |diabetes mellitus|*. Pre-coordinated concepts are identified by their defining relationships under the concept *246,061,005|attribute|*. Expressions will be represented using compositional grammar [9]. For example, diabetes mellitus is defined in SCT as follows.

Example 1

73211009 |Diabetes mellitus| <<< 126877002|disorder of glucose metabolism|, 362969004|disorder of endocrine system|, 363698007|finding site| 113331007|structure of endocrine system|.

where <<< is ⊑ and the comma represents *and*. Pre-coordinated concepts are determined in SCT concept files as either *primitive* (definitionStatusId = 900,000,000,000,074,008) concepts defined by subsumption operator⊑, or *fully defined* (definitionStatusId = 900,000,000,000,073,002) concepts defined by equivalence operator≡. Primitive concepts do not have unique relationships sufficient to distinguish them from their parents and sibling concepts. They only contain necessary relationships. In contrast, a fully defined concept has both necessary and sufficient relationships. Primitive concepts can only be used in post-coordinated expressions, whereas fully defined concepts can be used in pre-coordinated expressions. Users have to use a search engine, browser, or natural language processing to find the most suitable concept according to the concepts' fully specified names (FSNs), synonyms, and contexts.

Modeling of post-coordinated expressions

When the clinical idea is not stated on an "as is" basis in SCT, the user is able to compose already stated pre-coordinated concepts to form post-coordinated expressions [3]. SCM provides the rules that govern this process, and compositional grammar specifies the ways of this process [4, 9]. There are some main forms of post-coordination.

(1) The simplest form of a post-coordinated expression is the *combination* of multiple focus concepts. For example, *Needle biopsy of kidney* can be represented by an expression in compositional grammar.

Example 2

Needle biopsy of kidney === 7246002|Kidney biopsy|, 129249002 |Needle biopsy|.

where the comma represents the conjunction of these two concepts, and the new concept *Needle biopsy of kidney* is equivalent (===) to this conjunction; but the two concepts on the right side must come from only one top-level hierarchy, which can be inferred or managed through OWL axioms. Expressions can be written without terms [4, 9] to make normal forms that are used to measure expression equivalence and subsumption. The previous expression can be written in the following normal form (the *equivalent to* sign [===] is the default, so it can be removed):

129249002, 7246002

(2) The most common form of post-coordination is the *refinement*, which is characterized by refining the value of one or more of the defining attributes of the concept through the use of the form *<attribute name = attribute value>*, as follows [3].

- The *attribute name* is a concept that is a subtype of *246,061,005|attribute|.*
- The refinement *attribute value* is a concept or expression that is appropriate to the attribute name as specified by the SCM. In most cases, any subtype child or descendant of a concept that is permitted as an attribute value of an attribute is also permitted as an attribute value.
- Refinements may be grouped to represent interdependencies between them in the same way as super-type relationship groups.

For example, *radius fracture* can be represented as:

===125605004|Fracture of bone|: 363698007|Finding site| = 181940002|Radius|

In addition, the example in Fig. 1 describes the idea for *removal of an ovarian structure using a laser device*:

Example 3

===71388002 |procedure|: 405815000|procedure device| = 122456005 |laser device|,

260686004 |method| = 129304002 |excision - action|,

405813007 |procedure site - direct| = 15497006 |ovarian structure|

The word *and* is represented by the comma, meaning intersection or conjunction.

(3) A more complicated form of refinement is achieved by *attribute groups* (see Fig. 1). Grouping related attributes avoids ambiguities in complex expressions. There is no

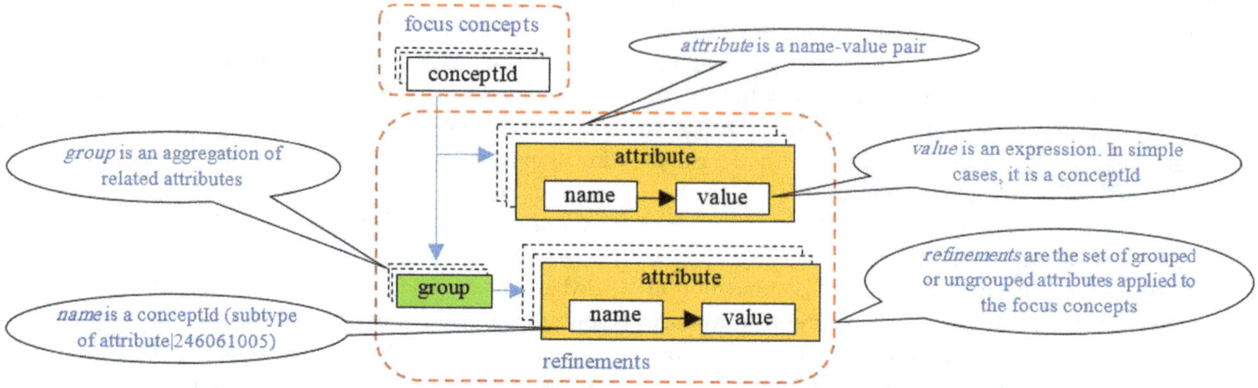

Fig. 1 Simple post-coordinated concept (expression) structure

limit on the number of groups and the number of attributes in each group. The following example describes a post-coordinated concept: *salpingo-oophorectomy, with laser excision of the right ovary and diathermy excision of the left fallopian tube.*

Example 4

As this example represents complex semantics, it will be illustrated using SCT diagramming guidelines [52], as seen in Fig. 2.

(4) Another more complicated form of refinement is modeled by *nested refinements* (see Fig. 3). Here, a complete expression can be enclosed in double parentheses and used to refine the attribute value of a refining attribute in another expression. This refinement is done by relationship group (RG). For example, the following expression describes a medication product that has a single-dose form, which is both a spray and a suspension:

Example 5

111613008|closed skull fracture with intracranial injury|===

451000119106|closed injury of head|, 371162008|closed fracture of skull,

(116676008|associated morphology|= 450695007|closed traumatic abnormality|, 363698007|finding site|= 128319008|intracranial structure|),

(116676008|associated morphology|= 20946005|fracture, closed|, 363698007|finding site|= 89546000|bone structure of cranium|)

Example 5 can be represented in a simplified way using DL syntax without identifiers, as follows:

closed skull fracture with intracranial injury ≡

closed injury of head ⊓ closed fracture of skull ⊓

∃RG (∃associated morphology.closed traumatic abnormality ⊓

∃finding site.intracranial structure) ⊓

∃RG (∃associated morphology.fracture, closed ⊓

∃finding site.bone structure of cranium)

(5) Expressions with *concrete values* have another form. In the previous expressions, attribute values are of concept types, but in current expressions, the attribute value is of primitive types, such as strings, floats, and integers. The expression shown below uses both concept values and concrete values to represent a capsule containing 500 mg of amoxicillin, where 111,115 is the identifier of an attribute.

Example 6

27658006 |amoxicillin|:

411116001 |has dose form| = 385049006 |capsule|,

{127489000 |has active ingredient| = 372687004 |amoxicillin|,

111115|has basis of strength| = (111115 |amoxicillin only|:

111115|strength magnitude| = #500, 111115|strength unit| = 258684004 |mg|)}

As with Example 5, the following is a simplified representation of Example 6 using DL syntax:

capsule containing 500 mg of amoxicillin ≡

amoxicillin ⊓

∃has dose form.capsule ⊓

∃RG (∃has active ingredient.amoxicillin ⊓

∃has basis of strength.(amoxicillin only ⊓

∃ strength magnitude.#500 ⊓

∃ strength unit.mg))

(6) The final type is the *qualification*, in which a concept is made more specific by applying to the permitted attributes some permitted values or qualifiers like episodicity, severity, and course [3]. The value of the qualifier is mainly a subconcept of *362,981,000|qualifier value|*. For example, the concept *periodic fever accompanied by chills* can be modeled as follows:

Example 7

periodic fever accompanied by chills === 274640006|fever with chills|: 246456000|episodicity| = 81591007|periodic|

Depending on the qualifiers used, the resulting concept can be a subtype of the focus concept. For example, *periodic fever accompanied by chills* is subsumed by *fever with chills*, but *known absent Asthma* is not an *Asthma*.

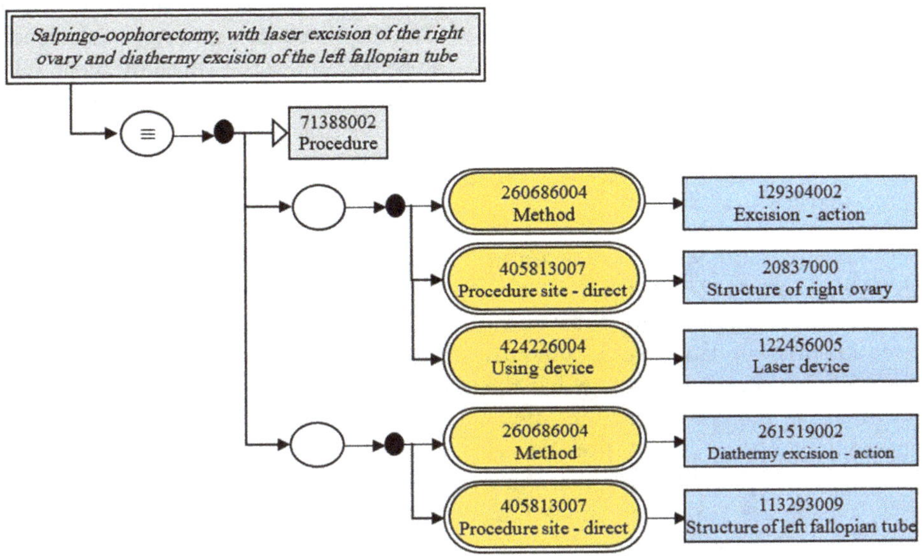

Fig. 2 Example 4 using SCT diagramming guidelines

A post-coordinated expression can be a simple expression or a complex expression. As shown in Fig. 1, a simple expression is an expression consisting of one or more conceptIds plus optional refinements. The refinements include any number of attributes, which are expressed as *name–value* pairs and may be applied either independently and/or as parts of groups [4]. The name part is a subclass of concept *246,061,005|attribute|*. It is the characteristic, which will be refined. The name part is defined based on SCM [4]. The value is a pre-coordinated conceptId.

Complex expressions are shown in Fig. 3. The main difference between complex and simple expressions is the

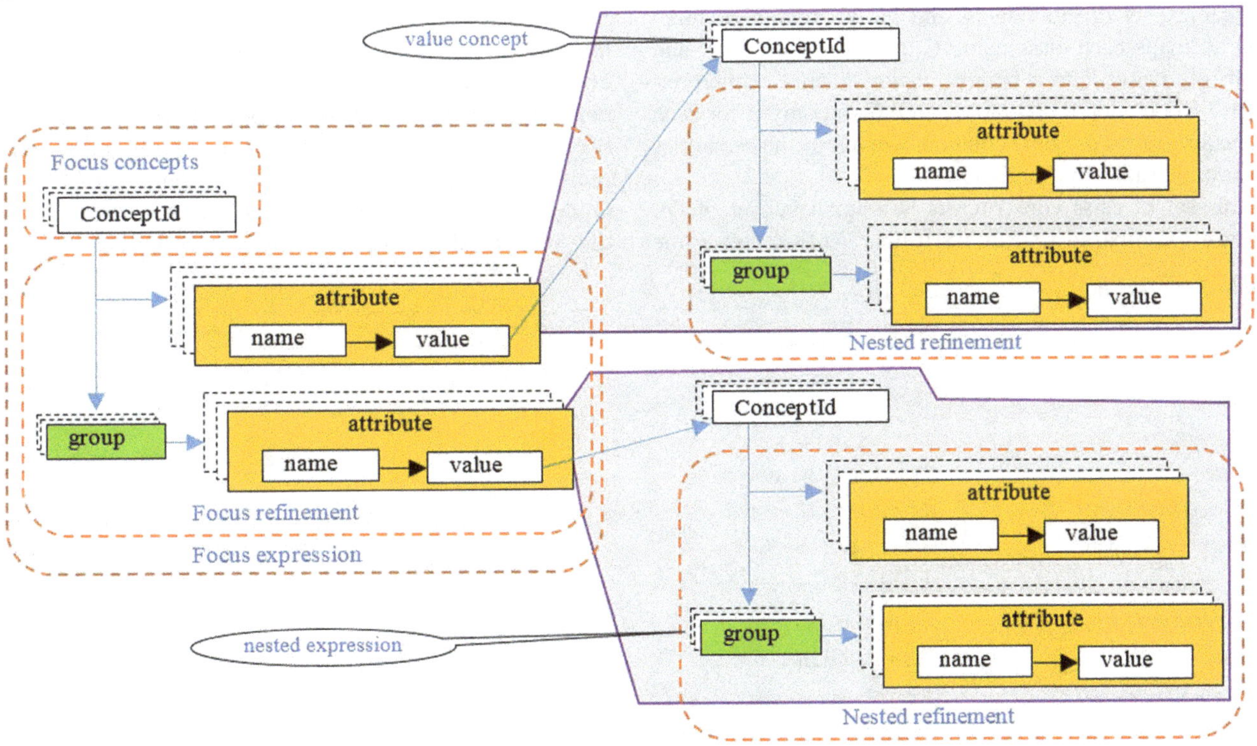

Fig. 3 Nested expressions in a complex post-coordinated concept structure

value of the name–value pair. This value can again be a nested expression, for example, *bacterial infectious disease* affecting the *left upper lobe of the lung* and caused by *Streptococcus pneumonia* is expressed as follows:

Example 8

87628006|bacterial infectious disease|:

246075003|causative agent|= 9861002|streptococcus pneumonia|,

363698007|finding site|= (45653009|structure of upper lobe of lung|,272741003|laterality|= 7771000|left|)

The resulting expressions can be stored for subsequent use in text files, extensible markup language documents, or relational databases [4]. However, an ontology has the features necessary to manage the consistency and flexibility of these expressions because it is based on formal description logic. This logic enables automatic reasoning and powerful analytic capabilities [26]. Expressions may be nested recursively, so there may be further levels of nested expressions with nested refinements.

Results

SCT description logic

In this section, we discuss the capabilities of SCT-based DL. SCT is based on a subset of EL++ formalism. EL++ is a restriction of ALC DL. The key axioms supported by EL++ DL [29] and implemented in SCT are represented in Table 1. The semantics of EL++ is defined in terms of interpretations $I=(\Delta^I, \cdot^I)$, where the domain Δ^I is a non-empty set of individuals, and the interpretation function, $\cdot^I$, maps each class name C to a subset C^I of Δ^I and each role name R to a binary relation R^I in Δ^I. Interpretation I is a model of an ontology, O, if and only if for each inclusion axiom in O the conditions given in the semantics column of Table 1 are satisfied.

This set of class constructors is a small subset of DL features, compared to ALC, SHOIN, SROIQ, etc. Some EL++ constructs are not implemented in SCT, including class disjointedness, property equivalence, transitive object properties, universal quantification (ONLY), disjunction (OR), class negation (NOT), and inverse object properties. These constructors are not supported owing to their complexity and high prerequisites in computation power and time.

SCT semantics and expressions are distributed in the form of compositional grammar [9]. To simplify the modeling of SCT expressions in DL and ontology terms, we suggest some mappings between the terminology of compositional grammar and constructs of OWL and DL (see Table 2). These mappings simplify the conversion of SCT expressions into OWL axioms.

Steps for building an SCT OWL 2 upper-level ontology

Medical terminologies have so many explicitly defined relationships between each other. In addition, there are many implicit pieces of information that can be inferred from these relationships. Modeling SCT semantics in the form of an ontology is better than using a relational data model because ontologies support consistency checking, and ontology reasoners can discover hidden knowledge [53]. An ontology has a dynamic nature, allowing new information to be added and existing information to be updated in a consistent way. The open world assumption facilitates the flexibility of SCT maintenance. The 2015 SCT version has 19 top-level concepts. To understand what each top-level concept means, we studied their children and read the SCT documentation concentrating on SCM and component structures [3, 30]. Moreover, universals or classes of BFO 2.0 and OGMS were studied to define the equivalences and subsumptions between SCT and OGMS [42]. As shown in Fig. 4, this study builds the SCTO using the following steps:

Table 1 Syntax and semantics of EL++ DL

Name	OWL syntax	Syntax	Semantics
Top	Thing	$\top$	Δ^I
Bottom	Nothing	$\bot$	$\varnothing$
Atomic class	Class	C	C^I
Primitive role	Object and data property	R	R^I
Existential quantification	ObjectSomeValuesFrom	$\exists R.\, C$	$\{x \in \Delta^I \mid \exists y \in \Delta^I : (x, y) \in R \wedge y \in C^I\}$
General class inclusion	SubClassOf	$C \sqsubseteq D$	$C^I \subseteq D^I$
Role inclusion	SubObjectPropertyOf	$R \sqsubseteq S$	$\{x, y \in \Delta^I \mid (x, y) \in R^I \rightarrow (x, y) \in S^I\}$
Class equivalence	EquivalentTo	$C \equiv D\ (C \sqsubseteq D, D \sqsubseteq C)$	$C^I = D^I$
Conjunction	ObjectIntersectionOf	$C \sqcap D$	$C^I \cap D^I$
Domain restriction	ObjectPropertyDomain	$\exists R.\ \top \sqsubseteq C$	$\{x \in \Delta^I \mid (x, y) \in R^I\} \subseteq C^I\}$
Range restriction	ObjectPropertyRange	$\top \sqsubseteq \forall R.\, C$	$\{y \in \Delta^I \mid (x, y) \in R^I\} \subseteq C^I\}$
Disjointedness	DisjointWith	$C \sqcap D \sqsubseteq \bot$	$C^I \cap D^I = \varnothing$

Table 2 Mapping between the SCT compositional grammar, ontology, and DL operators

SCT compositional grammar	OWL construct	DL construct
expression, subExpression	Axiom	Axiom
sctid = conceptReference = conceptid = term	String	String
numericalValue	Float/integer	Float/integer
Plus	objectIntersectionOf	$\sqcap$
definitionStatus (<<<, ===)	subClassOf, equivalentClasses	$\sqsubseteq, \equiv$
focusConcept	Class	C
refinement	some, objectIntersectionOf	$\exists, \sqcap$
attributeGroup	objectIntersectionOf	$\sqcap$
attributeSet	objectIntersectionOf	$\sqcap$
attributeValue	Data property, object property	Roles
expressionValue	objectIntersectionOf	$\sqcap$

(1) determine the SCT concepts that will be modeled in the ontology;
(2) determine the locations (universals) in OGMS where the SCT concepts will be modeled, either as equivalences or subsumptions;
(3) solve the problem of relationship and relationship group modeling;
(4) use the modeled relationship to add a set of axioms to refine the defined concepts in step 1; and
(5) specify how the ontology can model pre-coordination, post-coordination, and SCT constraints.

These steps are discussed in the following subsections.

Determining SCT top-level concepts

The 19 SCT concept hierarchies are organized into three main types: *object*, *value*, and *miscellaneous*. The main relationship in SCT is *116,680,003|is a|*, which organizes all concepts in a tree with one parent named *138,875,005|SNOMED CT Concept|*. Other relationships between concepts are formally managed by SCM, and they support the creation of the SCTO axioms. These relationships are represented as *object-attribute-value*. The *object* is the domain of the relationship and takes values from the hierarchies: *|clinical finding|*, *|procedure|*, *|observable entity|*, *|event|*, *|staging and scales|*, and *|specimen|*. The *value* is the range of the relationship and takes values from the hierarchies: *|body structure|*, *|organism|*, *|substance|*, *|pharmaceutical product|*, *|physical object|*, *|physical force|*, and *|environment or geographical location|*. The *attribute* is the name of the relationship and takes names from the hierarchies: *|qualifier value|*, *|record artifact|*, and *|linkage concept|*.

Organization of attributes in hierarchies enhances the semantics of the resulting ontology. For example, the attribute (property or relationship) *|associated with|* has three subtypes: *|after|*, *|due to|*, and *|causative agent|*. In addition, for each of the 19 hierarchies, SCM identifies its applicable attributes and values. For example, *|clinical finding|* is modeled with 16 attributes and 35 values [3], and any concept subsumed by *|clinical finding|* behaves in the same way. Our priority is to maintain all SCT content in the resulting ontology. However, some of the SCT top-level concepts are ambiguous, such as *Social Context*, *Situation with Explicit Context*, and *Special Concept*. These three concepts cannot be subsumed to BFO universals; therefore, they have no ontological relevance, and these concepts are not added in the SCTO. The other 16 concepts *are* modeled in the SCTO.

Determining the OGMS concepts

This step determines the mapping between SCT top-level concepts and the OGMS ontology universals [44]. Fig. 5 shows how the equivalences ($\equiv$) and subsumptions ($\sqsubseteq$) are achieved. These concepts are represented in another way in Fig. 5. The first column is the SCT concept; the second column is the OGMS classes; and the last column is the type of mapping. To preserve the logical appearance of SCT hierarchies, we prefer to add one class called *SNOMED CT Concept* $\sqsubseteq$ *entity*. All of the mapped concepts in Fig. 5 are sub-classes of *SNOMED CT Concept* as well.

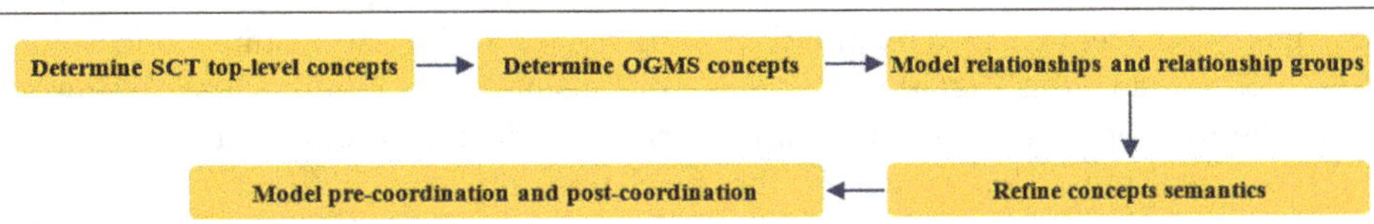

Fig. 4 SCTO development methodology

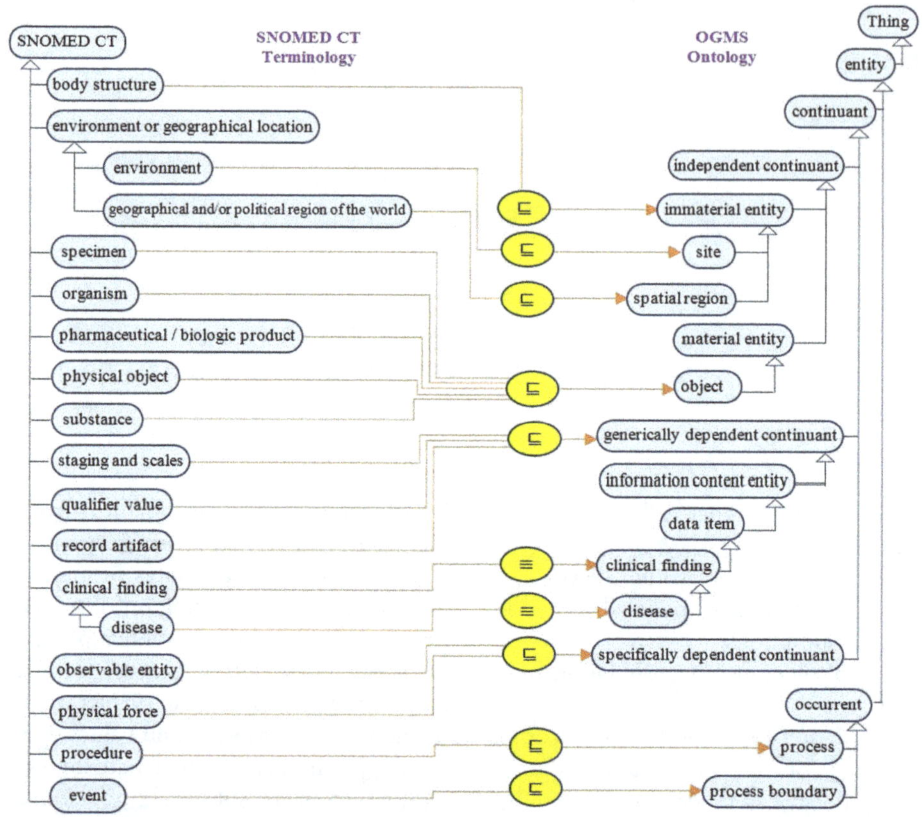

Fig. 5 Mapping of OGMS concepts to SCT concepts

The *Linkage Concept* has no medical meaning, but it is critical for modeling SCT relationships. As we will see in the next section, SCT relationships cannot be directly modeled as ontology object properties. As a result, this concept is added as a subclass of *SNOMED CT Concept* only. All concepts have a textual definition collected from SCT documentation [3]. All ontological SCT classes have identifiers with the format *SCTO_conceptId,* where *conceptId* is the SCT assigned conceptId for that concept. For example, *SCTO_123037004* is the identifier of the *body structure* concept.

Modeling SCT relationships and relationship groups

We classify SCT relationships into two main types: (1) classification relationships implemented by the *116,680,003|is a|* relationship, and (2) other attributes defined as sub-concepts of *410,662,002|concept model attribute|*. The IS_A relationship must not be implemented as an explicit IS_A object property. If source concept C1 is connected with destination concept C2 by a relationship with *typeId = 116,680,003,* then this relationship is mapped as C1⊑ C2 in the ontology. The Concept *definitionStatusId* from the concept table determines if the concept is defined by ⊑ (i.e. primitive) or by ≡ (fully defined). The IS_A relationship has a special nature: it is always ungrouped, so *relationshipGroup = 0.* Moreover, the other attributes have only one value, such as *characteristicTypeId = 900,000,000,000,011,006* and *modifierId = 900,000,000,000,451,002.* As a result, there is no need to repeat these data for all concepts. In order to implement other properties, we have two options. The first is to model SCT attributes in the *410,662,002|concept model attribute|* hierarchy directly as object properties. This option is straightforward, and facilitates the subsequent post-expression definition. However, much of the information about the relationships listed in the relationships file will be lost.

Concerning the second option, in order to preserve this information, we have two ways to put it into practise. Let us examine the first. In OWL 2,[6] properties (object or data) are binary relations, and OWL 2 and DL do not support the modeling of properties of properties (i.e. N-ary properties) [3]. There is a critical problem in modeling SCT relationships concerning how to describe the instances of relationships. Using an N-ary relationship–modeling process can solve this. For example, the relationship *56,265,001|heart disease| 363,698,007|finding site = 80,891,009|heart structure|* also has *relationshipId = 2,034,997,023, moduleId = 900,000,000,000,207,008, typeId* = *363,698,007*, *characteristicTypeId* = *900,000,000,000,011,006*, *modifierId* = *900,000,000,000,451,002*, *relationshipGroup* = *0*, and *active* = *1*.

This information must be preserved, because these attributes are important. For example, the active property helps with backward compatibility between SCT versions. We propose two ways to handle this modeling problem. One solution is to represent the relationship as a class (i.e. reification of the property) rather than a property, and create *n* new properties to represent an N-ary relation. For instance, the following example is modeled in Manchester syntax (*http://www.w3.org/TR/owl2-manchester-syntax/*) where we use the concept terms and not the conceptIds to facilitate readability (Fig. 6).

```
Class: 'heart disease'
SubClassOf:
'cardiac finding AND disorder of mediastinum AND disorder of cardiovascular system' AND
(has_finding_site ONLY 'finding site')
ObjectProperty: has_finding_site
Domain: 'clinical finding'
Range: 'finding site'
ObjectProperty: has_location
Domain: 'finding site'
Range: 'body structure'
Characteristics: Functional
class: 'finding site'
SubClassOf:
'concept model attribute' AND (has_location SOME 'heart structure') AND (has_relationshipId ONLY "2034997023") AND (has_moduleId ONLY '900000000000207008') AND (has_ typeId ONLY "363698007") AND (has_ characteristicTypeId ONLY '900000000000011006') AND (has_ modifierId ONLY '900000000000451002')
DataProperty: has_...
Domain: 'finding site'
Range: xsl:string
Characteristics: Functional
```

This way of modeling has important advantages. The relationship hierarchies are modeled in the same way as in SCT terminology, and all information distributed in SCT is preserved. However, the modeling of N-ary relationships has many limitations; see the SNOMED CT Technical Implementation Guide [3] for details.

The second way is to add a top-level concept named "SNOMED CT component" with three subclasses: *SNOMED CT Concept*, *SNOMED CT Description*, and *SNOMED CT Relationship* (see Fig. 7). The instances of *SNOMED CT Description* store the data in a description table for each concept using data properties. The instances of *SNOMED CT Relationship* will store relationship fields and connect SCT concepts. Many properties and inverse properties are not presented in Fig. 7 to simplify readability. Moreover, restrictions such as allValuesFrom, someValuesFrom, and functional are not represented. The modeling problem represented in Fig. 6 can be represented in Fig. 7 in a more formal and straightforward way.

Modeling of relationship groups A relationship group combines an *attribute–value pair* with one or more other *attribute–value pairs* (i.e. roles) to add clarity to concept definitions [3]. The purpose of relationship groups is to indicate that certain roles must go together, but their ordering is not required. The RGs add clarity to |*Clinical finding*| concepts by multiple |*Associated morphology*| and |*Finding site*| attributes, and add clarity to |*Procedure*|, which requires multiple |*Method*| and |*Procedure site*| attributes. Without relationship groups, class semantics is not correct. For example, the concept *86,299,006*|*tetralogy of Fallot*| is modeled without RGs, as shown in Fig. 8, where the five IS_A relationships are not modeled for simplification.

Tetralogy of Fallot is a disorder of the heart, which is characterized by five anatomic abnormalities, including a defect at the ventricular septum, stenosis at the pulmonary valve structure, overriding thoracic aorta, and hypertrophy at the right ventricular structure. Relationship definitions in SCT are able to relate tetralogy of Fallot to where these abnormalities are found using the "finding site" relations, and indicate what abnormality it is by using the "associated morphology." However, there is some confusion because of the many ways one can order the relationships together (see Fig. 8). RGs can solve this problem by grouping an associated morphology with its specific finding site. This process is shown in Fig. 9.

In the 2015 SCT version, there are 1,480,359 relationships defined with relationship groups (47.85%), i.e. with no *quantifiers* and IS_A relationships, and *RelationshipGroup* ≠ 0. *Finding Site* (20.97%), *Associated Morphology* (20.73%), and *Method* (20.82%) are the ones that use RGs the most.

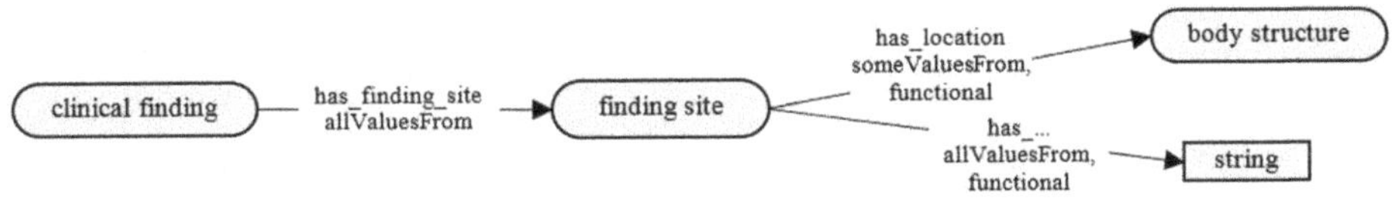

Fig. 6 Modeling of N-ary properties

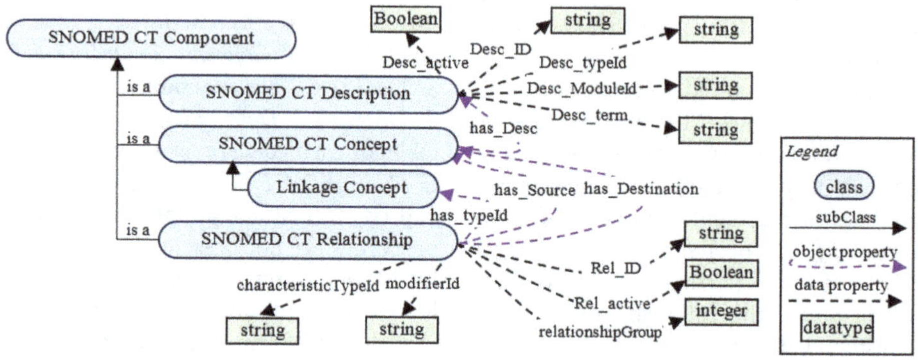

Fig. 7 Relationships and descriptions modeling

Attribute–value pairs are represented in DL using "exists-restrictions," denoted ($\exists R.\ C$), where R is the relationship's or attribute's name, and C is the expression representing the value concept. In DL, we can use braces, {}, as a symbol for role groups in order to represent the fact that two "exists-restrictions" should occur together. For example, the previously modeled concept *closed skull fracture with intracranial injury* can be normalized in DL notation as follows:

Example 9

$\equiv 451000119106 \sqcap 371162008 \sqcap$

$\{\exists 116676008.\ 450695007 \sqcap \exists 363698007.\ 128319008\} \sqcap$

$\{\exists 116676008.\ 20946005 \sqcap \exists 363698007.\ 89546000\}$

where the braces are used to model relationship groups.

Many reasoners support inference rules: for instance, Pellet supports OWL 2 profiles, including OWL EL [26]. In the SCTO, the authors added an SWRL rule to bind relationships that have the same relationshipGroup number, as follows:

Relationship_relationshipGroup(?r1, ?n1), Relationship_relationshipGroup(?r2, ?n2), equal(?n1, ?n2) -> Grouped_Relations(?r1, ?r2)

Many reasoners like Hermit and Pellet support rule reasoning [26]. The SCTO facilitates the creation of ontology groups. For example, the previous concept in Example 9 can be modeled in the SCTO as follows (see Fig. 7):

`Class:` *'closed skull fracture with intracranial injury'*

`EquivalentTo:` *'closed injury of head'* **and** *'closed fracture of skull'* **and**

{(`IsSourceOf some` (((`Relationship_destinationId some` *'intracranial structure'*) `and` (`Relationship_typeId some` *'finding site'*)) `and` `Grouped_Relations exactly 1` ((`Relationship_destinationId some` *'closed traumatic abnormality'*) `and` (`Relationship_typeId some` *'associated morphology'*))))

} **and**

{(`IsSourceOf some` (((`Relationship_destinationId some` *'bone structure of cranium'*) `and`

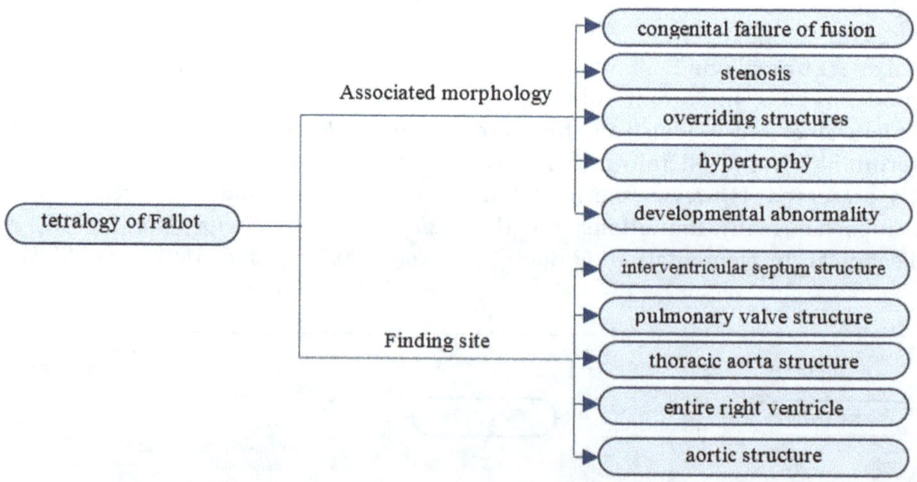

Fig. 8 Modeling tetralogy of Fallot without relationship groups

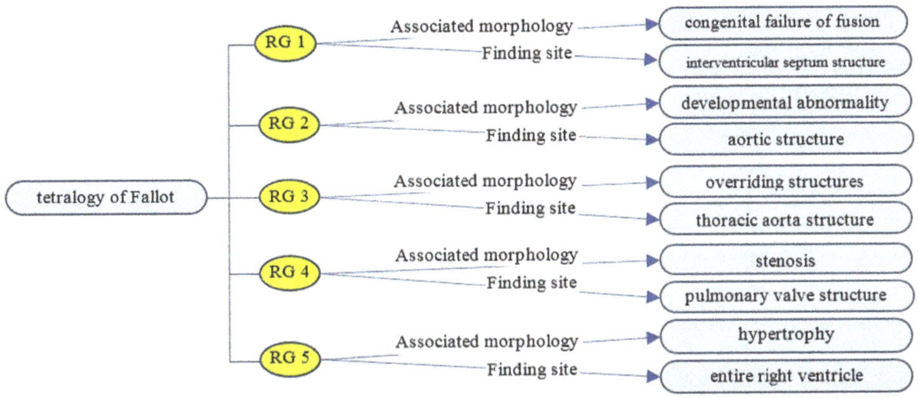

Fig. 9 Modeling tetralogy of Fallot with relationship groups

(`Relationship_typeId some` *'finding site'*)) `and Grouped_Relations exactly 1` ((`Relationship_destinationId some` *'fracture, closed'*) `and` (`Relationship_typeId some` *'associated morphology'*))))

One problem to solve with role grouping is the redundancy of expressions. Many authors proposed rules to eliminate redundancy [54]. The redundancy prevention axioms include (1) repeating ungrouped exists-restrictions ($\exists$**R.C** ⊓ {$\exists$**R.C** ⊓ $\exists$ S. D} = {$\exists$**R.C** ⊓ $\exists$ S. D}), (2) repeating a group with more general classes ({$\exists$**R.C$_1$** ⊓ $\exists$ S. D} ⊓ {$\exists$**R.C$_2$** ⊓ $\exists$ S. D} = {$\exists$**R.C$_2$** ⊓ $\exists$ S. D} when **C$_1$ ⊒ C$_2$**), and (3) repeating an exists-restriction with more general classes in the same group ({$\exists$**R.C$_1$** ⊓ $\exists$ **R.C$_2$** ⊓ $\exists$ S. D} = {$\exists$**R.C$_2$** ⊓ $\exists$ S. D} when **C$_1$ ⊒ C$_2$**), where *R, S* are relationships (i.e. object properties) and **C$_i$** represents a concept expression. All these axioms can be modeled in the SCTO in a straightforward way.

Refinement of concept semantics

One of the most important reasons for implementing SCT as an ontology is the ability to restrict semantics of concepts and relationships. In this section, we provide some examples from the added semantics for the SCTO. First, we assert that a class cannot be a subclass of more than one top-level hierarchy by the following axiom:

`DisjointClasses:` *'pharmaceutical / biologic product' 'physical force' 'linkage concept' 'environment or geographical location' 'qualifier value' 'observable entity' 'record artifact' procedure, event specimen substance 'staging and scales' 'physical object' 'clinical finding' organism*

Secondly, we try to convert the SCM semantics into axioms. The SCT documentation lists rules for permissible defining attributes for individual hierarchies and the permissible domains for each attribute, but these rules are not computable. Using the SCTO, these rules can be mapped to active axioms and SWRL rules. As a result, the ontology can preserve the consistency of SCT and facilitate its maintenance process. These axioms also support the checking of attribute ranges. Due to space restrictions, we give one example here, and the SCTO on BioPortal at *https://bioportal.bioontology.org/ontologies/SCTO* implements all of these axioms. The clinical finding class is defined in the SCM shown in Fig. 10. The semantics required by the model in Fig. 9 to implement the clinical finding term in Fig. 10 can be implemented as 15 disjunction (*or*) connected OWL axioms (`axiom`$_1$ `or ... or axiom`$_{15}$), one for each branch of Fig. 10. The axiom for the *finding site* of Fig. 10 can be represented as.

`axiom`$_1$ ≡ `(IsSourceOf some ((Relationship_destinationId some (`*`'acquired body structure'`* `or` *`'anatomical structure'`*`)) and (Relationship_typeId some` *`'finding site'`*`)))`

All of the other classes are handled in similar ways in the OWL ontology of the SCTO.

Modeling of pre-coordination and post-coordination

As discussed before, concept expressions in SCT can be:

- concept name ***C*** as primitive concept (*C* *C$_i$*) or defined concept (*C* ≡ *C$_i$*);
- conjunctions of concept names: C_1 C_2... C_n;
- conjunction of concept names with exists-restrictions and grouped exists-restrictions: C_1 C_2... C_n *R. C*... { *R. C* ...} ...

These types can easily be built by using SCTO classes, object properties, and data properties. The first two types are direct subsumptions, equivalences, and conjunctions of already existing classes, as shown before in Example 2. The third type is the most complex, so we are going to give an example.

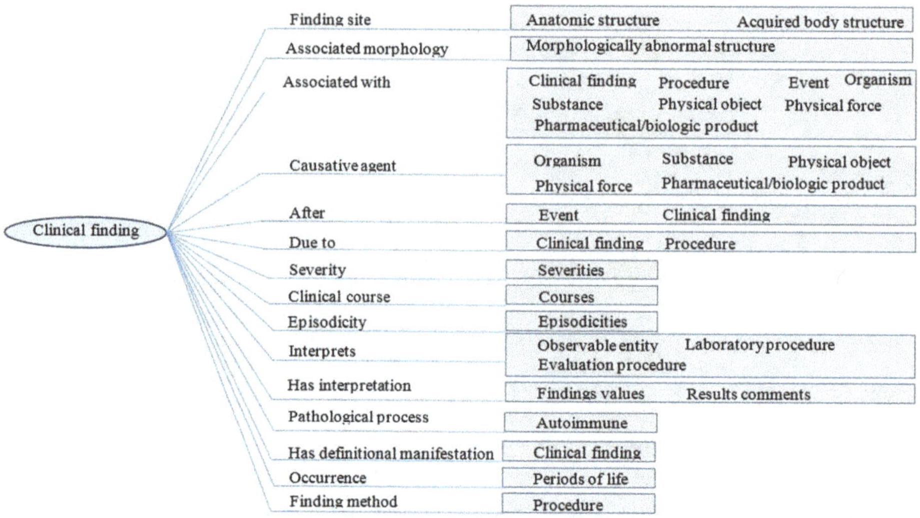

Fig. 10 SCT concept model for the clinical finding concept. Adapted from the SCT concept model [3]

Example 5 is similar to the previously modeled Example 9. Example 1 can be modeled as follows:

Class: *'Diabetes mellitus'*

SubClassOf: *'disorder of glucose metabolism'* **and** *'disorder of endocrine system'* **and**

(IsSourceOf some ((Relationship_destinationId some *'structure of endocrine system'*) and (Relationship_typeId some *'finding site'*)).

Examples 3, 4, and 7 are modeled in a similar way. Let us model the most complex one (Example 4) as follows:

Class: *'salpingo-oophorectomy, with laser excision of the right ovary and diathermy excision of the left fallopian tube'*

SubClassOf:

{

'procedure' and (IsSourceOf some ((((Relationship_destinationId some *'excision - action'*) and (Relationship_typeId some *'method'*)) and Grouped_Relations exactly 1 ((Relationship_destinationId some *'structure of right ovary'*) and (Relationship_typeId some *'procedure site - direct'*))) and Grouped_Relations exactly 1 ((Relationship_destinationId some *'laser device'*) and (Relationship_typeId some *'using device'*)))

} ***and***

{

'procedure' and (IsSourceOf some (((Relationship_destinationId some *'diathermy excision - action'*) and (Relationship_typeId some *'method'*)) and Grouped_Relations exactly 1 ((Relationship_destinationId some *'structure of left fallopian tube'*) and (Relationship_typeId some *'procedure site - direct'*))))

}

In this example, we repeated the class *Procedure* in both axioms to refine the selected concepts to be of the procedure type. Moreover, in the first group of this post-coordinated expression, we link three relationships with one relationship group. Due to space restrictions, we will not model the other examples, but they can be modeled in the same way.

The resulting SCTO

The overall result is a regular, standard, and uniform ontology more consistent than the SCT original ontology. The ontology is created with an OWL 2 format, which makes it easier to use, query, and ensure quality as the basis for the software. We focused on creating the SCTO's TBOX. Moreover, we designed the top-level classes only based on the BFO and OGMS ontologies. There are 14 subsumption mappings (82.35%), two equivalence mappings (11.77%), and concepts with no equivalence (5.88%). All of the 19 SCT hierarchies have been modeled in the SCTO under suitable BFO and OGMS universals, except three concepts: (1) *243796009|situation with explicit context*, which can be modeled with other existing classes; (2) *48176007|social context*, which has ambiguous semantics and cannot be mapped to any universal; and (3) *370115009|Special Concept*, which had not appeared in the SCM. The resulting ontology has no instances (i.e. ABOX) because the instantiation takes place for each individual's medical record. Actually, TBOX alone equals an ontology, but TBOX + ABOX is a knowledge base. Knowledge bases are used in specific systems for specific purposes, but they are outside the scope of this paper. The SCTO contains only the SCT top-level concepts, and focuses on modeling the semantics of these concepts in the form of

OWL2 axioms. Fig. 5 depicts the upper-level hierarchy of the SCTO based on OGMS at the topmost level.

The creation of all the SCT hierarchies can be automated by using the existing OWL API and reasoners such as Pellet, RacerPro, Hermit, etc. The SCTO implements the SCT formal and standard concept model and solves the modeling problems of pre-coordinated and post-coordinated concepts. OWL ontologies support the creation of more complex expressions built recursively from previously defined classes and properties using constructors provided by the ontology's language and logic. We used Protégé 5 to implement the SCTO.

Table 3 lists SCTO object properties, and their definitions, domains, and ranges. There are only eight object properties in the SCTO. By using only these properties, we have the ability to model SCT expressions, relationship groups, and constraints, as shown previously. The SCTO contains 20 data properties. Table 4 shows some examples from these properties.

Building a top-ontology–based SCTO has many benefits for new medical informatics. The resulting ontology is based on OGMS, which in turn uses BFO as its top-level ontology, a feature providing the unified and global semantics of SCT concepts. This way, SCT can be integrated with other ontologies, such as Logical Observation Identifiers Names and Codes (LOINC) and GO, etc. [40, 55], in a unique, logically, and medically consistent and applicable way. The SCTO can be integrated into the EHR healthcare environment with the Health Level 7 Reference Information Model to support semantic interoperability. Semantic queries using Simple Protocol and RDF (Resource Description Framework) Query Language (SPARQL) and Semantic Query-Enhanced Web Rule Language (SQWRL) can use reasoner inference capabilities to retrieve hidden information besides explicit information. The ontology can be used in clinical decision support systems as a means to determine levels of similarities and relationships between compared concepts. The SCTO is freely available on BioPortal, a web portal that provides a uniform mechanism to access biomedical ontologies and terminologies provided in different representation formats, including OBO and OWL. The following URL provides direct access to the SCTO on BioPortal: *https://bioportal.bioontology.org/ontologies/SCTO*, where it can be browsed, searched and visualized.

The SCTO is considered a first step towards a complete SCT OWL ontology. Table 5 provides a summary of the SCTO in terms of several statistical and quality-control metrics. The ontology currently incorporates 304 classes, 2400 axioms, 8 object properties, 20 data properties, and 1555 annotations. Each concept has a unique identifier with the format *SCTO_ConceptId*, such as *SCTO_90,708,001* for the *kidney disease* class. Each class and property has a standard definition from SCT documentation.

Consistency checking is syntactic-level evaluation. In order to confirm that the SCTO is consist and error-free, HermiT (version 1.3.8), Pellet, and FaCT++ reasoners were used with the Protégé 5 editor, and they revealed no discrepancies in the ontology. Moreover, the online tool Ontology Pitfall Scanner! (OOPS![7]) helped to detect some of the most common pitfalls appearing when developing ontologies. We ran OOPS! on the SCTO to ensure it is free of these pitfalls.

Table 3 Object properties of the SCTO

Property	Definition	Domain	Range
Has_description	Determines a description for a class.	SNOMED CT Concept	SNOMED CT Description
IsDescriptionOf	Is the inverse of Has_description.	SNOMED CT Description	SNOMED CT Concept
Relationship_destinationId	Identifies the class that is the destination of the relationship. Set to an identifier of a concept in the Concept file.	SNOMED CT Relationship	SNOMED CT Concept
Relationship_sourceId	Identifies the source concept of the relationship. Set to an identifier of a concept in the Concept file.	SNOMED CT Relationship	SNOMED CT Concept
Relationship_typeId	A concept enumeration value from the metadata hierarchy that identifies the semantic type of the relationship. It is a subtype of 410,662,002 |Concept model attribute|.	SNOMED CT Relationship	Linkage Concept
IsSourceOf	Determines the source of a relationship. It is the inverse of Relationship_sourceId.	SNOMED CT Concept	SNOMED CT Relationship
IsDestinationOf	Determines the destination of a relationship. It is the inverse of Relationship_destinationId.	SNOMED CT Concept	SNOMED CT Relationship
Grouped_Relations	Used to explicitly determine the grouped relationships	SNOMED CT Relationship	SNOMED CT Relationship
Total number of object properties			8

Table 4 Data properties of the SCTO

Property	Definition	Domain	Range
Concept_Id	The unique SNOMED CT Identifier for this Concept.	SNOMED CT Concept	String
Description_term	The description's text value, represented in UTF-8 encoding.	SNOMED CT Description	String
Description_typeId	Identifies whether the description is an FSN, synonym, or other description type.	SNOMED CT Description	String
Relationship_relationshipGroup	Groups together relationship versions that are part of a logically associated relationship group.	SNOMED CT Relationship	Integer
Relationship_active	Specifies whether the relationship's state is active or inactive.	SNOMED CT Relationship	Boolean
Relationship_characteristicTypeId	A concept enumeration value that identifies the characteristic type of the relationship.	SNOMED CT Relationship	String
...			
Total number of data properties			**20**

Discussion

We used SCT terminology to build some medical applications, and we experienced its current limitations discussed previously. We used SCT to build DDO [56], which is a diabetes diagnosis ontology, and DMTO [57], which is a diabetes mellitus treatment ontology. The resulting ontology enhances the semantics of SCT. Generally, there are some studies, which tried to enhance the semantics of SCT [31]. However, very few studies have unified its high-level concepts under suitable universals of top-level ontologies, and no studies have implemented the SCT concept model in OWL axioms using these top-level ontologies. Table 6 provides a comparison between these studies according to a set of metrics. In 2015, Souvignet and Rodrigues [58] followed a similar methodology to create a patient safety ontology by mapping the Patient Safety Categorical Structure data model to BFO 2. Héja et al. [32] mapped SCT to the DOLCE upper-level ontology, and they highlighted some ontological errors in SCT. However, they failed to propose an acceptable SCT ontology. As can be seen in Table 6, the SCTO is the most complete ontology, and combines the advantages of all the other studies.

Table 5 SCTO metrics

Metric	Value
Number of classes	304
Axioms	2400
Object properties	8
Data properties	20
Maximum number of parents	3
Average number of siblings	3.62
Maximum number of children	66
Average number of children	3
Classes with more than 25 children	1
Classes with a single child	25
Maximum number of siblings	66
Subclass axioms	330
Annotations	1555
Maximum depth	8

The immediate application of the resulting ontology is support for shared and unified understanding of SCT concepts and top-level universals. The defined classes have formal definitions based on DL, and they implement the SCM. SCTO supports the construction of distributed EHR systems and clinical decision support systems. It can be utilized in machine learning and natural language processing studies to understand the semantic meaning of medical concepts. This ontology can support information-retrieval applications by providing a vocabulary and a taxonomy that can be used for query expansion as well as semantic searches. As a result, the ontology supports the creation of semantically intelligent clinical decision–support applications. This version of the SCTO ontology has some limitations. It formally models the top-level classes of SCT hierarchy. After populating SCTO ontology with the other classes, relationships, and descriptions, the resulting ontology is expected to be more accurate, smaller in size, and interoperable with other ontologies. The resulting ontology needs to be tested in some real applications to measure its efficiency in the representation of complex semantics. These limitations will be covered in the future studies.

Conclusions

In this paper, we introduced the SCTO, which is based on the globally approved OGMS, which is in turn based on the BFO 2.0 top-level ontology. The 2015 SCT version's SCM was implemented in the form of OWL 2 axioms. The authors resorted to EL++ DL, which is

Table 6 A comparison between the SCTO and existing SCT studies

The study	Format	The base	Top-level ontology	Description logic	Modeled hierarchies	Publicly available	Size	Can model pre-coordinated concepts	Can model post-coordinated concepts	Handled semantics
Proposed SCTO	Ontology	SCM	BFO and OGMS	EL++	Whole SCT	OWL format	Top-level concepts	Yes	Yes	Complete OWL axioms for all top-level SCT concepts
SCT Perl script [3]	Ontology	No	No	EL++	Whole SCT	Perl script	Low-level concepts	Yes	No	SCT taxonomy
Schulz & Martínez-Costa [31]	Ontology	No	BioTopLite2	OWL DL	Whole SCT	No	Top-level concepts	Yes	No	SCT taxonomy and basic relations
Campbell et al. [20]	Graph database	No	No	No	Whole SCT	No	Low-level concepts	Yes	No	SCT taxonomy
Martínez-Costa and Schulz [59]	Ontology	SCT context model	BioTopLite	OWLDL	Clinical findings	No	Low-level concepts	Yes	Yes	SCT taxonomy and basic relations
Cheetham et al. [60]	Ontology	No	BioTopLite2	OWLDL	Disorders	No	Low-level concepts	Yes	Yes	SCT taxonomy and basic relations
Bodenreider [61]	Ontology	No	No	OWL EL	Disorders, procedures	No	Low-level concepts	Yes	No	SCT taxonomy
Hogan [62]	Ontology	No	BFO	OWL EL	Whole SCT	No	Top-level concepts	No	No	SCT taxonomy
Ochs et al. [63]	Abstraction network	No	No	No	Observable entity	No	Low-level concepts	Yes	No	SCT taxonomy

supported by SCT. The paper's main aim is to preserve all information released in SCT files, including concepts, descriptions, and relationships. All possible SCT expressions, including pre-coordinated and post-coordinated expressions, can be implemented using SCTO terminology (classes, object properties, and data properties). The SCTO contains 304 universals (classes and subclasses), 28 properties, 1555 annotations, and 2400 axioms. It is publicly available through BioPortal at *http://bioportal.bioontology.org/ontologies/SCTO/*. The resulting ontology can be used to integrate SCT with other terminologies, such as GO, LOINC, and RxNorm, because its concepts have unified semantics under OGMS ontology universals [40, 55].

In the future, we will use OWL 2 APIs to populate the SCTO with all of the SCT concepts, descriptions, and relationship instances. The SCT population has some tricky logical issues, such as whether or not the SCT terminology concept will be mapped to SCT ontology classes or individuals, and whether or not all classes should have at least one sibling, etc. Moreover, before population, the confusion between pathological structure, disposition, and process needs to be resolved, especially in the *clinical finding, procedure, event,* and *body structure* hierarchies: these issues will be identified and modeled. After population, ontology consistency checking will be performed, and the SCTO will be used for semantic queries taken from real healthcare environments. Moreover, we will solve the problem of situations that have an explicit context. The resulting ontology can be merged with other ontologies in specific domains, such as GO and LOINC [55]. As a result, SCT coverage will be enhanced.

Endnotes

[1]*https://www.w3.org/TR/owl2-primer/*

[2]*https://www.w3.org/2007/OWL/wiki/EL*

[3]*https://tu-dresden.de/ing/informatik/thi/lat/forschung/software/cel*

[4]*http://ifomis.uni-saarland.de/bfo/*

[5]*http://protege.stanford.edu/*

[6]*https://www.w3.org/TR/owl2-overview/*

[7]*http://oops.linkeddata.es/*

Abbreviations

DL: Description logic; EHR: Electronic health record; GO: Gene ontology; LOINC: Logical observation identifiers names and codes; OBO: Open biomedical ontologies; OGMS: Ontology for general medical science; OWL: Web ontology language; RDF: Resource description framework; SCT: SNOMED CT; SNOMED CT: Systematized nomenclature of medicine—clinical terms

Acknowledgements

This work was supported by a National Research Foundation of Korea grant funded by the Korean Government's Ministry of Science and ICT (NRF-2017R1A2B2012337).

The authors would like to thank Professor Barry Smith for his helpful comments and suggestions on the building of SCTO.

Funding

This work was supported by a National Research Foundation of Korea grant funded by the Korean Government's Ministry of Science and ICT (NRF-2017R1A2B2012337).

Authors' contributions

All authors participated equally in the SCTO design and implementation processes. They participated equally in drafting the article, revising it critically for important intellectual content, and proofreading the English. The final version to be submitted has been approved by all the authors. Author FF was responsible for the study of BFO and OGMS top-level ontologies and the definition of SCTO upper-level classes suitable for SCT main (upper level) concepts. Author SES studied the SCT documentation and technical specifications. He identified the main SCT concepts that needed to be mapped to BFO and OGMS universals, and defined the unified semantics of these concepts. Author FA and Author KSK wrote the semantics of the SCTO in OWL 2 format using the Protégé tool. All the authors participated equally in checking the ontology for consistency and completeness. Author SES uploaded the ontology to BioPortal. All authors read and approved the final manuscript.

Competing interests

The authors declare that they have no competing interests.

Author details

[1]Information Systems Department, Faculty of Computers and Informatics, Benha University, Banha, Egypt. [2]Department of Philosophy, University at Buffalo, Buffalo, NY, USA. [3]Department of Information and Communication Engineering, Inha University, Incheon, South Korea.

References

1. Arp A, Smith B, Spear A, Building ontologies with basic formal ontology, the MIT press, 2015.
2. Lee D, Cornet R, Lau F, De Keizer N. A survey of SNOMED CT implementations. J Biomed Inform. 2013;46(1):87–96.
3. IHTSDO (International Health Terminology Standards Development Organization), SNOMED CT Technical Implementation Guide. https://confluence.ihtsdotools.org/display/DOCANLYT/Data+Analytics+with+SNOMED+CT. Last seen 1 June 2017.
4. Bhattacharyya S. Introduction to SNOMED CT. Singapore: Springer Science. 2016.
5. Saitwal H, Qing D, Jones S, Bernstam E, Chute C, Johnson T. Cross-terminology mapping challenges: a demonstration using medication terminological systems. J Biomed Inform. 2012;45:613–25.
6. SNOMED CT Document Library, SNOMED international, Data Analytics with SNOMED CT, https://confluence.ihtsdotools.org/display/DOCANLYT/Data+Analytics+with+SNOMED+CT, Last seen 08 May 2017.
7. Ochs C, Case J, Perl Y. Analyzing structural changes in SNOMED CT's bacterial infectious diseases using a visual semantic delta. J Biomed Inform. 2017;67:101–16.
8. Perez-Rey D, Alonso-Calvo R, Paraiso-Medina S, Munteanu C, Garcia-Remesal M. SNOMED2HL7: a tool to normalize and bind SNOMED CT concepts to the HL7 reference information model. Comput Methods Prog Biomed. 2017; 149:1–9.
9. IHTSDO (International Health Terminology Standards Development Organization), SNOMED CT Compositional Grammar Specification and Guide. https://confluence.ihtsdotools.org/display/DOCSCG/Compositional+Grammar+-+Specification+and+Guide. Last seen 1 June 2017.
10. Ivanovic M, Budimac Z. An overview of ontologies and data resources in medical domains. Expert Syst Appl. 2014;41:5158–66.
11. Yamagata Y, Kozaki K, Imai T, Ohe K, Mizoguchi R. An ontological modeling approach for abnormal states and its application in the medical domain. Journal of Biomedical Semantics. 2014;5:23.
12. Isern D, Sanchez D, Antonio MA. Ontology-driven execution of clinical guidelines. Comput Methods Prog Biomed. 2012;107:122–39.
13. Gruber T. A translation approach to portable ontologies. Knowl Acquis. 1995;5(2):199–220.
14. Dentler K, Cornet R. Redundant elements in SNOMED CT concept definitions. AIME, Springer-Verlag Berlin Heidelberg. 2013:186–95.
15. Zhang M, Patrick J, Truran D, Innes K. Deriving a SNOMED CT data model. In Proceedings of the First Semantic Mining Conference on SNOMED CT. 2006:59–63.
16. Bodenreider O, Smith B, Kumar A, Burgun A. Investigating subsumption in SNOMED CT: an exploration into large description logic-based biomedical terminologies. Artif. Intell. Med. 2007;39(3):183–195.
17. Dentler K, Cornet R. Intra-axiom redundancies in SNOMED CT. Artif Intell Med. 2015;65:29–34.
18. Ceusters W. SNOMED CT's RF2: is the future bright? Stud Health Technol Inform. 2011;169:829–33. https://www.ncbi.nlm.nih.gov/pmc/articles/PMC3379709/
19. Oluoch T, de Keizer N, Langat P, Alaska I, Ochieng K, Okeyo N, Kwaro D, Cornet R. A structured approach to recording AIDS-defining illnesses in Kenya: a SNOMED CT based solution. J Biomed Inform. 2015;56:387–94.
20. Campbell W, Pedersen J, McClay J, Rao P, Bastola D, Campbell J. An alternative database approach for management of SNOMED CT and improved patient data queries. J Biomed Inform. 2015;57:350–7.
21. Bakhshi-Raiez F, de Keizer N, Cornet R, Dorrepaal M, Dongelmans D, Jaspers M. A usability evaluation of a SNOMED CT based compositional interface terminology for intensive care. Int J Med Inform. 2012;81:351–62.
22. Sir M, Bradac Z, Zdenek P. Ontology versus Database. IFAC. 2015;48(4):220–5.
23. Biskup J, Bring M, Bulinski M. Inference control of open relational queries under closed-world semantics based on theorem proving. Inf Syst. 2017;70:32–47.
24. Schadow G, Barnes M, McDonald C. Representing and querying conceptual graphs with relational database management systems is possible. in: Proc AMIA Symp. 2001:598–602.
25. National Health Services Snofyre, https://code.google.com/archive/p/snofyre/, Last seen 1 May 2017.
26. Dentler K, Cornet R, ten Teije A, de Keizer N. Comparison of Reasoners for large ontologies in the OWL 2 EL profile. Semantic Web Journal. 2011;2(2):71–87.
27. Souvignet J, Declerck G, Asfari H, Jaulent M, Bousquet C. OntoADR a semantic resource describing adverse drug reactions to support searching, coding, and information retrieval. J Biomed Inform. 2016;63:100–7.
28. Schulz S, Cornet R, Spackman K. Consolidating SNOMED CT's ontological commitment. Appl Ontol. 2011;6(1):1–11.
29. Penaloza R, Sertkaya B. Understanding the complexity of axiom pinpointing in lightweight description logics. Artif Intell. 2017;250:80–104.
30. Gao Y, Khazai R. SNOMED CT Concept Model: IHTSDO – International Health Terminology Standards Development Organization; 2015.
31. Schulz S, Martínez-Costa C. Harmonizing SNOMED CT with BioTopLite: An Exercise in Principled Ontology Alignment. MEDINFO 2015: eHealth-enabled Health, IMIA and IOS Press. 2015;216:-832.
32. Héja G, Surján G, Varga P. Ontological analysis of SNOMED CT. BMC Med Inform Decis Mak. 2008;8(Suppl 1):S8.
33. Lopez-Garcia P, Schulz S. Can SNOMED CT be squeezed without losing its shape? Journal of Biomedical Semantics. 2016;7:56.
34. Schulz S, Boeker M. BioTopLite: an upper level ontology for the life sciences evolution. Design and Application In GI-Jahrestagung. 2013:1889–99.
35. Rodrigues J, et al. ICD-11 and SNOMED CT common ontology: circulatory system. MIE. 2014:1043–7.
36. Chen C, Chang C, Peng Y, Poon S, Huang S, Li Y. Effect of implementation of a coded problem list entry subsystem. Comput Methods Programs Biomed. 2016;134:1–9.
37. Smith B, et al. The OBO foundry: coordinated evolution of ontologies to support biomedical data integration. Nat Biotechnol. 2007;25(11):1251–5.
38. Cimino J. Desiderata for controlled medical vocabularies in the twenty-first century. Methods Inf Med. 1998;37(4–5):394.
39. Rector A. Clinical terminology: why is it so hard? Methods Inf Med. 1999; 38(4/5):239–52.
40. BioPortal, http://bioportal.bioontology.org/, Last seen 15 May 2017.
41. BFO (Basic Formal Ontology), http://ifomis.uni-saarland.de/bfo/, Last seen 26 May 2017.
42. Ceusters W, Smith B. Biomarkers in the Ontology for General Medical Science. European Federation for Medical Informatics (EFMI). 2015;210:155–9.
43. Smith B, Aboutness C. Towards Foundations for the Information Artifact Ontology. In: Proceedings of the Sixth International Conference on Biomedical Ontology, July 27–30, 2015. Lisboa, Portugal; 2015. Available at http://ceur-ws.org/Vol-1515/regular10.pdf.
44. Scheuermann R, Ceusters W, Smith B. Toward an ontological treatment of disease and diagnosis. Summit Transl Bioinform. 2009;2009:116–20.
45. Dentler K, Cornet R, Teije A, de Keizer N. Comparison of Reasoners for large ontologies in the OWL 2 EL profile. IOS Press Semantic Web. 2011;1:1–5.

46. El-Sappagh S, El-Masri S, Elmogy M, Riad A. A diabetes diagnostic domain ontology for CBR system from the conceptual model of SNOMED CT. IEEE International Conference on Engineering and Technology (ICET). 2014:1–7.
47. Hussain M, et al. Cloud-based smart CDSS for chronic diseases. Health Technol. 2013;3:153–75.
48. Peleg M, et al. MobiGuide: a personalized and patient-centric decision-support system and its evaluation in the atrial fibrillation and gestational diabetes domains. User Model User-Adap Inter. 2017;27:159–213.
49. Rodrigues J, Schulz S, Rector A, Spackman K, Üstün T, Chute C, Mea V, Millar J, Persson K. Sharing ontology between ICD 11 and SNOMED CT will enable seamless re-use and semantic interoperability. Stud Health Technol Inform. 2013;192:343–6.
50. Cardillo E. Mapping between international medical terminologies, Annex 4 to SHN D3.3, 2015.
51. OWL 2 EL profile. OWL 2 Web Ontology Language Profiles, http://www.w3.org/TR/owl2-profiles/#OWL_2_EL, Last seen 15 May 2017.
52. IHTSDO, SNOMED CT Diagramming Guideline (v1.0), https://www.snomed.org/, last seen 10 November 2017.
53. He Z, Geller J, Chen Y. A comparative analysis of the density of the SNOMED CT conceptual content for semantic harmonization. Artif Intell Med. 2015;64:29–40.
54. Spackman K, Dionne R, Mays E, Weis J. Role grouping as an extension to the description logic of Ontylog motivated by concept modeling in SNOMED. In Proceedings of the AMIA Symposium. Am Med Inform Assoc. 2002:712–6.
55. Mary M, Soualmia L, Gansel X. Usability and Improvement of Existing Alignments: The LOINC-SNOMED CT Case Study: LNAI 10180, Springer International Publishing. 2017:145–8.
56. El-Sappagh S, Ali F. DDO: a diabetes mellitus diagnosis ontology. Applied Informatics. 2016;3(1):5.
57. El-Sappagh S, Kwak D, Ali F, Kwak KS. DMTO: a realistic ontology for standard diabetes mellitus treatment. Journal of biomedical semantics. 2018;9(1):8.
58. Souvignet J, Rodrigues J. Toward a Patient Safety Upper Level Ontology, 2015.
59. Martínez-Costa C, Schulz S. Ontology-based reinterpretation of the SNOMED CT context model, In ICBO; 2013:90–5.
60. Cheetham E, Gao Y, Goldberg B, Hausam R, Schulz S. Formal representation of disorder associations in SNOMED CT. Proceedings of the 2015 International Conference on Biomedical Ontology (ICBO2015). 2015:27–31.
61. Bodenreider O. Identifying missing hierarchical relations in SNOMED CT from logical definitions based on the lexical features of concept names. In ICBO/BioCreative, 2016.
62. Hogan W. Aligning the Top Level of SNOMED-CT with Basic Formal Ontology. KR-MED 2008. 2008;7:113.
63. Ochs C, Geller J, Perl Y, Chen Y, Agrawal A, Case J, Hripcsak G. A tribal abstraction network for SNOMED CT target hierarchies without attribute relationships. J Am Med Inform Assoc. 2015;22:628–39.

8

A semantics-oriented computational approach to investigate microRNA regulation on glucocorticoid resistance in pediatric acute lymphoblastic leukemia

Huiqin Chen[1], Dihua Zhang[2], Guoping Zhang[3], Xiaofeng Li[1], Ying Liang[1], Mohan Vamsi Kasukurthi[4], Shengyu Li[4], Glen M. Borchert[5] and Jingshan Huang[4,6,7*]

Abstract

Background: Acute lymphoblastic leukemia is the most prevalent neoplasia among children. Despite the tremendous achievements of state-of-the-art treatment strategies, drug resistance is still a major cause of chemotherapy failure leading to relapse in pediatric acute lymphoblastic leukemia. The underlying mechanisms of such phenomenon are not yet clear and subject to further exploration. Prior research has shown that microRNAs can act as post-transcriptional regulators of many genes related to drug resistance. However, details of microRNA regulation mechanisms in pediatric acute lymphoblastic leukemia are far from completely understood.

Methods: We utilized a computational approach based upon emerging biomedical and biological ontologies and semantic technologies to investigate the important roles of microRNA: mRNA regulation on glucocorticoid resistance in pediatric acute lymphoblastic leukemia. In particular, various filtering mechanisms were designed based on the user-provided MeSH term to narrow down the most promising microRNAs in an effective manner.

Results: During our manual search on background literature, we found a total of 18 candidate microRNAs that possibly regulate glucocorticoid resistance in pediatric acute lymphoblastic leukemia. After the first-round filtering using the Broader-Match option where both the user-provided MeSH term and its direct parent term were utilized, the number of targets for 18 microRNAs was reduced from 232 to 74. During the second-round filtering with the Exact-Match option where only the MeSH term itself was utilized, the number of targets was further reduced to 19. Finally, we conducted semantic searches in the OmniSearch software tool on the five likely regulating microRNAs and identified two most likely microRNAs.

Conclusions: We successfully identified two microRNAs, hsa-miR-142-3p and hsa-miR-17-5p, which are computationally predicted to closely relate to glucocorticoid resistance, thus potentially serving as novel biomarkers and therapeutic targets in pediatric acute lymphoblastic leukemia.

Keywords: Acute lymphoblastic leukemia (ALL), Drug resistance, microRNA (miRNA or miR), Glucocorticoids (GC), miRNA target, Biomedical and biological ontology (bio-ontology), Semantic integration, Semantic search

* Correspondence: huang@southalabama.edu
[4]School of Computing, University of South Alabama, Mobile, AL 36688, USA
[6]College of Math and Computer Science, Fuzhou University, Fuzhou, Fujian, China
Full list of author information is available at the end of the article

Background

Acute lymphoblastic leukemia (ALL) is the most common childhood malignant tumor and accounts for about 80–85% of acute leukemia in children. During the last four decades, great achievements have been made in ALL treatment, and the disease-free survival rates have increased to approximately 85% in developed countries [1–3]. Glucocorticoids (GCs) such as prednisone and dexamethasone (DEX) are essential drugs for ALL chemotherapy, and response to GC treatment is a strong independent factor of ALL prognosis. Currently, the 10-year event-free survival rate is about 80% for pediatric ALL patients with good response to prednisone. Unfortunately, there are still 57% of patients who have poor response to prednisone, and resistance to prednisone has become one of the main obstacles to achieve successful treatment outcomes in pediatric ALL [1–4]. As a result, there is an urgent need to investigate the mechanisms underlying GC resistance and thereby to explore novel therapeutic strategies to reverse GC resistance, which will help achieve full treatment potential and significantly improve prognosis.

Prior research [5, 6] showed that abnormal expression of microRNAs (miRNAs or miRs) is closely associated with GC resistance in pediatric ALL. Understanding miRNA regulation mechanisms in the modulation of GC response can potentially result in the discovery of novel molecular markers by which to predict GC resistance and thus to design therapeutic targets. Unfortunately, the exploration of miRNA: mRNA regulation is not trivial, which requires: (1) querying PubMed database [7] to look for biologically validated miRNA targets; (2) finding computationally putative miRNA targets by inquiring on numerous prediction databases such as miRDB [8], TargetScan [9], and miRanda [10]; and (3) obtaining additional information for each candidate target from data sources such as Gene Ontology (GO) [11] annotations, RNAcentral sequence annotations [12], pathway analysis by Protein ANalysis THrough Evolutionary Relationships (PANTHER) Classification System [13], the National Center for Biotechnology Information (NCBI) Gene database [14], and the Medical Headings (MeSH) database [15]. These data sources have heterogeneous semantics, and conventional, non-semantics-oriented knowledge discovery approaches are not suitable to properly handle complex semantics embedded in such big data. Therefore, it is critical to seek assistance from emerging semantic technologies, if more flexible, effective, and efficient miRNA knowledge acquisition is desired. In this paper, we introduce the utilization of OmniSearch software [16–18], a semantic search tool based upon biomedical and biological ontologies (bio-ontologies) and semantic technologies, to help better investigate miRNA regulation mechanisms in GC-resistant pediatric ALL. Note that our research efforts were initially reported in our BIBM 2017 proceeding paper [19]. Compared with the conference paper, this extended journal version has at least 75% new contents. To be more specific, all sections were significantly extended, detailed as follows. In "Background" Section, we added 17 papers into the background literature and gave a thorough discussion on our research background as well as related work. In "Methods" Section, we described all steps in our methods with significantly greater details. In particular, the manual search was described in detail along with 11 new references; and the MeSH-term filtering mechanisms were explained in detail along with a new figure. In "Results and Discussion" Section, we added greater details of results obtained from our methods, including detailed explanation and discussion in text, two new figures, and five new tables. In addition, we also conducted effectiveness and efficiency analysis in the OmniSearch software and reported these results. In "Conclusions" Section, we enriched it by adding details of our plan for future work.

Methods

Approach overview

We first performed a manual background literature search to identify an initial set of miRNAs that might be involved in the regulation of GC resistance in pediatric ALL. Next, we used the OmniSearch tool and user-provided MeSH terms to filter out more likely regulating miRNAs. Finally, we conducted semantic searches on this smaller set of miRNAs and obtained federated knowledge including putative and/or validated targets, associated GO annotations, related PubMed publications, RNAcentral sequence annotations, and pathway analysis. Based on such comprehensive search results, we disclosed the most promising miRNAs, along with their respective targets, as candidate novel biomarkers in GC-resistant pediatric ALL.

Bio-ontologies underlying OmniSearch

Being a semantic integration & search software system, OmniSearch was built upon Ontology for MicroRNA Target (OMIT) [20] and Non-Coding RNA Ontology (NCRO) [21]. Technical details of these two Basic Formal Ontology (BFO)-compliant bio-ontologies were included in our previously published work [20, 21]. In this paper, we want to emphasize the well-structured MeSH terms defined in the OMIT ontology. As shown in Fig. 1: (1) all ontological terms are organized under the is_a hierarchy; (2) the left portion illustrates the term MeSH term along with its direct parent, all ancestors, some siblings, and some offspring terms; and (3) the right portion shows the entire set of offspring terms for the term *Leukemia*.

Semantics-oriented MeSH-term filtering mechanisms

Technical details of the OmniSearch software tool were reported in our earlier work [16–18]. In this study, we

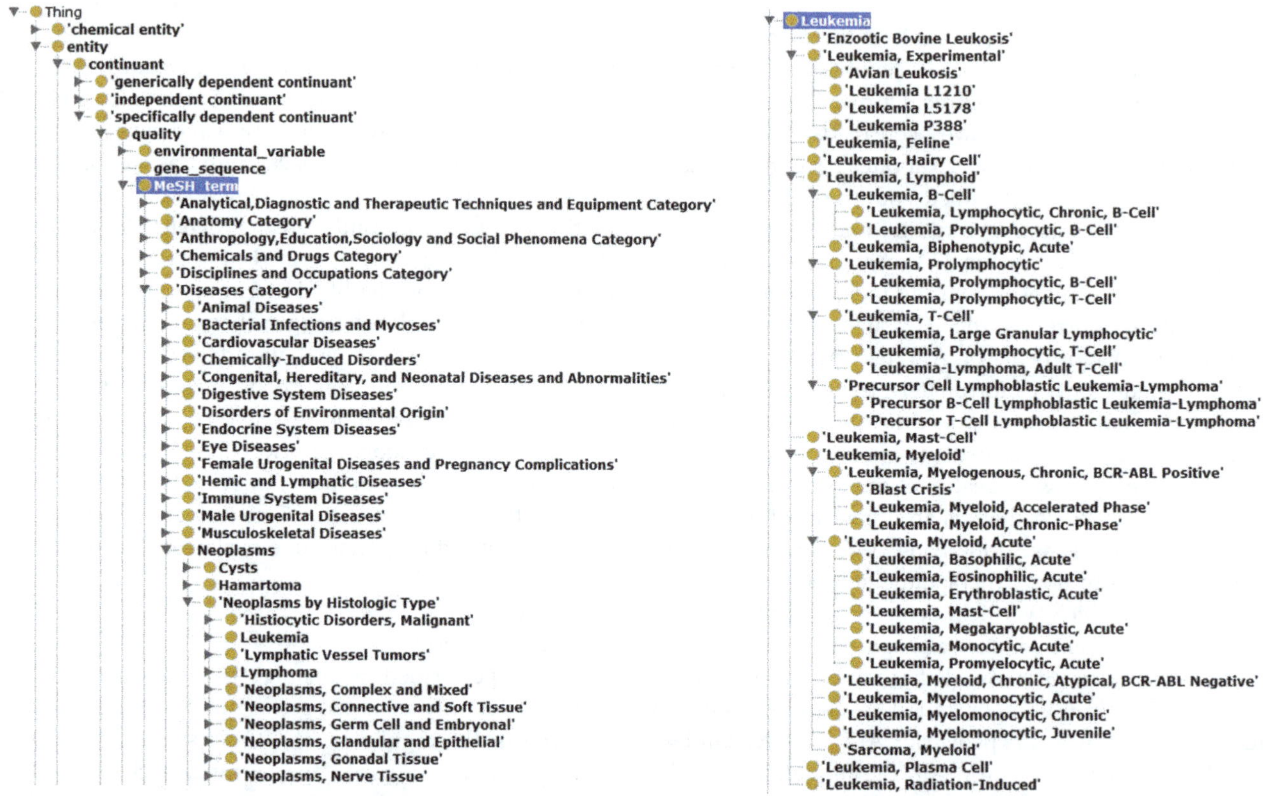

Fig. 1 BFO-compliant, well-structured MeSH terms in the OMIT ontology presented in Protégé, an ontology development tool from Stanford. Left: the term MeSH term along with its direct parent, all ancestors, some siblings, and some offspring terms. Right: the entire set of offspring terms for the term *Leukemia*

have implemented user-friendly and highly flexible filtering mechanisms through user-provided MeSH terms. First of all, users can input any portion of a MeSH term that is related to their semantic search query. Depending on the user selection of "Match from the beginning" or "Match anywhere," OmniSearch will return a list of relevant MeSH terms. This feature is user-friendly and convenient, especially to those users who are either not familiar with MeSH terms or not sure about the accurate spelling of a specific MeSH term.

Once a MeSH term is included into the user search query, there are three different filtering options: Exact-Match, Broader-Match, or Narrower-Match. The default selection is the Exact-Match option, where a record will be retrieved only if it contains the exact user-provided MeSH term. The other two filtering options are both based upon the semantics formally encoded in the OMIT ontology, detailed as follows.

Under the Broader-Match option, both the user-provided MeSH term and all of its parent terms will be used to filter out records. A record will be retrieved if it contains the MeSH term itself or any of its parent terms. For example, suppose the user supplies in the search query a MeSH term Leukemia, B-Cell, whose parent term is Leukemia, Lymphoid; all records containing either B-Cell leukemia or lymphoid leukemia will be returned. This option is useful in situations where the user-provided MeSH term is too specific (e.g., Leukemia, B-Cell), which will result in excluding records that are actually relevant (e.g., related to some lymphoid leukemia other than B-Cell leukemia) and should not be filtered out.

On the contrary, under the Narrower-Match option, both the user-provided MeSH term and all of its offspring terms will be utilized. A record will be retrieved if it contains the MeSH term itself or any of its offspring terms. For example, suppose the user supplies a MeSH term Leukemia, T-Cell, which has three offspring terms: Leukemia, Large Granular Lymphocytic; Leukemia, Prolymphocytic, T-Cell; and Leukemia-Lymphoma, Adult T-Cell; any records containing T-Cell leukemia or any of its subtypes will be returned. The motivation of having this option available is to deal with situations where the user-provided MeSH term is too general.

In summary, whereas the Exact-Match option is appropriate for users who are confident on their selected MeSH terms, both the Broader-Match and Narrower-Match options, when deemed necessary, are able to effectively expand original search queries and, in a user-friendly and highly flexible manner.

Results

Results from manual background literature search

During our manual search on background literature, we found a total of 18 candidate miRNAs that possibly regulate GC resistance in pediatric ALL: hsa-miR-124-3p [22], hsa-miR-124-5p [22], hsa-miR-128-3p [23], hsa-miR-142-3p [24], hsa-miR-15b-3p [25], hsa-miR-17-5p [26], hsa-miR-18a-3p [27], hsa-miR-182-5p [28], hsa-miR-193a-3p [27], hsa-miR-218-5p [27], hsa-miR-221-3p [29], hsa-miR-335-5p [30], hsa-miR-532-5p [27], hsa-miR-550a-3p [27], hsa-miR-625-5p [27], hsa-miR-633 [27], hsa-miR-638 [27], and hsa-miR-708-5p [31, 32]. GC response can be mediated by miRNAs through their influence on GC signaling pathway, leading to diverse GC responsiveness. On the other hand, GCs can regulate the function of some miRNAs, thus suggesting a bidirectional influence between GCs and miRNAs. We have reviewed and searched PubMed literature related to the effects of miRNAs on GC responsiveness in vivo or in vitro experiments, and the terms that we used in the manual search included: miRNAs, glucocorticoid response, glucocorticoid resistance, glucocorticoid receptors, and acute lymphoblastic leukemia. All the acquired miRNAs in the background literature search were selected as potential target miRNAs for further investigation.

Table 1 Number of targets retrieved in OmniSearch without applying the MeSH-term filtering

miRNA	Number of reporting databases	Number of total targets supported by at least one publication
hsa-miR-124-3p	3	15
hsa-miR-124-5p	2	0
hsa-miR-128-3p	3	5
hsa-miR-142-3p	4	69
hsa-miR-15b-3p	2	0
hsa-miR-17-5p	3	84
hsa-miR-18a-3p	3	4
hsa-miR-182-5p	3	16
hsa-miR-193a-3p	4	17
hsa-miR-218-5p	3	2
hsa-miR-221-3p	3	1
hsa-miR-335-5p	3	8
hsa-miR-532-5p	3	5
hsa-miR-550a-3p	2	0
hsa-miR-625-5p	2	1
hsa-miR-633	2	0
hsa-miR-638	2	3
hsa-miR-708-5p	3	2
Average	3	13
Total	–	232

More likely regulating miRNAs through two rounds of the MeSH-term filtering

Before applying the MeSH-term filtering, a large number of targets (either computationally putative or biologically validated) were retrieved for each of the 18 miRNAs. As exhibited in Table 1, the total number of targets for these 18 miRNAs is 232; that is, more than 2 hundred miRNA: target pairs need to be further investigated, which would simply be, if not impossible, too time-consuming and labor-intensive.

As detailed in Section "Methods," OmniSearch supplies users with flexible, semantics-oriented filtering on relevant MeSH terms. After the first-round filtering using the Broader-Match option where both the user-provided MeSH term (Leukemia in this study) and its direct parent term (Neoplasms by Histologic Type) were utilized, the number of targets for each miRNA was significantly reduced, as exhibited in Table 2 (note that the numbers of predicted and validated targets in both Table 2 ad Table 3 were obtained from the OmniSearch user interface). In particular, there are six miRNAs (hsa-miR-221-3p, hsa-miR-633, hsa-miR-550a-3p, hsa-miR-638, hsa-miR-124-5p, and hsa-miR-15b-3p, all italicized in the table) that had no retrieved targets after the filtering. That is, no putative and/or validated targets of these six miRNAs are yet discovered to be related to either leukemia or some other neoplasms of various histologic types. Therefore, it is less likely that these miRNAs have some regulation on GC resistance in pediatric ALL. Consequently, these miRNAs were removed from further consideration.

During the second-round filtering with the Exact-Match option where only the MeSH term Leukemia itself was utilized, the number of targets for each miRNA was further reduced, as shown in Table 3. Seven miRNAs (hsa-miR-124-3p, hsa-miR-182-5p, hsa-miR-335-5p, hsa-miR-708-5p, hsa-miR-625-5p, hsa-miR-218-5p, and hsa-miR-532-5p, all italicized in the table) had no retrieved targets. In other words, no putative and/or validated targets of these seven miRNAs are yet discovered to be directly related to leukemia even though they are related to some neoplasms other than leukemia. Therefore, these seven miRNAs were excluded from further analysis.

After two rounds of the MeSH-term filtering, we obtained a set of five likely regulating miRNAs: hsa-miR-142-3p, hsa-miR-17-5p, hsa-miR-18a-3p, hsa-miR-128-3p, and hsa-miR-193a-3p, along with a total of 19 respective targets, for further analysis. Note that if not for the effective filtering

Table 2 Targets retrieved after applying the first-round MeSH-term filtering (broder-match on "leukemia")

miRNA	Number of predicted targets	Number of validated targets
hsa-miR-142-3p	12	11
hsa-miR-17-5p	7	11
hsa-miR-18a-3p	2	2
hsa-miR-128-3p	4	0
hsa-miR-193a-3p	4	1
hsa-miR-124-3p	0	7
hsa-miR-182-5p	4	4
hsa-miR-335-5p	1	0
hsa-miR-708-5p	0	1
hsa-miR-625-5p	1	0
hsa-miR-218-5p	1	0
hsa-miR-532-5p	0	1
hsa-miR-221-3p	*0*	*0*
hsa-miR-633	*0*	*0*
hsa-miR-550a-3p	*0*	*0*
hsa-miR-638	*0*	*0*
hsa-miR-124-5p	*0*	*0*
hsa-miR-15b-3p	*0*	*0*
Total	36	38

mechanisms provided in the OmniSearch software tool, we would have had to analyze 232 rather than 19 miRNA: target pairs. Up to this point, almost a 92% reduction in human efforts was already achieved. We will continue our discussion in Section "Discussion" on the efficiency feature in the OmniSearch software.

Table 3 Targets retrieved after applying the second-round MeSH-term filtering (exact-match on "leukemia")

miRNA	Number of predicted targets	Number of validated targets
hsa-miR-142-3p	5	4
hsa-miR-17-5p	3	3
hsa-miR-18a-3p	2	0
hsa-miR-128-3p	1	0
hsa-miR-193a-3p	0	1
hsa-miR-124-3p	*0*	*0*
hsa-miR-182-5p	*0*	*0*
hsa-miR-335-5p	*0*	*0*
hsa-miR-708-5p	*0*	*0*
hsa-miR-625-5p	*0*	*0*
hsa-miR-218-5p	*0*	*0*
hsa-miR-532-5p	*0*	*0*
Total	11	8

Discussion

Analysis of miRNA: Target regulation via semantic search

We conducted semantic searches in the OmniSearch software tool on the five likely regulating miRNAs. Federated knowledge was obtained for each miRNA: (1) computationally predicted and/or biologically validated targets; (2) associated GO annotations; (3) supporting PubMed publications; (4) RNAcentral sequence annotations for involved ncRNA molecules; and (5) pathway analysis results on relevant targets. Table 4 lists both predicted and validated targets for these five miRNAs, where each target name is followed by its formal gene name (in square brackets). Figures 2 and 3 are screenshots of the results when conducting semantic searches on hsa-miR-142-3p and hsa-miR-17-5p, respectively. Screenshots for the other three miRNAs are not included due to the space limit.

We speculated that **hsa-miR-142-3p** and **hsa--miR-17-5p** are the two most promising miRNAs related to GC resistance in pediatric ALL. Our observations on comprehensive knowledge retrieved in OmniSearch are summarized below.

According to the research reported in [33], hsa-miR-142-3p was originally identified as a hematopoietic specific miRNA and expressed in various hematopoietic cell lineages. Lv M et al. [34] reported that T-cell ALL patients with high expression of hsa-miR-142-3p had a significantly shorter survival time than those with low expression. The poor prognosis was closely correlated to the oncogenic role of hsa-miR-142-3p that was mediated by decreasing CAMP levels, promoting T-leukemic cell growth, and inducing resistance to GC treatment through targeting GC receptor-α. To date, whether hsa-miR-142-3p is involved in B-cell ALL remains unknown. Ding S et al. confirmed that hsa-miR-142-3p was significantly down-regulated in SLE CD4+ T cells compared with healthy controls; in addition, the hsa-miR-142-3p level was inversely correlated with the putative SLE-related targets signaling lymphocytic activation molecule-associated protein (SAP), CD84, and interleukin-10 (IL-10). The reduced hsa-miR-142-3p expression in CD4+ T cells can significantly increase protein levels of these target genes and causes B cell hyperstimulation.

In 2012, Harada M et al. [26] examined the effect of DEX treatment on the miRNA profile of B-ALL cell lines and found the down-regulation of a group of miRNAs that were most notable members of the miR-17 cluster. Furthermore, experiments on primary ex vivo ALL cells found that apoptosis induced by DEX was related to down-regulated hsa-miR-17-5p levels. On the contrary, up-regulation of hsa-miR-17-5p resulted in a decrease in Bim protein levels and DEX-induced cell

Table 4 Putative and validated targets for each of the more likely regulating miRNAs

More likely regulating miRNAs	Computationally predicted targets	Biologically validated targets
hsa-miR-142-3p	• ASH1L [ash1 (absent, small, or homeotic)-like (Drosophila)] • CP [ceruloplasmin (ferroxidase)] • MLLT1 [myeloid/lymphoid or mixed-lineage leukemia; translocated to, 1] • MLLT4 [myeloid/lymphoid or mixed-lineage leukemia; translocated to, 4] • SAG [S-antigen; retina and pineal gland (arrestin)]	• CCNT2 [cyclin T2] • EGR2 [early growth response 2] • HOXA10 [homeobox A10] • HOXA7 [homeobox A7]
hsa-miR-17-5p	• AGO2 [argonaute 2, RISC catalytic component] • BCR [breakpoint cluster region] • NPM1 [nucleophosmin (nucleolar phosphoprotein B23, nunatrin)]	• E2F1 [E2F transcription factor 1] • RUNX1 [runt related transcription factor 1] • TP53 [tumor protein p53]
hsa-miR-18a-3p	• ARHGAP26 [Rho GTPase activating protein 26] • IMPACT [impact RWD domain protein]	None
hsa-miR-128-3p	• PHF6 [PHD finger protein 6]	None
hsa-miR-193a-3p	None	• MCL1 [myeloid cell leukemia 1]

death. Therefore, hsa-miR-17-5p and other miR-17 members might play important roles in GC-induced cell death and GC resistance in B-ALL.

In addition, we further analyzed two targets of hsa-miR-142-3p: SAG [S-antigen; retina and pineal gland (arrestin)] and EGR2 [early growth response 2]. Arrestins (β-arrestin-1 and β-arrestin-2) are gene produts of SAG. The non-visual arrestins are multi-functional scaffolding proteins that play critical roles in G protein-coupled receptors (GPCRs) signaling. Upon binding activated GPCRs at the plasma membrane, β-arrestin terminates G protein-dependent responses (desensitization) and stimulates β-arrestin-dependent signaling pathways. Alteration of β-arrestin levels was confirmed in many human diseases, including Parkinson's disease with dementia, multiple sclerosis, type 2 diabetes, coronary artery disease, and various cancers. However, very little is known about the β-arrestin levels and factors that control β-arrestin gene expression in ALL. GCs enhance the expression of β-arrestin-1 and repress the expression of β-arrestin-2 at the transcriptional level by the binding of GC receptor (GR) to intragenic GC response elements (GREs). The increased expression of β-arrestin-1 after GC treatment impairs G protein-dependent activation of inositol phosphate signaling, thereby enhancing β-arrestin-1-dependent stimulation of the MAPK pathway by protease-activated receptor 1. Despite all the aforementioned findings, whether SAG plays a role in the regulation of β-arrestin expression and GC resistance in childhood ALL still remains to be elucidated.

EGRs were initially identified as immediate early genes functioning as a convergence point from many stimuli such as growth factors, hormones, and neurotransmitters. EGR2 has been widely studied in hindbrain development; peripheral nerve myelination; cognitive processes; and T-cell activation, induction of anergy, and development. Interestingly, EGR2 was identified as a crucial mediator for epidermal growth factor (EGF)-induced osteoprogenitor proliferation and survival. In addition, EGR2 was also one of the most strongly inhibited genes in GC-treated MC3T3 cells. GC treatment leads to a drastic decrease in bone marrow osteoprogenitor number and an increase in osteoblast and osteocyte apoptosis in mice. Furthermore, EGR2-stimulated survival was due to increasing the amount of antiapoptotic protein MCL1. However, whether EGR2 is directly involved in regulating GC-resistance of childhood ALL is still not known.

Based on the above comprehensive analysis, it is reasonable to consider **hsa-miR-142-3p** and **hsa-miR-17-5p** as the two most likely regulating miRNAs in GC-resistant pediatric ALL. Therefore, these two miRNAs as well as their respective targets can potentially serve as novel biomarkers and therapeutic targets in pediatric ALL treatment.

Effective and efficient analysis in OmniSearch

OmniSearch is highly effective and efficient to help users to obtain their desired search results.

1. During our previous investigation [16–18], both effectiveness and efficiency features of the OmniSearch software tool were demonstrated in an objective and unbiased manner when tested among domain experts from numerous institutions.
2. As discussed earlier in Section "Results," after applying the MeSH-term filtering, we only needed to focus on 19 rather than 232 miRNA: target pairs, giving us a 91.8% reduction in human efforts.
3. We asked five domain experts to further test OmniSearch efficiency. These experts are the first five co-authors of this paper, who are clinical investigators in pediatric ALL and/or biomedical scientists in miRNA research. Once the set of five likely regulating miRNAs was obtained, these experts were advised to use two different approaches, i.e., their conventional search methods vs. the OmniSearch tool, to explore potential miRNA: target regulation mechanisms in pediatric ALL. Time spent in each approach was recorded for each expert and then averaged among all experts. Details of efficiency evaluation on searching all five miRNAs are

Rows per page 100 | 9 Total Targets | « ‹ Page 1 of 1 › » | Go to Page Go

☐ All	Candidate Target ♦	Target Functional Annotations ♦	miRDB ▾	TargetScan ♦	miRanda ♦	miRTarBase ♦	Publications ♦	Weighted Score ♦
☐ 1	CCNT2	cyclin T2	95	99	1.2744	🔗	22493297	65.02
☐ 2	ASH1L	ash1 (absent, small, or homeotic)-like (Drosophila)	78	87	1.1161	-	25238203	55.31
☐ 3	EGR2	early growth response 2	70	85	0.5845	🔗	23602969	51.75
☐ 4	MLLT1	myeloid/lymphoid or mixed-lineage leukemia; translocated to, 1	-	49	-	-	23581416 + 3 More	16.33
☐ 5	SAG	S-antigen; retina and pineal gland (arrestin)	-	-	0.2405	-	23602969	0.08
☐ 6	HOXA10	homeobox A10	-	-	-	🔗	24057258	-
☐ 7	HOXA7	homeobox A7	-	-	-	🔗	24057258	-
☐ 8	CP	ceruloplasmin (ferroxidase)	-	-	0.8770	-	24629639	0.29
☐ 9	MLLT4	myeloid/lymphoid or mixed-lineage leukemia; translocated to, 4	-	-	0.3446	-	23581416 + 3 More	0.11

Fig. 2 OmniSearch semantic search results for hsa-miR-142-3p (with the MeSH term *Leukemia* and the Exact-Match option)

provided in Table 5. The data in the table clearly demonstrate that efficiency in OmniSearch is satisfactory – a large portion of user time was saved on: (1) obtaining search results (67% on average); (2) conducting pathway analysis (57% on average); and (3) comparing results across four miRNA target databases (63% on average).

Conclusions

ALL is the most important neoplasia among children. Although great progress has been made in clinical

Rows per page 100 | 6 Total Targets | « ‹ Page 1 of 1 › » | Go to Page Go

☐ All	Candidate Target ♦	Target Functional Annotations ♦	miRDB ▾	TargetScan ♦	miRanda ♦	miRTarBase ♦	Publications ♦	Weighted Score ♦
☐ 1	E2F1	E2F transcription factor 1	95	97	-	🔗	20013804	63.89
☐ 2	NPM1	nucleophosmin (nucleolar phosphoprotein B23, numatrin)	-	98	-	-	22681934	32.67
☐ 3	AGO2	argonaute 2, RISC catalytic component	-	90	-	-	24263100	30
☐ 4	BCR	breakpoint cluster region	-	83	-	-	20842500	27.67
☐ 5	TP53	tumor protein p53	-	-	-	🔗	19347736 + 1 More	-
☐ 6	RUNX1	runt related transcription factor 1	-	82	-	🔗	24263100 + 1 More	27.33

Fig. 3 OmniSearch semantic search results for hsa-miR-17-5p (with the MeSH term *Leukemia* and the Exact-Match option)

Table 5 OmniSearch efficiency analysis: saved time for end users

miRNA under search	Percentage of saved time on obtaining search results	Percentage of saved time on conducting pathway analysis	Percentage of saved time on comparing results across different target databases
hsa-miR-142-3p	69%	59%	57%
hsa-miR-17-5p	71%	53%	63%
hsa-miR-18a-3p	53%	63%	59%
hsa-miR-128-3p	68%	58%	70%
hsa-miR-193a-3p	73%	51%	64%
Average for five miRNAs	67%	57%	63%

treatment during the past decades, drug resistance still remains a major cause of chemotherapy failure and relapse in pediatric patients. In particular, GC resistance is a critical clinical problem causing treatment failure in pediatric ALL patients. Therefore, there exists an urgent need to further understand the mechanisms of GC resistance and, in turn, to explore novel therapeutic strategies to improve treatment outcomes and disease prognosis. Overwhelming evidence illustrates that miRNAs act as post-transcriptional regulators of genes related to drug resistance, and deregulated miRNA expression might contribute to different GC treatment response in ALL. However, functions of individual miRNAs and their potential mechanisms involved in GC response are still largely unknown. In the present study, we introduced the utilization of OmniSearch, a semantic integration and search software tool, to facilitate the exploration of important roles of miRNAs performed on GC-resistant pediatric ALL. Our methodologies were demonstrated to be promising to significantly assist with unraveling miRNA regulation mechanisms. Specifically, the OmniSearch software is user-friendly, effective, and highly efficient. Using OmniSearch, we successfully disclosed two miRNAs, hsa-miR-142-3p and hsa-miR-17-5p, which likely regulate GC resistance in pediatric ALL. These two miRNAs as well as their respective targets can potentially serve as novel biomarkers and therapeutic targets.

An immediate piece of future work is to conduct wet-lab validation of biological functions of miRNAs along with their putative targets reported in this paper. We plan to perform luciferase reporter assays to confirm the suppression of target mRNAs by their paired miRNAs, followed by soft agar assays to assess the role of these miRNA: mRNA pairs in the regulation of GC resistance in pediatric ALL. Such wet-lab validation is supposed to improve the whole research pipeline and to reduce type I and II errors as well. Another promising research direction is to use semantic data mining techniques to explore both direct and indirect data associations among originally heterogeneous data sources. Such data associations, especially those indirect ones, will supply us with additional clues in further understanding miRNA regulation in pediatric ALL.

Abbreviations

ALL: Acute lymphoblastic leukemia; BFO: Basic formal ontology; bio-ontologies: Biomedical and biological ontologies; DEX: Dexamethasone; GC: Glucocorticoid; GO: Gene ontology; GPCRs: G protein-coupled receptors; GR: GC receptor; GREs: GC response elements; IL-10: Interleukin-10; MeSH: Medical Headings; miRNA/miR: microRNA; NCBI: National Center for Biotechnology Information; NCI: National Cancer Institute; NCRO: Non-Coding RNA Ontology; NIH: National Institutes of Health; OMIT: Ontology for MicroRNA Target; PANTHER: Protein ANalysis THrough Evolutionary Relationships; SAP: SLE-related targets signaling lymphocytic activation molecule-associated protein

Acknowledgements

See "Funding" Section for details.

Funding

This study was partially supported by The National Cancer Institute (NCI) of The National Institutes of Health (NIH), under the Award Number U01CA180982. The views contained in this paper are solely the responsibility of the authors and do not represent the official views, either expressed or implied, of the NIH or the U.S. government. Publication of this article was supported through other resources.

Authors' contributions

HC and DZ collected the dataset and drafted the manuscript together. HC, DZ, GZ, XL, YL, and GMB performed the data analysis and helped with making the tables and figs. JH conceived the study and revised the manuscript. MVK and SL participated in the manuscript preparation. All authors have read and approved the final manuscript.

Competing interests

The authors declare that they have no competing interests.

Author details

[1]Department of Pediatrics, The Third Affiliated Hospital, Sun Yat-sen University, Guangzhou, Guangdong, China. [2]Department of Nephrology, The First Affiliated Hospital, Sun Yat-sen University, Guangzhou, Guangdong, China. [3]Department of Oncology, Yuebei People's Hospital, Shaoguan, Guangdong, China. [4]School of Computing, University of South Alabama, Mobile, AL 36688, USA. [5]College of Medicine, University of South Alabama, Mobile, AL 36688, USA. [6]College of Math and Computer Science, Fuzhou University, Fuzhou, Fujian, China. [7]School of Information, Qilu University of Technology (Shandong Academy of Sciences), Jinan, Shandong, China.

References

1. Schrappe M, Reiter A, Zimmermann M, Harbott J, Ludwig WD, Henze G, Gadner H, Odenwald E, Riehm H. Long-term results of four consecutive trials in childhood ALL performed by the ALL-BFM study group from 1981 to 1995. Berlin-Frankfurt-Munster. Leukemia. 2000;14(12):2205–22.

2. Bhadri VA, Trahair TN, Lock RB. Glucocorticoid resistance in paediatric acute lymphoblastic leukaemia. J Paediatr Child Health. 2012;48(8):634–40.
3. Dördelmann M, Reiter A, Borkhardt A, Ludwig WD, Götz N, Viehmann S, Gadner H, Riehm H, Schrappe M. Prednisone response is the strongest predictor of treatment outcome in infant acute lymphoblastic leukemia. Blood. 1999;94(4):1209–17.
4. Möricke A, Reiter A, Zimmermann M, Gadner H, Stanulla M, Dördelmann M, Löning L, Beier R, Ludwig WD, Ratei R, Harbott J, Boos J, Mann G, Niggli F, Feldges A, Henze G, Welte K, Beck JD, Klingebiel T, Niemeyer C, Zintl F, Bode U, Urban C, Wehinger H, Niethammer D, Riehm H, Schrappe M. Risk-adjusted therapy of acute lymphoblastic leukemia can decrease treatment burden and improve survival: treatment results of 2169 unselected pediatric and adolescent patients enrolled in the trial ALL-BFM 95. Blood. 2008;111(9):4477–89.
5. Rainer J, Ploner C, Jesacher S, Ploner A, Eduardoff M, Mansha M, Wasim M, Panzer-Grümayer R, Trajanoski Z, Niederegger H, Kofler R. Glucocorticoid-regulated miRNAs and mirtrons in acute lymphoblastic leukemia. Leukemia. 2009;23(4):746–52.
6. Lewis BP, Burge CB, Bartel DP. Conserved seed pairing, often flanked by adenosines, indicates that thousands of human genes are miRNA targets. Cell. 2005;120(1):15–20.
7. Lu Z. PubMed and beyond: a survey of web tools for searching biomedical literature. Database. 2011:1–13.
8. miRDB. [Online]. Available: http://mirdb.org/miRDB/. (Date accessed: 04/05/2018).
9. TargetScan. [Online]. Available: http://www.targetscan.org. (Date accessed: 04/05/2018).
10. miRanda. [Online]. Available: http://www.miRNA.org. (Date accessed: 04/05/2018).
11. Ashburner M, Ball CA, Blake JA, Botstein D, Butler H, Cherry JM, Davis AP, Dolinski K, Dwight SS, Eppig JT, Harris MA, Hill DP, Issel-Tarver L, Kasarskis A, Lewis S, Matese JC, Richardson JE, Ringwald M, Rubin GM, Sherlock G. Gene ontology: tool for the unification of biology. The Gene Ontology Consortium. Nat Genet. 2000;25(1):25–9.
12. RNAcentral. [Online]. Available: http://rnacentral.org/. (Date accessed: 04/05/2018).
13. Mi H, Muruganujan A, Thomas PD. PANTHER in 2013: modeling the evolution of gene function, and other gene attributes, in the context of phylogenetic trees. Nucleic Acids Res. 2013;41(Database issue):D377–86.
14. NCBI Gene [Online]. Available: http://ncbi.nlm.nih.gov/gene/. (Date accessed: 04/05/2018).
15. Medical Subject Headings (MeSH) Database [Online]. Available: https://www.nlm.nih.gov/mesh/. (Date accessed: 04/05/2018).
16. Huang J, Gutierrez F, Strachan HJ, Dou D, Huang W, Smith B, Blake JA, Eilbeck K, Natale DA, Lin Y, Wu B, Silva N, Wang X, Liu Z, Borchert GM, Tan M, Ruttenberg A. OmniSearch: a semantic search system based on the ontology for MiRNA target (OMIT) for miRNA-target gene interaction data. J Biomed Semant. 2016;7:25.
17. Huang J, Dou D, She J, Limper AH, Yang Y, Yang P. A comprehensive (biological and computational) investigation on the role of microRNA: mRNA regulations performed in chronic obstructive pulmonary disease and lung cancer. Proceedings of the 2016 IEEE International Conference on Bioinformatics and Biomedicine (BIBM-2016). Shenzhen: IEEE Computer Society Press; 2016. p. 1067–72.
18. Huang J, Gutierrez F, Dou D, Blake JA, Eilbeck K, Natale DA, Smith B, Lin Y, Wang X, Liu Z, Tan M, Ruttenberg A. A semantic approach for knowledge capture of miRNA-target gene interactions. Proceedings of the 2015 IEEE International Conference on Bioinformatics and Biomedicine (BIBM-2015). Washington D.C.: IEEE Computer Society Press; 2015. p. 975–82.
19. Chen H, Zhang D, Zhang G, Li X, Liang Y, Kasukurthi M, Borchert GM, and Huang J. MeSH term-based semantic analysis of microRNA regulation on glucocorticoid resistance in pediatric acute lymphoblastic leukemia. Proceedings of the 2017 IEEE International Conference on Bioinformatics and Biomedicine (BIBM-2017). Kansas City: IEEE Computer Society Press; 2017. p. 1233–4.
20. Huang J, Dang J, Borchert GM, Eilbeck K, Zhang H, Xiong M, Jiang WJ, Wu H, Blake JA, Natale DA, Tan M. OMIT: dynamic, semi-automated ontology development for the miRNA domain. PLoS One. 2014;9(7);1–16.
21. Huang J, Eilbeck K, Smith B, Blake JA, Dou D, Huang W, Natale DA, Ruttenberg A, Huan J, Zimmermann MT, Jiang G, Lin Y, Wu B, Strachan HJ, He Y, Zhang S, Wang X, Liu Z, Borchert GM, Tan M. The non-coding RNA ontology (NCRO): a comprehensive resource for the unification of non-coding RNA biology. J Biomed Semant. 2016;7(24):1–12.
22. Liang YN, Tang YL, Ke ZY, Chen YQ, Luo XQ, Zhang H, Huang LB. MiR-124 contributes to glucocorticoid resistance in acute lymphoblastic leukemia by promoting proliferation, inhibiting apoptosis and targeting the glucocorticoid receptor. J Steroid Biochem Mol Biol. 2017;172:62–8.
23. Kotani A, Ha D, Schotte D, den Boer ML, Armstrong SA, Lodish HF. A novel mutation in the miR-128b gene reduces miRNA processing and leads to glucocorticoid resistance of MLL-AF4 acute lymphocytic leukemia cells. Cell Cycle. 2010;9(6):1037–42.
24. Lv M, Zhang X, Jia H, Li D, Zhang B, Zhang H, Hong M, Jiang T, Jiang Q, Lu J, Huang X, Huang B. An oncogenic role of miR-142-3p in human T-cell acute lymphoblastic leukemia (T-ALL) by targeting glucocorticoid receptor-α and cAMP/PKA pathways. Leukemia. 2012;26(4):769–77.
25. Lovat F, Fassan M, Gasparini P, Rizzotto L, Cascione L, Pizzi M, Vicentini C, Balatti V, Palmieri D, Costinean S, Croce CM. miR-15b/16-2 deletion promotes B-cell malignancies. Proc Natl Acad Sci U S A. 2015;112(37):11636–41.
26. Harada M, Pokrovskaja-Tamm K, Söderhäll S, Heyman M, Grander D, Corcoran M. Involvement of miR17 pathway in glucocorticoid-induced cell death in pediatric acute lymphoblastic leukemia. Leuk Lymphoma. 2012;53(10):2041–50.
27. Yang A, Ma J, Wu M, Qin W, Zhao B, Shi Y, Jin Y, Xie Y. Aberrant microRNA-182 expression is associated with glucocorticoid resistance in lymphoblastic malignancies. Leuk Lymphoma. 2012;53(12):2465–73.
28. Kotani A, Ha D, Hsieh J, Rao PK, Schotte D, den Boer ML, Armstrong SA, Lodish HF. miR-128b is a potent glucocorticoid sensitizer in MLL-AF4 acute lymphocytic leukemia cells and exerts cooperative effects with miR-221. Blood. 2009;114(19):4169–78.
29. Yan J, Jiang N, Huang G, Tay JL, Lin B, Bi C, Koh GS, Li Z, Tan J, Chung TH, Lu Y, Ariffin H, Kham SK, Yeoh AE, Chng WJ. Deregulated MIR335 that targets MAPK1 is implicated in poor outcome of paediatric acute lymphoblastic leukaemia. Br J Haematol. 2013;163(1):93–103.
30. Han BW, Feng DD, Li ZG, Luo XQ, Zhang H, Li XJ, Zhang XJ, Zheng LL, Zeng CW, Lin KY, Zhang P, Xu L, Chen YQ. A set of miRNAs that involve in the pathways of drug resistance and leukemic stem-cell differentiation is associated with the risk of relapse and glucocorticoid response in childhood ALL. Hum Mol Genet. 2011;20(24):4903–15.
31. Zhang H, Luo XQ, Zhang P, Huang LB, Zheng YS, Wu J, Zhou H, Qu LH, Xu L, Chen YQ. MicroRNA patterns associated with clinical prognostic parameters and CNS relapse prediction in pediatric acute leukemia. PLoS One. 2009;4(11):e7826.
32. Xu L, Liang YN, Luo XQ, Liu XD, Guo HX. Association of miRNAs expression profiles with prognosis and relapse in childhood acute lymphoblastic leukemia. Zhonghua Xue Ye Xue Za Zhi. 2011;32(3):178–81.
33. Chen CZ, Li L, Lodish HF, Bartel DP. MiRNAs modulate hematopoietic lineage differentiation. Science. 2004;303(5654):83–6.
34. Lv M, Zhang X, Jia H, Li D, Zhang B, Zhang H, Hong M, Jiang T, Jiang Q, Lu J, Huang X, Huang B. An oncogenic role of miR-142-3p in human T-cell acute lymphoblastic leukemia (T-ALL) by targeting glucocorticoid receptor-alpha and cAMP/PKA pathways. Leukemia. 2012;26(4):769–77.

9

Real-time location system-based asset tracking in the healthcare field

Sooyoung Yoo[1†], Seok Kim[1†], Eunhye Kim[1], Eunja Jung[2], Kee-Hyuck Lee[1] and Hee Hwang[1*]

Abstract

Background: Numerous hospitals and organizations have recently endeavored to study the effects of real-time location systems. However, their experiences of system adoption or pilot testing via implementation were not shared with others or evaluated in a real environment. Therefore, we aimed to share our experiences and insight regarding a real-time location system, obtained via the implementation and operation of a real-time asset tracking system based on Bluetooth Low Energy/WiFi in a tertiary care hospital, which can be used to improve hospital efficiency and nursing workflow.

Methods: We developed tags that were attached to relevant assets paired with Bluetooth Low Energy sensor beacons, which served as the basis of the asset tracking system. Problems with the system were identified during implementation and operation, and the feasibility of introducing the system was evaluated via a satisfaction survey completed by end users after 3 months of use.

Results: The results showed that 117 nurses who had used the asset tracking system for 3 months were moderately satisfied (2.7 to 3.4 out of 5) with the system, rated it as helpful, and were willing to continue using it. In addition, we identified 4 factors (end users, target assets, tracking area, and type of sensor) that should be considered in the development of asset tracking systems, and 4 issues pertaining to usability (the active tag design, technical limitations, solution functions, and operational support).

Conclusions: The successful introduction of asset tracking systems based on real-time location in hospitals requires the selection of clear targets (e.g., users and assets) via analysis of the user environment and implementation of appropriate technical improvements in the system as required (e.g., miniaturization of the tag size and improvement of the sensing accuracy).

Keywords: Asset tracking, Efficiency, Healthcare, Real-time locating system, System implementation

Background

The appropriate placement and supply of commodities in hospitals not only improves the quality of patient treatment but also influences the outcomes of treatment in emergency situations. Therefore, commodity management could be considered an exceedingly important task that should not be neglected by hospitals [1–4]. Nurses are generally tasked with the management of commodities in medical sites, and when their shifts end, they transfer responsibility for the equipment in their departments and wards to nurses on the next shift. Therefore, the effective management of commodities and a reduction in the time required to transfer them between nurses would not only increase the time available to nurses for the provision of patient care but also improve care quality [5–9].

One method of improving commodity management involves real-time location systems (RTLSs), which are used to manage assets efficiently in other industries. Interest in the introduction of these systems to the healthcare field is increasing, [10] albeit gradually [5, 11].

* Correspondence: neoroandy@snubh.org; neuroandy@snubh.org
†Sooyoung Yoo and Seok Kim contributed equally to this work.
[1]Office of eHealth Research and Businesses, Seoul National University Bundang Hospital, 166, Gumi-ro, Bundang-gu, Seongnam-si 436-707, South Korea
Full list of author information is available at the end of the article

In healthcare, RTLS solutions are used mainly to track medical staff, patients, and assets. The introduction of these solutions has been shown to provide hospitals with certain benefits [5, 7, 10, 12–16] including cost reduction, improvements in medical care quality and work processes, and increased patient satisfaction.

Recently, the healthcare sector has adopted the barcode, radio-frequency identification (RFID), WiFi, and Bluetooth sensing technology in the development of tracking systems. Barcode technology, in particular, has been widely adopted by nurses to reduce medication administration errors and the related costs and to improve patient safety [17]. Furthermore, previous studies have shown that these systems are effective in reducing costs, improving the quality of medical services, enhancing work processes, and boosting patient satisfaction, by tracking medical professionals and patients [6, 8, 10, 12–16, 18, 19]. RTLS technology is based mainly on the use of WiFi and RFID, although some research has examined whether Bluetooth could be used as the basis of RTLSs [5, 6, 20]. Researchers in the healthcare field have demonstrated strong interest in localization systems; however, these systems are still in their infancy. Given the differences between sensors in terms of trackable distance, cost, and accuracy, people should consider the pros and cons of sensors to ensure selection of the most appropriate product [21]. In addition, the user interface, security, and effects of interference need to be considered [22, 23]. Therefore, system users should share their experiences of implementation with others to aid medical institutions that are willing to adopt the technology in developing the most suitable systems [6, 11].

Therefore, this study aimed to share considerations and insights and to provide information regarding the adoption of an RTLS in a medical environment, obtained via the implementation and operation of a real-time Bluetooth Low Energy (BLE)/WiFi-based asset tracking system in a tertiary general university hospital.

Methods

Development of the BLE/WiFi-based asset tracking system

The development of the asset tracking system initially involved obtaining the definition of the asset management process by various medical professionals including a medical doctor, 4 nurses, a medical informatics professor, and 2 staff members from the asset management department at the tertiary general university hospital to which the authors are affiliated. Thirty developers ultimately participated in the development process, which took place over the course of 13 months, from November 2013 to November 2014. For approximately 2 months thereafter, we stabilized the system and performed tests to improve the software used to develop the BLE beacon, active tags, and web-based asset management application during the 13-month period.

The asset tracking system tracked the locations of assets throughout every ward in the hospital using the existing WiFi infrastructure; however, we used separate BLE beacons to provide location measurements with greater accuracy in the emergency room and the storage areas of the wards. The location of each asset and the status of the active tag battery could be checked using the hospital information system, into which the asset management system was integrated. Figure 1 shows the overall architecture of the BLE/WiFi-based asset tracking system.

The asset management application consisted of 2 applications: 1 for users (i.e., nurses) and 1 for system administrators. In the user application, the types and positions of the assets on each floor were depicted as a bird's eye view of the entire hospital, with the detailed locations marked clearly on a floor plan (see Fig. 2). The user application also provided detailed location information according to the asset status (i.e., onsite, offsite, or borrowed) for each department. In contrast, the administrator application provided information regarding the registration and management of target assets, the assets' most recent locations and location histories, whether assets were onsite or offsite, and battery power levels for the tags. In addition, administrators could check the status of specific assets and all assets in a registered department using the search filter.

Active tags and BLE beacons

The active tags and BLE beacons were designed in consideration of the characteristics of the medical environment and RTLS-based tracking system. Because the active tags were used to track highly mobile assets, they were battery operated and able to transmit their own location information based on data received from the beacon. Battery capacity was prioritized during the production stage, with the aim of maximizing the convenience of the tags. We ultimately selected tags that were 66 × 40 × 25 mm in size and required 2 AA batteries (3000 mAh, 3.0 V). We attached tags to a total of 400 instruments, including 4 iPads and 21 oxygen holders in the emergency room, 200 infusion pumps in the emergency room and 3 intensive care units (ICUs), and 160 patient monitors and 15 bladder scanners in all departments. The tag locations were selected to minimize interference with the equipment and prioritized according to improvements in nursing workflow and relocation frequency.

The beacons relied on BLE, which is a low-power, low-cost solution that has been used widely in recent years. They operated with replaceable batteries to obviate the need for separate power supplies. The beacons

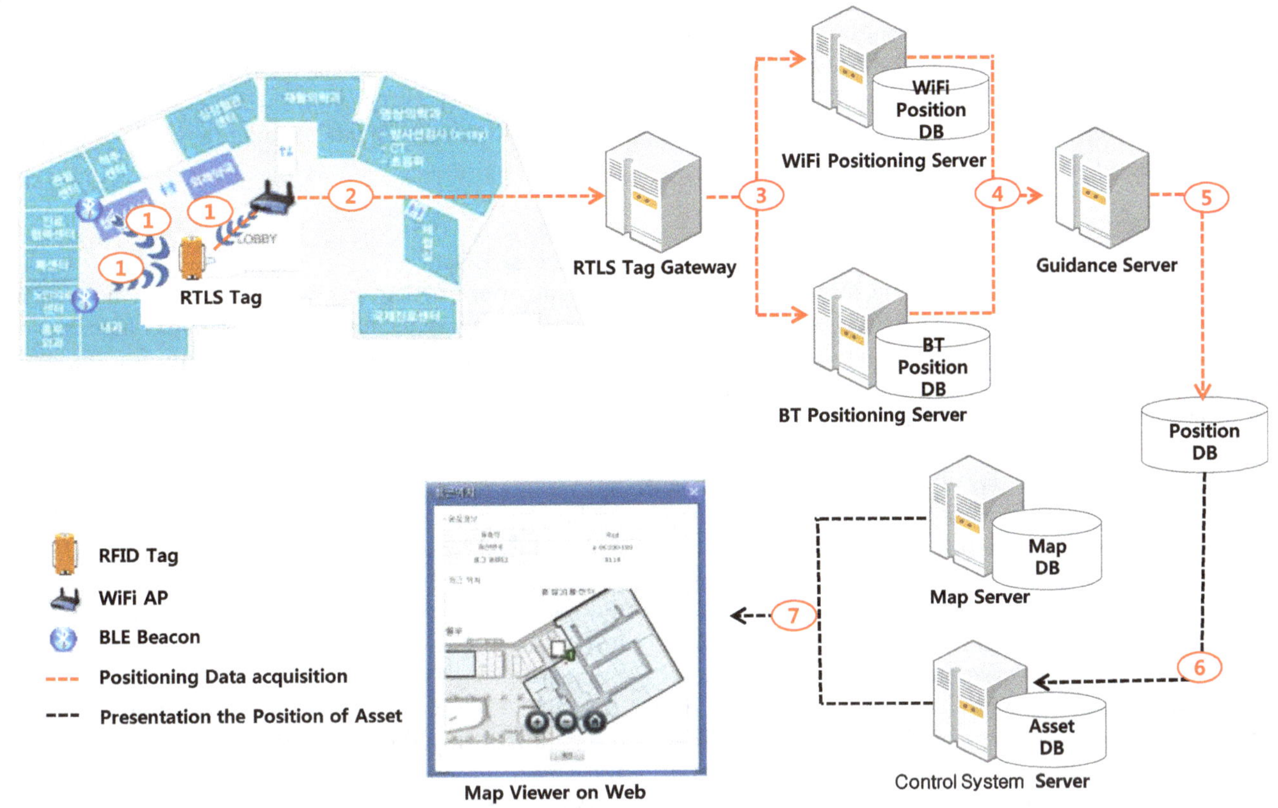

Fig. 1 Overall architecture of the asset tracking system

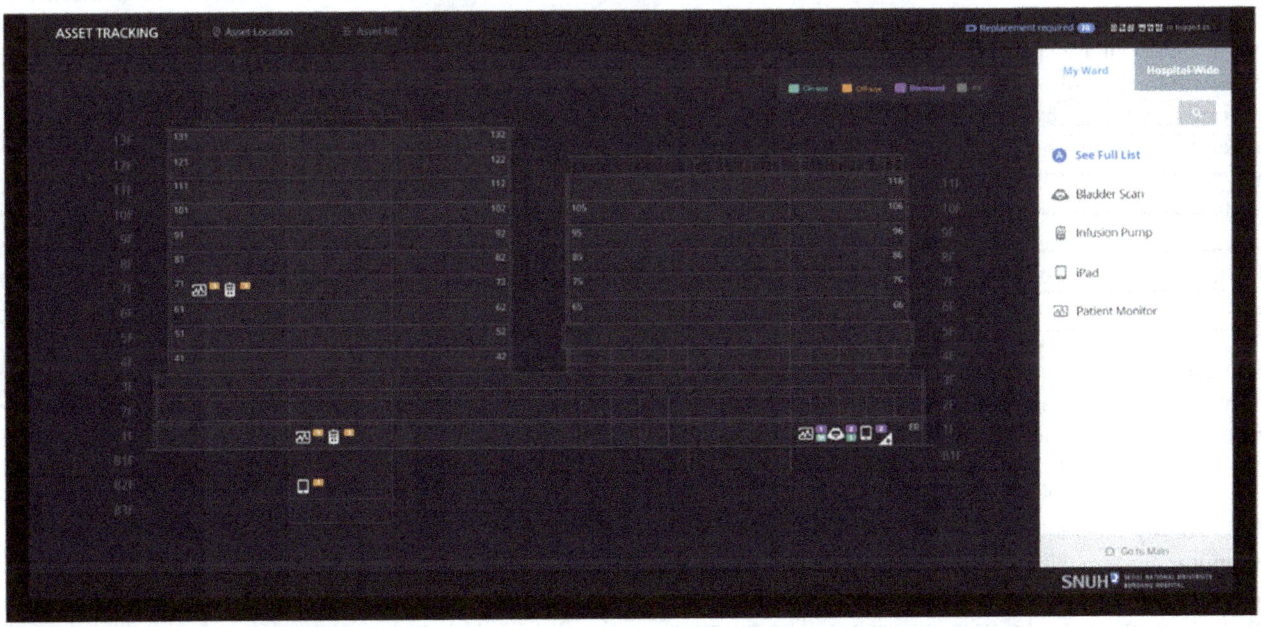

Fig. 2 Interface of the asset tracking system for users (Nurses)

were 120 × 120 × 30 mm in size, with an estimated battery life expectancy of a year. In total, 98 BLE beacons were created; of these, 53, 31, 4, and 9 were positioned in the emergency room, the wards, the ICUs, and other hospital areas, respectively. The beacons were installed on the ceiling of each location.

Setting asset tracking periods

The continuous transmission and reception of location information is essential for real-time location confirmation. However, because the active tags were battery powered and attached to mobile equipment, real-time transmission of the location information caused a battery drainage problem. Accordingly, in consideration of the battery life, we set each tag to transmit location information 16 times per day within a different period, mainly during the nurses' work shifts, to avoid the burden of frequent battery replacement. Specifically, tag location signals were emitted at 30-min intervals throughout the nurses' work shifts and at 2-h intervals during other hours. This setting was determined after consulting nurses who worked in the field and considering the system's operational efficiency according to the battery performance of the tags. The 16 specific times per day were finally set as 06:00, 06:30, 07:00, 09:00, 11:00, 13:00, 13:30, 14:00, 14:30, 15:00, 17:00, 19:00, 21:00, 21:30, 22:00, and 23:00. Tracking 16 times per day was a rule that we implemented upon introducing the system, but the tracking intervals can be modified to provide optimal settings that reflect the users' needs.

Satisfaction questionnaire for the end users

Following the development of the asset tracking system, a survey was conducted to examine the perceived quality and usability of the pilot system and to determine the end users' overall satisfaction over the course of 2 months starting from December 2014. Nurses were the end users for the asset tracking system. Although the system was installed in the emergency room and all wards and ICUs, the self-report satisfaction survey was conducted only in the 3 wards with the highest numbers of users, 3 ICUs (i.e., surgical, internal medicine, and neonatal), and the emergency room. In total, 280 nurses completed the survey over the course of a month (February 16 to March 16, 2015). We received 244 anonymous responses (response rate: 87.1%), and the final dataset contained data for 117 nurses following data cleansing and the exclusion of data for nurses who had not used the system (Fig. 3).

The survey questionnaire was developed based on the Computer System Usability Questionnaire to assess the overall system, and the Questionnaire for User Interface Satisfaction to assess the user experience. The questionnaire consisted of 17 items divided between 5 categories, with responses provided on a 5-point scale. The questionnaire data were analyzed via frequency analysis and the Kruskal-Wallis test, using SAS 9.3 (SAS Institute, Cary, NC, USA) to determine whether the results were affected by the participants' demographic characteristics.

Results

End-user satisfaction

The end user participants who completed the satisfaction questionnaire were primarily women, which is probably due to the nature of the nursing profession, and a large proportion were general duty nurses. In addition, the participants were evenly distributed between departments (i.e., wards, ICUs, and the emergency room) and were primarily in their 20s and 30s (Table 1).

The participants' mean satisfaction ratings for the 17 items ranged from 2.7 (for the tag size) to 3.4 (for the provision of the information required for nursing work, the need for the system, and intention regarding its future use).

As shown in Table 2, the ICU nurses generally exhibited higher levels of satisfaction than the emergency room nurses. In addition, statistically significant differences were observed for all items in the expectancy effects category, which pertained to the system's expected effects with constant use in the future, and for 3 of the 4 items in the information quality category, which reflected the accuracy and display of information. In other words, while the nurses' acceptance of the system's practical functions differed between departments, they gave similar responses regarding whether the asset tracking system provided functions that were necessary on the ground, and they intended to use the system.

Table 3 shows the participants' other subjective opinions (provided via free text in the questionnaire) of the ways in which the asset tracking system could be improved based on their 2-month pilot use. These opinions were classified according to whether they pertained to location accuracy, the tag, asset tracking, or user education. The most frequently observed comments concerned location accuracy in the system. In addition, we classified the content of the categories into subcategories and found that comments regarding expansion of the range of target assets for tracking were expressed frequently. Issues regarding the size of the active tag were also noted.

Discussion

The following discussion considers the lessons that were learned during the introduction and pilot operation of the BLE/WiFi-based asset tracking system, based on the end users' opinions.

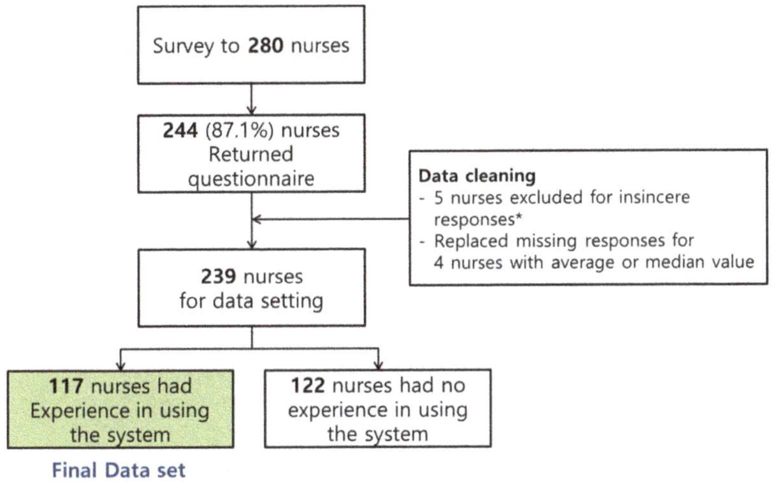

Fig. 3 Participant flow in the user satisfaction survey. * The insincere response means respondents having same answers for all questionnaires

Scope of asset tracking

Medical institutions that intend to develop and introduce RTLSs are required to define the end users, target assets, tracking areas, and sensor types via thorough discussion prior to implementation [14, 20]. In the present study, nurses were selected as the end users of the system. Most nurses in South Korea are responsible for a higher number of patients relative to nurses in other advanced countries; nevertheless, they undertake various duties in addition to patient care. This additional work includes the management of assets between work shifts in order to ensure continuous care. A considerable amount of time is spent performing these duties. For example, in the present study, nurses managed 44 assets in 11 categories on the wards, 118 assets in 11 categories in the ICUs, and 265 assets in 33 categories in the emergency room. Furthermore, nurses are required to confirm the locations of all assets managed by their departments during handover to nurses on other shifts [14, 20].

Table 1 Participants' demographic characteristics

Classification		*n*	%
Sex	Male	4	3.4
	Female	113	96.6
Position	Head nurse	8	6.8
	Nurse	109	93.2
Department	Ward	32	27.4
	Intensive care unit	45	38.5
	Emergency room	40	34.2
Age group	20s	59	50.4
	30s	52	44.4
	40s	6	5.1
Work experience	< 1 year	28	23.9
	1–3 years	38	32.5
	3–5 years	12	10.3
	> 5 years	39	33.3
Total		117	100.0

The selection of the target assets for the pilot system's implementation involved the creation of a list of all types of equipment managed by the nurses, which resulted in the selection of the most meaningful 5 assets (Fig. 4). Because of their high levels of mobility between departments, tracking the locations of these instruments was expected to increase nursing efficiency. The end-user satisfaction survey indicated that the asset tracking system was more helpful in managing/transferring/locating the assets than the manual management, with a satisfaction score that was above average. Considering the limited technology and limited tracking items used during the pilot, it seems that nursing work efficiency will be improved with the wider adoption of the system. Some examples of the practical use by the nurses in this study are as follows.

> *"In the ward, it is not easy to trace the movement of patients who need various tests (MRI, CT, etc.), many procedures (emergency hemodialysis, angiography, etc.), and consultation. However, using the system, we were able to easily identify and collect the assets that the patient needed."*

> *"When it is urgent to inject an emergency patient with many medications, such as fluid, dopamine, dobutamine, Lasix, and albumin through an infusion pump, an asset tracking system can be used to quickly locate available devices. As such, medical staff can provide intervention to patients more quickly."*

Table 2 Comparison of the mean satisfaction ratings according to the department (Intensive Care Unit, Emergency Room, and Ward)

Survey items			*M (SD)*				*P*
			Total	ER	ICU	Ward	
Information quality	1	Does the asset tracking system provide the information necessary to perform nursing work?	3.4 (0.785)	3.3 (0.716)	3.5 (0.661)	3.3 (0.991)	0.201
	2	Is the information provided by the asset tracking system accurate?	2.9 (0.928)	2.4 (0.781)	3.3 (0.793)	2.9 (1.014)	< .0001*
	3	Is the information provided by the asset tracking system expressed using appropriate terminology and in an appropriate format?	2.9 (0.844)	2.6 (1.005)	3.2 (0.712)	2.9 (0.641)	0.006*
	4	Does the asset tracking system provide up-to-date information appropriate for the current situation?	2.9 (0.908)	2.6 (0.868)	3.3 (0.733)	2.8 (1.019)	0.002*
System quality	1	Is the asset tracking system easy to use?	3.1 (0.902)	3.0 (0.974)	3.2 (0.773)	3.1 (0.976)	0.297
	2	Are you satisfied with the speed of the asset tracking system?	3.0 (0.904)	2.6 (0.838)	3.2 (0.735)	3.0 (1.078)	0.010*
	3	Do you need a separate user manual for the asset tracking system?	3.6 (0.993)	3.5 (1.132)	3.7 (0.905)	3.6 (0.948)	0.824
	4	Are you satisfied with using the asset tracking system through the electronic medical record?	3.2 (0.886)	3.1 (0.841)	3.3 (0.879)	3.2 (0.954)	0.371
Active tag	1	Are you satisfied with the size of the tag affixed to the device?	2.7 (0.992)	2.6 (0.979)	2.7 (0.953)	2.9 (1.070)	0.712
	2	You can replace the battery by pushing open the top part of the tag cover. Do you think this method of opening and closing the tag is appropriate?	3.0 (0.895)	2.7 (0.905)	2.9 (0.915)	3.3 (0.745)	0.014*
Expectancy effects	1	Is the asset tracking system more helpful for asset management than the previous method (i.e., manual management)?	3.2 (0.928)	2.9 (0.810)	3.5 (0.894)	3.4 (1.008)	0.007*
	2	Is the asset tracking system more helpful for transferring the nursing instruments than the previous method (manual management)?	3.2 (0.952)	2.9 (0.778)	3.4 (0.957)	3.3 (1.085)	0.033*
	3	Is the asset tracking system more helpful for locating mobile equipment than the previous method (manual management)?	3.3 (0.972)	2.8 (0.813)	3.5 (0.894)	3.5 (1.078)	0.001*
	4	Do you think the equipment will be used more efficiently with the asset tracking system than with the previous method (manual management)?	3.3 (0.927)	3.0 (0.832)	3.5 (0.894)	3.5 (0.983)	0.017*
Overall satisfaction	1	Are you satisfied with the overall use of the asset tracking system?	3.1 (0.834)	2.7 (0.716)	3.3 (0.780)	3.3 (0.902)	0.002*
	2	Do you need the asset tracking system for your nursing work?	3.4 (0.884)	3.1 (0.883)	3.5 (0.815)	3.4 (0.946)	0.083
	3	Do you intend to continue using the asset tracking system?	3.4 (0.811)	3.2 (0.747)	3.5 (0.815)	3.6 (0.833)	0.068

$^*p < .05$; comparisons were performed between 3 departments. *ER* emergency room, *ICU* intensive care unit

> *"In the past, we had to check all of the assets we were managing, including the quantity and the location of the assets at the end of the shift. However, after using the asset tracking system, we can check the location and quantity at once by looking at the dashboard, which can save a lot of time."*

The main reasons for equipment to be excluded were as follows: it was not needed by the end users, the tag influenced the usability of the asset, poor return on investment, and it did not fulfill the criteria for the tracking area (Table 4).

Location vs. positioning

RTLSs use both access points (APs) and beacons, which are typically placed indoors, to ensure tracking accuracy. In the present study, locations were tracked using an existing WiFi infrastructure that covered all of the hospital wards, while the location positioning of greater accuracy in the emergency and storage rooms was measured via BLE beacons. Because errors begin to occur at a distance of 10 m for WiFi or 5 m for BLE, it is necessary to choose an appropriate type of sensor for each target asset and area [21, 24].

Table 3 Participants' subjective opinions

Major classification	*n*	Sub-classification	*n*	Opinion
Locating/positioning	30	Detailed locations	7	I wish that the system showed more detailed locations in the ward
		Location accuracy	18	The item is not in the location indicated The location information is unreliable Location errors occur depending on the strength of the WiFi signal
		Tracking period	5	Real-time location identification would be nice
Active tag	18	Tag loss	7	The tags fall off the assets due to weak adhesion, and having to find the lost tags is burdensome
		Tag size	9	I wish the tag was smaller
		Battery cover	1	The battery cover falls off easily
		Battery life	1	The battery drains too quickly
Target assets	21	Tracking additional assets	10	I wish we could add tags to other equipment I wish that all the equipment in the asset categories (e.g., patient monitors) was included in the system[a]
		Asset identification method	11	In addition to the asset identifier being automatically assigned to each asset for the system to recognize, a manual method of managing asset identifiers would be nice
Education	4	Need for user education	4	An explanation of the purpose and use of the system is needed

Comments were provided via free text in the questionnaire
[a]Some assets (e.g., patient monitors) used by some departments were not tracked in the study

The system had several technical limitations. For example, the most important aspect of asset tracking is the ability to determine the precise location of a piece of equipment. However, the sensors do not always provide accurate locations in indoor tracking due to interference from other radio waves. Indeed, in the present study, users occasionally reported that assets were located on a different floor or in a different room to that shown in the tracking application; this is likely to have occurred because of the AP signal strength. In addition, we noted a problem with the batteries in the tags. As mentioned earlier, batteries were used in the tags and beacons to ensure their portability; however, periodical battery replacement for the beacons (once per year) and tags (every 100 days) would be difficult because of the sheer number of assets. Therefore, with respect to the tags, it would be necessary to decide whether to miniaturize them for greater usability or fit them with large-capacity batteries for greater operational efficiency. The sensing period for location identification would also require adjustment. This could be achieved using either signals generated by the tags or call signals from the beacon and AP; however, the provision of real-time measurements would require the generation of signals by the tags every 5 to 10 s, which would be fatal for battery life. In the present study, signal generation was limited to 16 times per day and focused on the nurses' shifts. However, because the emergency room typically requires frequent movement of equipment, the generation of location information only 16 times per day might have

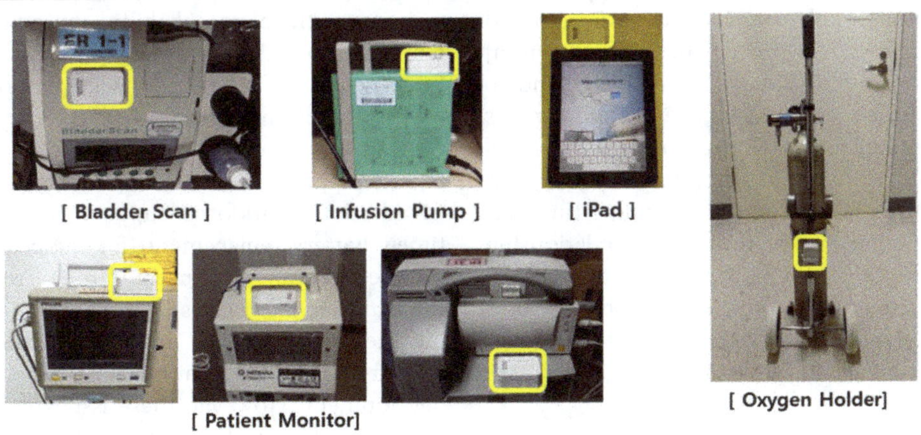

Fig. 4 Five types of asset targeted for tracking. Locations at which the active tags were attached to the 5 types of equipment selected as asset tracking targets

Table 4 Reasons for excluding assets from the real-time tracking

Asset	Reason for exclusion
Patient tracking	Little need for tracking at the site (e.g., psychiatric patients, neonates)
Laryngoscopy handle	Reduces the usability of intubation devices (i.e., it is difficult to affix the tag because it could hinder visibility) Difficulty in managing intubation devices (e.g., disinfection following each use)
Sandbag and ice pack	While necessary, the return on investment is low (i.e., the tag cost is high relative to the unit cost for these items)
Operating room items	The mobility of expensive medical instruments in the operating room is markedly low, so there is little need for tracking
Wheelchairs	While necessary, they were excluded because they are not for indoor use only (e.g., they are used outdoors frequently at medical institutions)

been insufficient. The fact that the number of assets managed by the emergency room was higher, relative to those managed by other departments, could also explain the low satisfaction levels observed in the study.

This configuration increased the difficulty in providing real-time identification of asset locations, which was inconvenient for the end users. The limitations concerning accuracy and battery life coincide with technical limitations noted in other studies [5, 11, 14, 20, 25] and are expected to improve gradually. However, accurate location positioning using BLE may not be easily solved due to the frequency hopping of the BLE beacon [26]. Therefore, each site will be required to develop solutions to these issues as they arise. In addition, given the recent expansion of services based on wireless communication, and considering the interference caused by each signal, a more suitable method should be used to track assets [22, 23, 27].

Design of the active tags

We developed the BLE/WiFi-based tags because the target assets did not include a signal-sensing function. However, this increased the size of the tags, which reduced their adhesive power and led to the loss of some tags. This occurred because we ultimately selected non-rechargeable AA batteries during the production process to increase the duration of the battery replacement cycle (i.e., lithium polymer [26 × 35 × 15 mm] and alkaline or manganese [AA size of 66 × 40 × 25 mm] batteries last for 20 and 100 days, respectively), and to ensure greater management efficiency. Although tag loss disrupted the continuity of asset tracking and incurred ongoing costs, the prioritization of battery capacity over tag size was unavoidable considering the long-term management efficiency. Because of this inverse relationship between the efficiency of the tag size and management, the needs of the site and the organization's policy standards should be established and reflected in the production and introduction of the active tags.

System functionality and usability

The interface used in the asset tracking system was integrated with the hospital information system, which allowed the end user to use the system while checking patient records. However, after 3 months of pilot use, the end users required a function to modify the names of assets since we displayed the names that were managed by the logistics department with a read-only mode for end users. This function could be integrated into the interface easily and would probably increase user satisfaction. Notably, the emergency room nurses' satisfaction levels were considerably lower than those of nurses at the other sites, despite the higher location accuracy in the emergency room, which contained 53 beacons, while each storage room in the ICUs and wards contained a single beacon. It seems that the emergency room nurses had a higher expectation and a higher need initially, resulting in low satisfaction due to the accuracy problem. Okoniewska et al. also suggested that the RTLS system should improve the accuracy of location tracking and visualization in response to the converging opinions of nurses [20]. Furthermore, regarding the patients' satisfaction with the patient tracking system, Stubig et al. found that their satisfaction improved when the medical staff also used the location information compared to when their location information was only tracked [11].

Education and operational support

Users reported that sufficient support would be needed to improve the approachability and efficiency of the system. Educational efforts and a larger management workforce would be major factors in providing this support [20]. In addition, it would be necessary to supply sufficient information regarding the system operation and to provide appropriate education to ensure its smooth use. In addition, workforce support is required to ensure timely battery replacement (for the beacon and tags). In the present study, end users were not required to replace the batteries themselves because it was unnecessary during the 3-month pilot period, and the study was conducted during the maintenance period of the system development. However, these issues will require consideration in future; therefore, end users should be provided with the necessary information regarding battery replacement [20].

Limitations

The main limitations of the present study were that it was conducted in a single medical institution, and the study design excluded the general outpatient environment. In addition, the tracking method was limited to WiFi and Bluetooth, and only some of the assets were tracked, which did not allow maximization of the benefits of tracking the assets used by nurses. Future research should be conducted in consideration of the issues highlighted in the present study. Moreover, future studies should not only involve the collection of data regarding end users' subjective experiences but also include usability tests and time-motion studies.

Conclusions

The results of the study demonstrated that BLE/WiFi-based asset tracking systems are needed in medical organizations and that they are helpful for nursing work. However, several technical and managerial issues were identified and should be addressed to ensure effortless use of the system and improve user convenience. In addition, the development and introduction of an asset tracking system in consideration of the lessons learned from the present study is required.

Abbreviations

AP: Access point; BLE: Bluetooth Low Energy; ICU: Intensive care unit; RFID: Radio-frequency identification; RTLS: Real-time location system

Funding

This work was supported by the Information Technology Research and Development program at Seoul National University Bundang Hospital and SK Telecom.

Authors' contributions

SY and S designed the study and wrote the manuscript. EK, EJ, and KL contributed to the data categorization and analysis. H contributed to the discussion and reviewed the manuscript. All authors read and approved the final manuscript.

Competing interests

The authors declare that they have no competing interests.

Author details

[1]Office of eHealth Research and Businesses, Seoul National University Bundang Hospital, 166, Gumi-ro, Bundang-gu, Seongnam-si 436-707, South Korea. [2]Nursing Department, Seoul National University Bundang Hospital, 166, Gumi-ro, Bundang-gu, Seongnam-si 436-707, South Korea.

References

1. Castro L, Lefebvre E, Lefebvre LA. Adding intelligence to mobile asset management in hospitals: the true value of RFID. J Med Syst. 2013;37(5):9963.
2. Gastaldi L, Mangiaracina R, Miragliotta G, Perego A, Tumino A. Measuring the benefits of tracking medical treatment through RFId. Int J Product Perform Manag. 2015;64(2):175–93.
3. Roper KO, Sedehi A, Ashuri B. A cost-benefit case for RFID implementation in hospitals: adapting to industry reform. Facilities. 2015;33(5/6):367–88.
4. Sato K, Kuroda T, Seiyama A. Visualization and quantitative analysis of nursing staff trajectories based on a location system. In: Innovation in medicine and healthcare 2015: Springer; 2016. p. 25–35.
5. Fisher JA, Monahan T. Evaluation of real-time location systems in their hospital contexts. Int J Med Inform. 2012;81(10):705–12.
6. Hopkins CW. Measuring leadership rounding performance in a hospital environment using real time location systems. Greenville: East Carolina University; 2015.
7. Jones TL, Schlegel C. Can real time location system technology (RTLS) provide useful estimates of time use by nursing personnel? Research in nursing & health. 2014;37(1):75–84.
8. Prathiba SA, Jain D: Hospital Management System Using RFID. 2015.
9. Stubig T, Suero E, Zeckey C, Min W, Janzen L, Citak M, Krettek C, Hufner T, Gaulke R. Improvement in the workflow efficiency of treating non-emergency outpatients by using a WLAN-based real-time location system in a level I trauma center. J. Am. Med. Inform. Assoc. 2013;20(6):1132–6.
10. Ward DR, Ghali WA, Graham A, Lemaire JB. A real-time locating system observes physician time-motion patterns during walk-rounds: a pilot study. BMC medical education. 2014;14:37.
11. Stubig T, Zeckey C, Min W, Janzen L, Citak M, Krettek C, Hufner T, Gaulke R. Effects of a WLAN-based real time location system on outpatient contentment in a level I trauma center. Int J Med Inform. 2014;83(1):19–26.
12. Cagle R, Darling E, Kim B. Identifying healthcare activities using a real-time location system. J. Med. Pract. Manage. 2014;30(2):128–30.
13. Fernandez-Llatas C, Lizondo A, Monton E, Benedi JM, Traver V. Process mining methodology for health process tracking using real-time indoor location systems. Sensors (Basel). 2015;15(12):29821–40.
14. Kamel Boulos MN, Berry G. Real-time locating systems (RTLS) in healthcare: a condensed primer. Int J Health Geogr. 2012;11:25.
15. Li J: Just-in-time Management in Healthcare Operations. 2015.
16. Wamba SF, Ngai EW. Importance of the relative advantage of RFID as enabler of asset management in the healthcare: results from a Delphi study. In: System Science (HICSS), 2012 45th Hawaii International Conference on: 2012: IEEE; 2012. p. 2879–89.
17. Voshall B, Piscotty R, Lawrence J, Targosz M. Barcode medication administration work-arounds: a systematic review and implications for nurse executives. J. Nurs. Adm. 2013;43(10):530–5.
18. Dimitrov DV. Medical internet of things and big data in healthcare. Healthcare informatics research. 2016;22(3):156–63.
19. Baek M, Koo BK, Kim BJ, Hong KR, Kim J, Yoo S, Hwang H, Seo J, Kim D, Shin K. Development and utilization of a patient-oriented outpatient guidance system. Healthcare informatics research. 2016;22(3):172–7.
20. Okoniewska B, Graham A, Gavrilova M, Wah D, Gilgen J, Coke J, Burden J, Nayyar S, Kaunda J, Yergens D, et al. Multidimensional evaluation of a radio frequency identification wi-fi location tracking system in an acute-care hospital setting. J. Am. Med. Inform. Assoc. 2012;19(4):674–9.
21. Dardari D, Closas P, Djurić PM: Indoor tracking: theory, methods, and technologies. IEEE Transactions on Vehicular Technology 2015, 64(4): 1263–1278.
22. Yearp A, Newell D, Davies P, Wade R, Sahandi R. Wireless remote patient monitoring system: effects of interference. In: Innovative Mobile and Internet Services in Ubiquitous Computing (IMIS), 2016 10th International Conference on: 2016: IEEE; 2016. p. 367–70.
23. Frisby J, Smith V, Traub S, Patel VL. Contextual computing: a Bluetooth based approach for tracking healthcare providers in the emergency room. J Biomed Inform. 2017;65:97–104.
24. Yoo S, Jung SY, Kim S, Kim E, Lee KH, Chung E, Hwang H. A personalized mobile patient guide system for a patient-centered smart hospital: lessons learned from a usability test and satisfaction survey in a tertiary university hospital. Int J Med Inform. 2016;91:20–30.
25. No-authors. Asset tracking systems. Health devices. 2006;35(11):397–419.
26. Faragher R, Harle R. An analysis of the accuracy of bluetooth low energy for indoor positioning applications. In: Proceedings of the 27th international technical meeting of the satellite division of the Institute of Navigation (ION GNSS+'14): 2014; 2014. p. 201–10.
27. Hurstel J, Guivarc'h M, Pommel L, Camps J, Tassery H, Cohen S, Bukiet F. Do cell phones affect establishing electronic working length? J Endod. 2015; 41(6):943–6.

Discovering and identifying New York heart association classification from electronic health records

Rui Zhang[1,2*], Sisi Ma[1,3], Liesa Shanahan[4], Jessica Munroe[4], Sarah Horn[4] and Stuart Speedie[1]

Abstract

Background: Cardiac Resynchronization Therapy (CRT) is an established pacing therapy for heart failure patients. The New York Heart Association (NYHA) class is often used as a measure of a patient's response to CRT. Identifying NYHA class for heart failure (HF) patients in an electronic health record (EHR) consistently, over time, can provide better understanding of the progression of heart failure and assessment of CRT response and effectiveness. Though NYHA is rarely stored in EHR structured data, such information is often documented in unstructured clinical notes.

Methods: We accessed HF patients' data in a local EHR system and identified potential sources of NYHA, including local diagnosis codes, procedures, and clinical notes. We further investigated and compared the performances of rule-based versus machine learning-based natural language processing (NLP) methods to identify NYHA class from clinical notes.

Results: Of the 36,276 patients with a diagnosis of HF or a CRT implant, 19.2% had NYHA class mentioned at least once in their EHR. While NYHA class existed in descriptive fields association with diagnosis codes (31%) or procedure codes (2%), the richest source of NYHA class was clinical notes (95%). A total of 6174 clinical notes were matched with hospital-specific custom NYHA class diagnosis codes. Machine learning-based methods outperformed a rule-based method. The best machine-learning method was a random forest with *n*-gram features (F-measure: 93.78%).

Conclusions: NYHA class is documented in different parts in EHR for HF patients and the documentation rate is lower than expected. NLP methods are a feasible way to extract NYHA class information from clinical notes.

Keywords: Clinical notes, Electronic health records, New York heart association (NYHA), Natural language processing

Background

Heart Failure (HF) is a progressive condition associated with high morbidity and mortality rates. Approximately 8% of the population in developed countries over the age of 75 [1] is affected by HF. The estimated 5.7 million Americans with heart failure account for more than 1 million hospital admissions annually [2]. Cardiac Resynchronization Therapy (CRT) is an established pacing therapy for patients with HF. Despite multiple clinical trials demonstrating the safety and efficacy of CRT, an estimated 25–30% of CRT patients do not experience clinical benefits [3–5].

Patient response to CRT is often measured using a composite score of several clinical outcomes, including mortality, heart failure hospitalization, ejection fraction (EF) measurements, and New York Heart Association (NYHA) functional classification [4–7]. NYHA class (I-IV) is a system for evaluating the severity of functional limitations from a patient's heart failure condition (Table 1) [5]. Classification is based on the symptoms a patient experiences during activity and is

* Correspondence: zhan1386@umn.edu
[1]Institute for Health Informatics, University of Minnesota, Minneapolis, MN, USA
[2]College of Pharmacy, University of Minnesota, Minneapolis, MN, USA
Full list of author information is available at the end of the article

Table 1 Definition of NYHA classification. (adapted from [14])

NYHA Class	Patient Symptoms
I	No limitation of physical activity. Ordinary physical activity does not cause undue fatigue, palpitation, dyspnea (shortness of breath).
II	Slight limitation of physical activity. Comfortable at rest. Ordinary physical activity results in fatigue, palpitation, dyspnea (shortness of breath).
III	Marked limitation of physical activity. Comfortable at rest. Less than ordinary activity causes fatigue, palpitation, or dyspnea.
IV	Unable to carry on any physical activity without discomfort. Symptoms of heart failure at rest. If any physical activity is undertaken, discomfort increases.

most often documented in clinical dictation/notes thereby limiting computational access.

Electronic health record systems are primarily designed to support the process of clinical care and billing for the services provided and contain both structured and unstructured clinical data. Some of the information such as diagnoses, procedures, or medications exists in the form of standard codes such as International Classification of Diseases, Ninth and Tenth Revision (ICD9/ ICD10), Current Procedural Terminology (CPT) or RxNorm (a normalized name system for generic and branded drugs from the National Library of Medicine) which have nationally agreed upon meanings. Typically, such systems also support structured information in the form of local codes that have been created for internal use by the organization supporting the EHR. In addition to structured data, most EHRs contain clinical notes created during clinical care to document detailed patient information for billing and communication purposes. Such unstructured clinical notes are another source of valuable information that often goes well beyond the structured EHR data in characterizing patients' medical conditions. However, as they are intended for human use rather than computational analysis, it is a considerable challenge to extract information for the purpose of secondary analyses or clinical research.

Identifying NYHA class from clinical notes in an EHR system in a systematic way could change clinical practice in several ways. Capturing NYHA class consistently over time may inform a better understanding of the progression of HF to assess CRT effectiveness and its benefit-risk profile versus other therapies and how to improve the response rate and effectiveness of CRT. A patient's NYHA class assessment over time provides the potential to better understand why some patients benefit from CRT while others do not [3–5]. Additionally, if NYHA class can be reliably derived from other EHR values, it may provide more consistent and objective measure of an HF patient's functional status. In our prior study [8], we have demonstrated the feasibility of leveraging NLP techniques to extract NYHA class from clinical notes.

To the best of our knowledge, there has been no study investigating the sources of NYHA class in the EHRs and assessing the data availability for NYHA class pre- and post-implant of CRT devices. We further improved the performance of NLP algorithms, comparing with our prior work, to extract specific outcome data (NYHA class) for patients with a CRT device from electronic health records. This study explores the possibility of monitoring CRT effectiveness as measured by NYHA class more efficiently and potentially improve health care for HF patients.

Methods

Data sources

The patient population for this study was drawn from clinical data documented between December 1, 2011 and January 1, 2016 by Fairview Health Services (FHS). Data containing approximately 2.6 million patients extracted from FHS's EHR resides in a Clinical Data Repository (CDR) maintained by the University of Minnesota Academic Health Center.

Study overview

As shown in Fig. 1, we undertook the following steps to execute this study: 1) retrieved EHR data for heart failure patients; 2) identified sources of NYHA classifications; 3) selected local diagnosis codes that corresponded to an NYHA classification; 4) retrieved clinical notes with explicit mentions of NYHA; 5) collected a subset of clinical notes as reference standard; 6) developed and evaluated NLP methods. We will describe each step, in detail below.

Retrieving EHR for heart failure patients

In this study, we focused on a heart failure patient cohort identified using diagnosis codes associated with a heart failure. All patients who had at least one diagnosis of heart failure (as defined by the list of International Classification of Diseases, Ninth and Tenth Revisions (i.e., ICD9 and ICD10 codes) in Table 2 were included. Associated with each encounter were age at encounter, ICD9 or ICD10 encoded diagnoses, local coding that informed the standard diagnostic codes, procedures with associated narrative comments, and clinical notes. The resultant information was organized into a datamart of related tables within the secure environment that were employed to carry out the research activities for the above objectives. All start dates were approximate and depended on the date for the adoption of the EHR at each particular site.

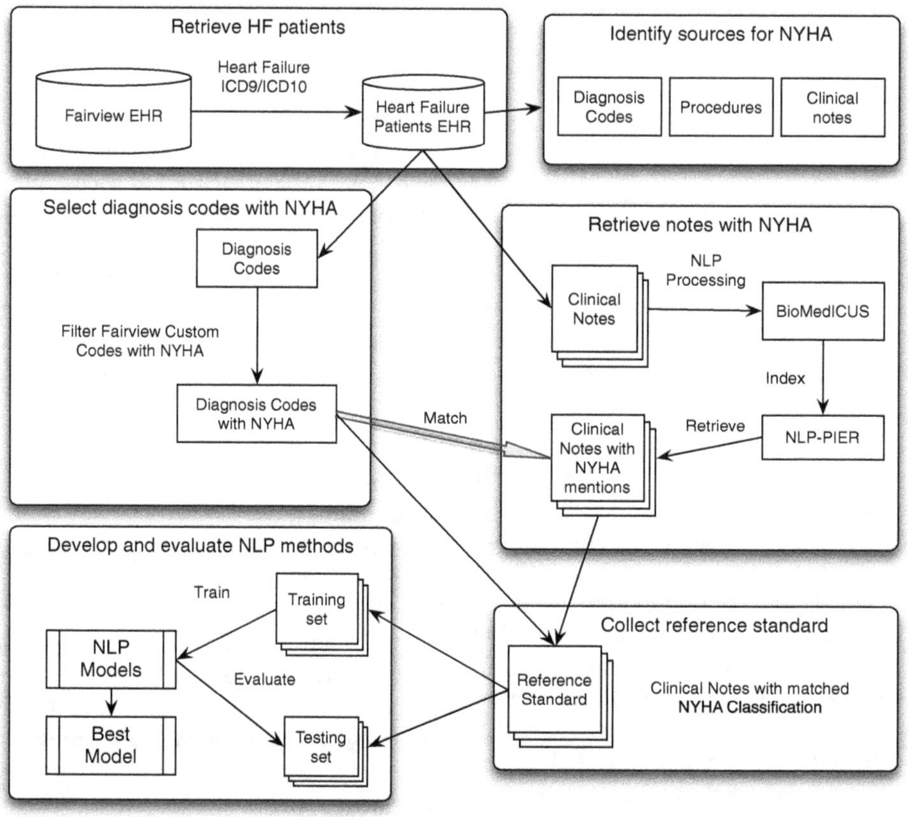

Fig. 1 Overview of methodology

Identifying sources of NYHA classifications

The first step in the process was to investigate the possible sources of NYHA Class within the datamart. This involved a systematic search for explicit mentions of NYHA Class in the custom diagnostic codes' descriptive names, both local and standard, as well as in all the descriptive information (such as "Narratives") associated with procedures and observations. Any mention of NYHA class or its synonyms (e.g., New York Heart Association, etc.) was noted. The availabilities of NYHA class in the various EHR data sources were compared. All sources of NYHA class were identified and characterized in terms of frequency of occurrence. Furthermore, since NYHA Class is often used as a clinical outcome measure for CRT patients, its availability for these patients over a five-year timespan was also examined. The subset of patients who had a CRT implant and at least one NYHA Class was used for the purpose of developing a model for estimating NYHA Class for a patient encounter from structured data available from the EHR for that encounter.

Table 2 A list of diagnosis codes for identifying health failure patients

ICD Revisions	ICD codes
ICD9	398. 91, 428. *, 402. 01, 402. 11, 402. 91, 404. 01, 404. 03, 404. 11, 404. 13, 404. 91, 404. 93, 428. 1–428. 4, 428. 9
ICD10	I11. 0, I13. 0, I13. 2, I50. 1-I50. 4, I50. 9, I97. 13, I50. 4, I50. 9

Selecting diagnosis codes with NYHA classification

To collect NYHA class labels, we selected patients having encounters associated with Fairview custom diagnosis codes with NYHA information. Such Fairview custom codes, with labels like "Congestive heart failure with left ventricular diastolic dysfunction, NYHA class 3 (H)" indicated a NYHA classification III in this case. These local custom code strings with NYHA information were extracted and mapped to the corresponding NYHA classification (I – IV) based on the statements in the code names.

Retrieving clinical notes with NYHA mentions

To collect the corpus of text notes for this study, the NLP web-based search engine, Patient Information Extraction from Researchers (PIER) [9] was used to search clinical notes containing NYHA concepts. Before the searching, clinical notes in the CDR were first processed by BioMedICUS (BioMedical Information Collection and Understanding System) [10], which is an NLP system based on the Unstructured Information Management Architecture – Asynchronous Scaleout (UIMA-AS) architecture. BioMedICUS identifies Unified Medical Language System (UMLS) Metathesaurus concepts associated with a note that are stored in an Elasticsearch cluster along with the source note itself. This allows PIER to search notes through UMLS concept unique identifiers (CUIs) or keywords for NYHA. To retrieve clinical notes with NYHA mentions, we searched for the CUIs listed in Fig. 2 that were obtained using the UMLS Metathesarus browser. We also conducted keyword searching using "New York heart association", "NYHA", "New York heart classification", "NY classification", "NY class" to cover the lexical variations for NYHA.

Developing a reference standard

We refer the reference standard as the clinical notes with their associated NYHA classes. To create such a NYHA reference standard to train and evaluate the NLP algorithms, we matched the clinical notes that were documented to encounters with at least one Fairview NYHA Class diagnosis code (where NYHA class can be determined) for the same patient and same date. It is assumed that the notes should mention the same NYHA classification as associated NYHA Fairview diagnosis code within a single patient encounter. We then assigned the NYHA class associated with Fairview custom codes to the clinical notes in the same encounter. The notes with the assigned NYHA as labels were selected as a reference standard for developing and evaluating our NLP methods. A total of 6174 clinical notes with an associated NYHA classification were obtained.

Developing NLP methods to identify NYHA classes in clinical notes

To select the best method, we evaluated and compared a rule-based method with machine learning-based methods to extract NYHA class from clinical notes. We split the corpus into 3700 notes as a training data set and 2474 notes as a testing set.

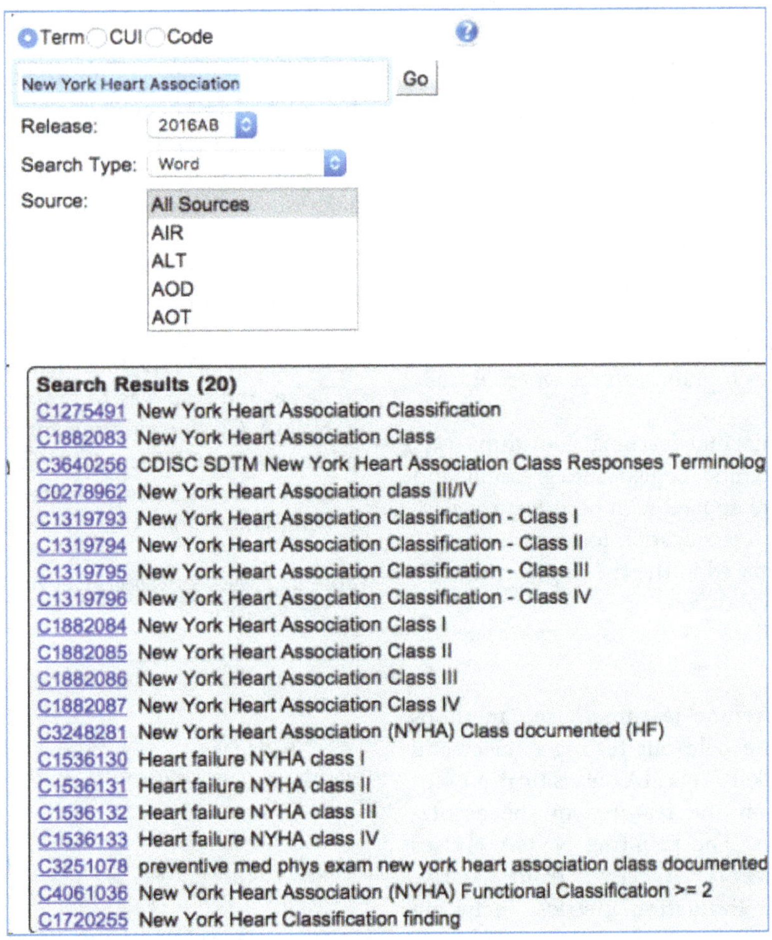

Fig. 2 UMLS CUIs associated with NYHA classification used for retrieving clinical notes

Rule-based method

Rules were created by iteratively reviewing the notes to discover patterns. The training set was used to refine the patterns to capture most expressions for NYHA classes. Co-occurring NYHA classes such as "NYHA II/III" were also recognized. Listed below are summarizations of the patterns to identify classifications that appeared within 40 characters after a NYHA string such as "NY class":

- Single digit 1, 2, 3, and 4;
- Single Roman numeral I, II, III, and IV;
- Two digits or Roman numerals (between range 1 to 4, inclusive), separated by single character '-' or '/'. Space can be inserted/omitted between characters. Only patterns related to two contingency classes, such as NYHA 1–2 and NYHA II–III, were considered.

Machine learning-based methods

Clinical notes were pre-processed and features were generated. Details in each step are described below:

- The classic stopwords [11] (such as "of", "as") were removed from the texts. This step deemphasizes these less important words for building the model.
- To normalize lexically different forms of the same term as equivalent, lexical variant generation (LVG) was used.
- The words based on their term frequency in the corpus were ranked. The words within the lowest 1% of the rank were discarded. This step removes the least frequently used words from the model development process.
- Feature set 1 includes "bag-of-words" features.
- Feature set 2 includes n-gram features where n was from 2 to 5.
- Three widely used machine learning algorithms (Support Vector Machine, Logistical Regression, and Random Forest) were applied with both feature sets to determine NYHA classification for each encounter, and compared in the training corpus using 10-fold cross validation.

Evaluation

Both rule-based and machine learning-based methods were applied to the same held-out testing dataset and generated the most likely NYHA classification for each encounter based on the features in the associated set of clinical notes. The resulting NYHA classes were compared with the NYHA classes from the reference standard corpus. Evaluation metrics, including precision, recall, and F-measure, were used for each class and overall NYHA class assignment for three machine learning methods with each of the two features sets.

Results

Identifying sources of NYHA classifications

Examination of the datamart data elements revealed that there was one structured data item that contained NYHA class information. That was the local diagnosis code that was generated in the system and used to determine the standard ICD9/ICD10 diagnosis code. There was a total of 260 such codes associated with ICD9/ICD10 codes for HF. A typical code description was "CHF (NYHA class III, ACC/AHA stage C) (H)". A second source of NYHA Class information was in the Impression/Narrative field associated with procedures. These fields were examined with a straightforward string searching approach to identify NYHA information. No NYHA Class information was found in the table of observations. The most productive source of information about NYHA class was the clinical note.

We initially identified 36,276 patients that met the inclusion criteria (a diagnosis of HF or evidence of a CRT device). 35,900 of those had a HF diagnosis and 376 had evidence of a CRT without a HF diagnosis. Descriptive statistics for various patient cohorts was summarized in Table 3. In addition, The NYHA Class sources and frequencies results per patient are summarized in Fig. 3. Among all three resources, the richest information was from clinical notes (95.6%) as opposed to diagnosis local codes (31.3%) and narrative filed with procedures (2.1%). There are few patients (0.6%) who can be identified from all three resources. NYHA class was available for 6907 patients with a HF diagnosis, i.e., 19.2% of all HF patients. Those with a CRT device had a 72.9% rate of NYHA documentation per patient.

The second step was to examine the documentation of an NYHA Class over time for a group of patients who had received a CRT implant. The group consisted of 696 patients with 51,138 encounters over a five-year period post-implant. Table 4 summarized the frequency of this

Table 3 Statisics for various patient cohorts

Cohort definition	Number of patients
Patients who have a diagnosis of HF or evidence of a CRT device	32,276
Patinets who have a HF diagnosis	35,900
Patients who have evidence of a CRT device without a HF diagnosis	376
Patients with a HF diagnois having NYHA mentions	6907
Patients who have evicence of a CRT device (with or without a HF diagnosis) and NYHA mentions	696
Patients who have NYHA mentions in clinical notes and corresponding local diagnosis codes	1370

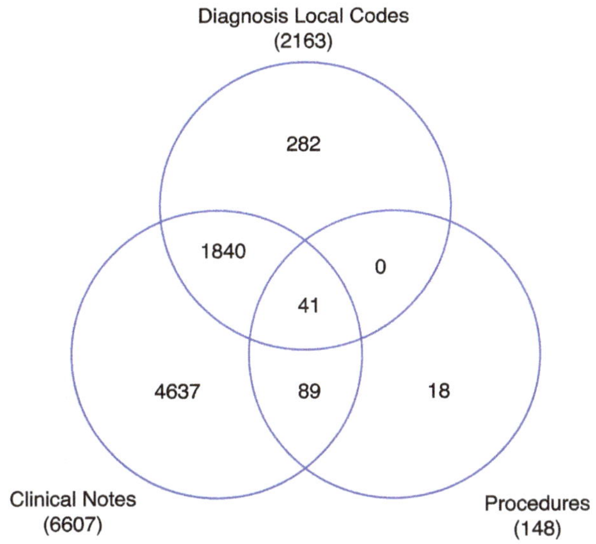

Fig. 3 Overlap of number of patients for various NYHA classification sources in the EHR

documentation before and after implantation. The percentage of patients with at least one instance of a documented NYHA class ranged from 51.6% for the pre-implant period to 30.0% for year 5 post implant. The proportion of encounters with an associated NYHA Class remained fairly similar over the post-implant years (range: 16.7 to 25.5%). As expected both the number of CRT patients and their instances of NYHA Classification declined over time likely due to both the patient survival rate and to movement to other health care organizations. The observed lower rate of NYHA Class per encounter in the pre-implant period was quite possibly due to the larger number of encounters during that period.

Evaluating NLP methods to identify NYHA classification from clinical notes

A total of 6174 clinical notes from 6039 encounters for 1370 patients was obtained as reference standard. Table 5 lists the distribution of NYHA classes in the entire corpus as well as the training and testing sets. Overall, NYHA class II had the largest proportion (22%) and class IV the smallest (8%).

The rule-based method performed well overall (F-measure: 93.54%), with its performance varying from the lowest of 86.16% for Class IV to the highest of 96.41% for Class II (See Table 6). The best machine learning-based method random forest with *n*-gram features (overall F-measure: 93.78%) slightly outperformed the rule-based method and significantly outperformed those with bag-of-word features (Table 7). The performance is slightly lower than its performance (F-measure: 96.0%) in the training set using 10-fold cross validation. This is also a better performance compared with our prior work [8]. We also compared the various n-grams ranges and found the best performance with the features from bigram to five-grams (Fig. 4). On both feature sets, the random forest method performed the best among three machine learning algorithms. The F-measures for extracting NYHA class I, II and III are over 92% with respect to the reference standard for both rule-based and machine learning-based methods with *n*-gram features. Table 8 lists the top bag-of-words and *n*-gram features for those methods. For all methods, they were most accurate in identifying Class II and least in identifying Class IV.

Discussion

NYHA class for HF patients proved to be rather elusive. It was documented in heterogeneous types of data, including diagnostic local codes, clinical notes and the description component of procedures, none of which comprehensively documented NYHA class. Clinical notes appeared to be the best source for NYHA data in the EHR though local diagnostic information identified approximately 27% more patients with NYHA documentation. Extraction of NYHA class from unstructured notes required significant NLP data analysis and we demonstrate the feasibility and accuracy of using such methods to automatically identify existing NYHA class in those notes.

We conclude that it is possible to retrieve a significant amount of NYHA class information for HF patients from the EHR using a combination of clinical notes and local diagnosis codes. The use of local diagnosis codes is somewhat problematic as it is not a particularly generalizable approach across EHRs. However, the extent to which the overlap between clinical notes and the local diagnostic codes is driven by the coding process of Health Information Management coding specialists may

Table 4 NYHA documentation over time for CRT patients

	Pre Implant	Post Implant				
		Year 1	Year 2	Year 3	Year 4	Year 5
CRT Patients	696	600	485	405	310	212
CRT Patients with NYHA Class	51.6%	35.7%	27.4%	25.3%	24.6%	30.0%
Encounters	11,844	5550	3984	3171	2174	1740
Encounters with NYHA Class	10.5%	25.5%	18.3%	16.7%	19.9%	20.7%

Table 5 Number of clinical notes in training and testing set

NYHA Classification	Training Set	Testing Set	Total
I	843	524	1367
II	1506	996	2502
III	1045	745	1790
IV	306	209	515
Total	3700	2474	6174

serve as a guidepost to further extraction of NYHA Class from notes.

The overall rate of NYHA Class documentation for HF patients was slightly less than 1 in five (19%). The American College of Cardiology recommends that "NYHA Class should occur at each office visit to quantify the degree of functional limitation imposed by HF" [12]. It is obvious that the documentation rate falls far short of this recommendation for the population of HF patients in this study. While there are numerous possible reasons why NYHA Class might be missing including patient attrition from the health system and documentation in locations other than the EHR, it is certainly possible that providers are not yet consistently following this recommendation. Further investigation of this observation is required.

As was expected, NYHA class was documented with a much higher frequency in CRT patients. Almost four out of every five (79.2%) of these patients had at least one instance of an NYHA class recorded. Examination of the pre-implant period when it was available indicated that about half of the patients (51.9%) had an NYHA class documented prior to the date of implant. Through manual inspection we observed that this did not always occur during the encounter in which the implant was performed. This higher rate is to be expected as a NYHA class is one of the factors used to determine the need for CRT as well as a measure of effectiveness once the implant takes place. Yet the rate still falls short of the expected 100% for these patients. While there are a range of explanations similar to those for the general HF population, further investigation is required.

The more detailed examination of the rate of NYHA Class documentation over time revealed that it remained fairly constant over the five-year time span post-implant at a rate of approximately 16–25% of annual patient encounters. Since these encounters were limited to those identified as "face-to-face" encounters with clinicians, it is reasonable to assume that they would provide opportunities for documenting NYHA class. We did observe an expected decline

Table 6 Performance of rule-based method

NYHA Classification	Precision	Recall	F-Measure
I	95.07%	97.39%	96.21%
II	95.72%	97.10%	96.41%
III	94.34%	95.07%	94.70%
IV	94.83%	78.95%	86.16%
Overall	94.99%	92.13%	*93.54%*

Italics indicate the best performance

Table 7 Performances of machine learning-based methods

NYHA Classification	Precision	Recall	F-Measure
Feature Set 1: bag-of-words			
Support Vector Machine			
I	84.71%	82.06%	83.36%
II	88.30%	91.80%	90.01%
III	88.34%	88.46%	88.40%
IV	80.00%	70.81%	75.13%
Overall	85.34%	83.28%	84.23%
Logistic Regression			
I	83.61%	79.97%	81.75%
II	86.87%	91.99%	89.36%
III	87.66%	88.46%	88.06%
IV	80.72%	64.11%	71.47%
Overall	84.72%	81.13%	82.66%
Random Forest			
I	87.54%	86.93%	87.24%
II	91.23%	94.40%	92.79%
III	91.83%	90.40%	91.11%
IV	79.89%	72.25%	75.88%
Overall	87.63%	86.00%	86.75%
Feature Set 2: n-gram			
Support Vector Machine			
I	95.05%	93.73%	94.39%
II	95.71%	96.81%	96.26%
III	94.95%	95.20%	95.08%
IV	89.66%	87.08%	88.35%
Overall	93.84%	93.21%	93.52%
Logistic Regression			
I	93.09%	91.46%	92.27%
II	94.74%	95.66%	95.20%
III	93.12%	94.81%	93.96%
IV	87.18%	81.34%	84.16%
Overall	90.03%	90.82%	90.42%
Random Forest			
I	97.02%	96.52%	96.77%
II	97.58%	97.49%	97.54%
III	93.01%	96.63%	94.78%
IV	93.99%	82.30%	87.76%
Overall	95.40%	92.23%	93.78%

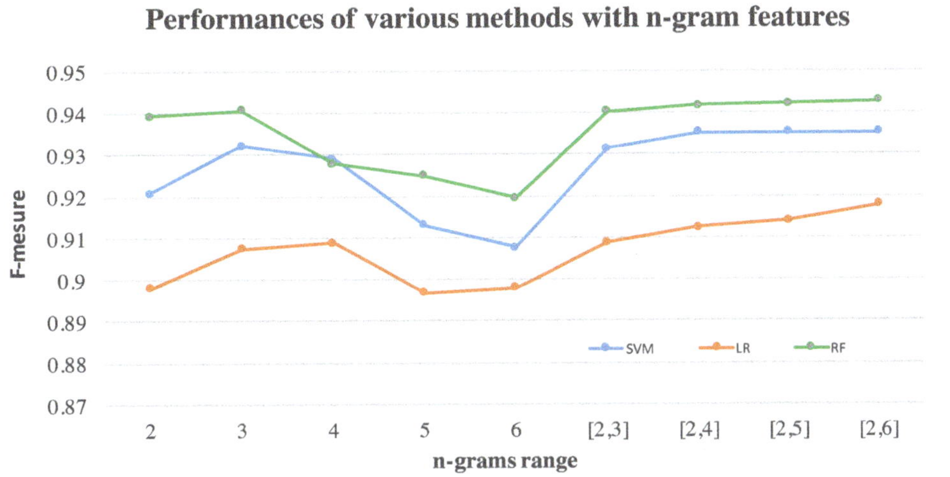

Fig. 4 Performance comparison of machine learning methods with various n-gram ranges. Notes: [2, 5] indicates the n-grams feature where range for *n* is from 2 to 5

in the numbers of CRT patients with encounters over the five-year period certainly due in part to the survival rate of CRT patients which has been reported as a median of 6–8 years [13], but also quite possibly due to patients leaving the health system for a variety of non-clinical reasons. It is important to note that we did not distinguish between encounters with cardiologists and other clinical specialties including primary care. It is possible and reasonable that the documentation rate was higher for cardiology encounters than for other specialists which would at least partially account for the lower than expected overall rate for encounters.

Table 8 Top 15 n-gram features from feature sets 1 and 2

Rank	Feature set 1: Bag of words	Feature set 2: n-grams
1	ii	nyha class ii
2	iii	class ii
3	iv	nyha class iii
4	b	class iii
5	428.0dd	nyha class iv
6	428.0db	class iv
7	chf	nyha class ii
8	congestive	nyha class 2
9	428.0 dc	nyha class 3
10	lvad	class
11	systolic	chf
12	diastolic	class 3
13	428.0bm	class 2
14	c	congestive heart failure
15	stage	nyha class

Applying NLP algorithms to those associated notes indicated that for over 95% of the encounters where NYHA was mentioned in the clinical notes, it matched the custom code NYHA class. This is to be expected given that these local diagnosis codes were assigned by experts after they reviewed clinical notes. Similar to the rule-based method, machine learning-based methods performed well on NYHA class I-III. Performance of machine learning-based algorithms with *n*-grams performed better, due to the fact that bag-of-word features miss the ordering information of words like *n*-grams. With such context information, the performance generally improved about 8%. The smaller proportion (only 8%) of NYHA class IV mentions, compared with other NYHA classes that were better represented in the dataset, may have led to a lower performance on both NLP methods for this class. Further investigation is needed to identify other possible reasons for the low recall for class IV.

After carefully reviewing some wrongly identified instances, we found two categories of error. One was from the cases where the NYHA class was ambiguous, such as "NYHA 1 or 2". The rules only allowed the contiguous classes with the AND logic link, such as "NYHA 1–2". Some NYHA mentions were not a diagnosis statement, but from the section of recommendation or history. Our method currently cannot differentiate between historical NYHA class and current NYHA class in the notes. Our reference standard is built from the local diagnosis codes on the same encounter, which usually reflect the current NYHA classes during the encounter.

There are limitations which need further investigation. We focused solely on a matched set of notes and NYHA local codes for the same patients. The generalizability of algorithms across the larger and more varied body of clinical notes available in a typical EHR will need further validation, although the machine learning models with *n*-gram features perform exceptionally well. Further work employing NLP techniques with notes in which NYHA class is not explicitly identified may well lead to a higher rate of identification based on other relevant data in those notes. Information relating to NYHA class was also found in various text-based comment fields throughout the record. Future work would include those text fields to explore their value in further improving the performance of the NLP model.

Conclusions

NYHA classification is not well-documented in structured data but rich NYHA information is stored in unstructured clinical notes. We developed a rule-based method and compared it to machine learning methods to identify NYHA class I-IV from those notes. The Random Forest method with n-gram features performed best in identifying NYHA I-III Class. Further validation of these results and methods is required.

Abbreviations

CDR: clinical data repository; CRT: Cardiac Resynchronization Therapy; EHR: electronic health records; FHS: Fairview Health Services; HF: heart failure; NLP: natural language processing; NYHA: New York heart association

Acknowledgments

The clinical data was provided by the University of Minnesota's Clinical Translational Science Institute (CTSI) Informatics Consulting Service. The authors thank John Herre, MD of Cardiology and Electrophysiology, Sentara Norfolk General Hospital, Norfolk Virginia for providing clinical expertise, Gretchen Sieger and CTSI Best Practice Informatics Consulting (BPIC) team for their data support for this study.

Funding

This research and publication of this article were supported by the Medtronic, Inc.

Authors' contributions

RZ, SM, and SS conceived the study idea and design, and retrieved the data. All authors participated in writing and reviewed the manuscript. All authors read and approved the final manuscript.

Authors' information

Described in the title page.

Competing interests

The authors declare that they have no competing interests.

Author details

[1]Institute for Health Informatics, University of Minnesota, Minneapolis, MN, USA. [2]College of Pharmacy, University of Minnesota, Minneapolis, MN, USA. [3]Department of Medicine, University of Minnesota, Minneapolis, MN, USA. [4]Medtronic, Inc., Minneapolis, MN, USA.

References

1. Redfield MM, Jacobsen SJ, Burnett JC, Mahoney DW, Bailey KR, Rodeheffer RJ. Burden of systolic and diastolic ventricular dysfunction in the community: appreciating the scope of the heart failure epidemic. JAMA. 2003;289(2):194–202.
2. Mozaffarian D, Benjamin EJ, Go AS, Arnett DK, Blaha MJ, Cushman M, Das SR, de Ferranti S, Després JP, Fullerton HJ, et al. Heart disease and stroke Statistics-2016 update: a report from the American Heart Association. Circulation. 2016, 133(4):e38–360.
3. Ghio S, Freemantle N, Scelsi L, Serio A, Magrini G, Pasotti M, Shankar A, Cleland JG, Tavazzi L. Long-term left ventricular reverse remodelling with cardiac resynchronization therapy: results from the CARE-HF trial. Eur J Heart Fail. 2009;11(5):480–8.
4. Linde C, Gold MR, Abraham WT, St John Sutton M, Ghio S, Cerkvenik J, Daubert C, Group RrRiSlvdS. Long-term impact of cardiac resynchronization therapy in mild heart failure: 5-year results from the REsynchronization reVErses remodeling in systolic left vEntricular dysfunction (REVERSE) study. Eur Heart J. 2013;34(33):2592–9.
5. Packer M. Proposal for a new clinical end point to evaluate the efficacy of drugs and devices in the treatment of chronic heart failure. J Card Fail. 2001;7(2):176–82.
6. Zannad F, Garcia AA, Anker SD, Armstrong PW, Calvo G, Cleland JG, Cohn JN, Dickstein K, Domanski MJ, Ekman I, et al. Clinical outcome endpoints in heart failure trials: a European Society of Cardiology Heart Failure Association consensus document. Eur J Heart Fail. 2013;15(10):1082–94.
7. Neaton JD, Gray G, Zuckerman BD, Konstam MA. Key issues in end point selection for heart failure trials: composite end points. J Card Fail. 2005;11(8): 567–75.
8. Zhang R, Ma S, Munroe J, Horn S, Speedy S: Automatic methods to extract New York heart association classification from clinical notes. In: IEEE International conference on Bioinformatics and Biomedicine 2017: 1277–80.
9. McEwan R, Melton GB, Knoll B, Wang Y, Hultman G, Dale J, Meyer T, Pakhomov S. NLP-PIER: a scalable natural language processing, indexing, and searching architecture for clinical notes. AMIA Jt Summits Transl Informatics. 2016:150–9.
10. BioMedICUS [http://athena.ahc.umn.edu/biomedicus/index.jsp. Accessed 10 Jan 2018.
11. Stopword List. http://www.textfixer.com/resources/common-english-words.txt. Accessed 10 Jan 2018.
12. American College of Cardiology Toolkit. http://www.acc.org/tools-and-practice-support/clinical-toolkits/heart-failure-practice-solutions. Accessed 10 Jan 2018.
13. Gasparini M, Leclercq C, Yu CM, Auricchio A, Steinberg JS, Lamp B, Klersy C, Leyva F. Absolute survival after cardiac resynchronization therapy according to baseline QRS duration: a multinational 10-year experience: data from the Multicenter International CRT Study. Am Heart J. 2014;167(2):203–209.e201.
14. Dolgin M, Committee NYHAC. In: Dolgin M, editor. Nomenclature and criteria for diagnosis of diseases of the heart and great vessels. 9th ed. Boston: Little, Brown; 1994.

11

Leveraging text skeleton for de-identification of electronic medical records

Yue-Shu Zhao[1†], Kun-Li Zhang[2*†], Hong-Chao Ma[2*] and Kun Li[2]

Abstract

Background: De-identification is the first step to use these records for data processing or further medical investigations in electronic medical records. Consequently, a reliable automated de-identification system would be of high value.

Methods: In this paper, a method of combining text skeleton and recurrent neural network is proposed to solve the problem of de-identification. Text skeleton is the general structure of a medical record, which can help neural networks to learn better.

Results: We evaluated our method on three datasets involving two English datasets from i2b2 de-identification challenge and a Chinese dataset we annotated. Empirical results show that the text skeleton based method we proposed can help the network to recognize protected health information.

Conclusions: The comparison between our method and state-of-the-art frameworks indicates that our method achieves high performance on the problem of medical record de-identification.

Keywords: De-identification, Text skeleton, PHI

Background

Electronic Medical Records (EMRs), due to the large amount of information they contain, are valuable resources worth studying. However, because of the large number of Protected Health Information (PHI) existing in EMR, it is difficult for researchers or organizations to obtain these records. Therefore, de-identification of such records is an essential step for using EMRs outside hospitals. Figure 1 shows a sample record with private information, including name, age and record number of patients (highlighted in Fig. 1).

Dorr et al. [1] have evaluated the time cost to manually de-identify narrative text notes (87.2 ± 61 s per note). They concluded that the problem of de-identification was time-consuming. Therefore, a de-identification system is required to automatically detect the personal identifiers. Most of the state-of-the-art systems adopted heuristic or hand-made rules for improving the performance, but the rules are difficult to generalize.

In early 1996, a system named Scrub was proposed by Sweeney [2], through a rule-based approach to hide PHI. In the same year in United States, the Health Insurance Portability and Accountability Act (HIPAA) was passed, 18 categories of information, such as the patients names, ID numbers, dates, locations, etc., were defined within the scope of its protection and must be removed from the clinical data before it can be safely de-identified. Since then, many pattern-matching-based and data-driven systems have been introduced [3–6].

To accelerate automated de-identification research, a unified platform to evaluated different systems was firstly provided by the 2006 i2b2 de-identification challenge [7].

* Correspondence: ieklzhang@zzu.edu.cn; ma-hc@foxmail.com
[†]Equal contributors
[2]School of Information Engineering, Zhengzhou University, Science Avenue, Zhengzhou, Henan 450001, China
Full list of author information is available at the end of the article

Record date: **2060-10-11**

BCH EMERGENCY DEPT VISIT

HESS, CLARENCE **643-65-59-5** VISIT DATE: **10/11/60**

HISTORY OF PRESENTING COMPLAINT: The patient is a **46**

Fig. 1 A snippet of an EMR

In this challenge, eight PHI categories, Patients, Doctors, Hospitals, IDs, Dates, Locations, Phone numbers and Ages, were used to annotate Partner Healthcare data. The competing systems employed rule-based [8] and statistic-based methods. Some researchers considered the challenge as a problem of classification, while others considered it as a sequence labeling problem. These methods include Hidden Markov Models (HMM), Conditional Random Fields (CRFs) [9], Support Vector Machines (SVM) [10], and Decision Trees [11]. Compared with other researches, the results manifested that machine learning-based systems were the best [7].

Along with some recent studies [12], researchers reached an agreement that it is necessary to build a stricter standard than HIPAA. To achieve the goal, the 2014 i2b2 de-identification challenge for longitudinal clinical narratives focused on 25 PHI types, inclusive of 12 types as defined by HIPAA [13, 14]. Some well performing systems submitted to the 2014 i2b2 de-identification track, employed CRFs mixed with dictionaries and regular expressions [15–17].

Li et al. [18] introduced a Stackelberg game to balance risk and utility in EMRs de-identification, they believe their approach is a clear example of risk management approaches to medical data de-identification. Dernoncourt et al. [19] introduced the first de-identification system based on artificial neural network (ANN) and achieved state-of-the-art results on two English datasets.

In this paper, we propose a novel method, which has strong generalization ability, to figure out the de-identification challenge. The method combines text skeleton (TS) and recurrent neural network (RNN) to identify private information in EMRs. The framework, without any structure changed, does well on 2006 i2b2 de-identification challenge, 2014 i2b2 de-identification challenge and a Chinese EMRs dataset annotated by ourselves. The experimental results show that our method is competitive and outperforms the state-of-the-art frameworks at binary token-level. Specifically, the performance on two different i2b2 datasets as well as the Chinese dataset demonstrated an F-score of about 0.98 consistently.

Methods

Datasets

We evaluate our model on three datasets: two English datasets from the 2006 i2b2 [7] and the 2014 i2b2 [14] de-identification challenges, one Chinese dataset we annotate by ourselves. The Chinese EMRs come from a maternal and child health-care hospital consisting of 9700 medical records of 485 gravidas. The PHI categories which include dates, IDs, patients, doctors, locations, hospitals and ages are the same as the 2006 i2b2 de-identification dataset. In this work, our dataset is annotated after Chinese word segmentation. Hence the PHIs would not be sliced by mistake. The sizes of the datasets and the distributions of primary PHI categories are presented in Table 1.

RNN model

We first present a de-identification system based on RNN as a challenging baseline. RNN is a class of artificial neural network architecture which uses iterative function loops to store information [19]. The long-distance history is stored in a recurrent hidden vector which is dependent on the immediate previous hidden vector. Long Short-Term Memory (LSTM) [20] is one of the most popular variations of RNN. There are several multiplicative gates in LSTM memory cells which can store and access

Table 1 Overview of the datasets

	i2b2–2006	i2b2–2014	Chinese
Number of records	669	1304	9700
Number of tokens	560,852	1,005,582	3,026,944
Number of PHIs	19,498	28,862	48,072
Number of PHI tokens	29,917	38,435	137,496
Vocabulary Size	20,254	41,879	32,265
Percentage of ID	24.6%	3.6%	8.8%
Percentage of DATE	36.4%	43.2%	38.9%
Percentage of HOSPITAL	12.3%	8.0%	2.2%
Percentage of DOCTOR	19.2%	16.6%	14.7%
Percentage of PATIENT	4.7%	7.6%	17.3%
Percentage of AGE	0.1%	6.9%	16.1%

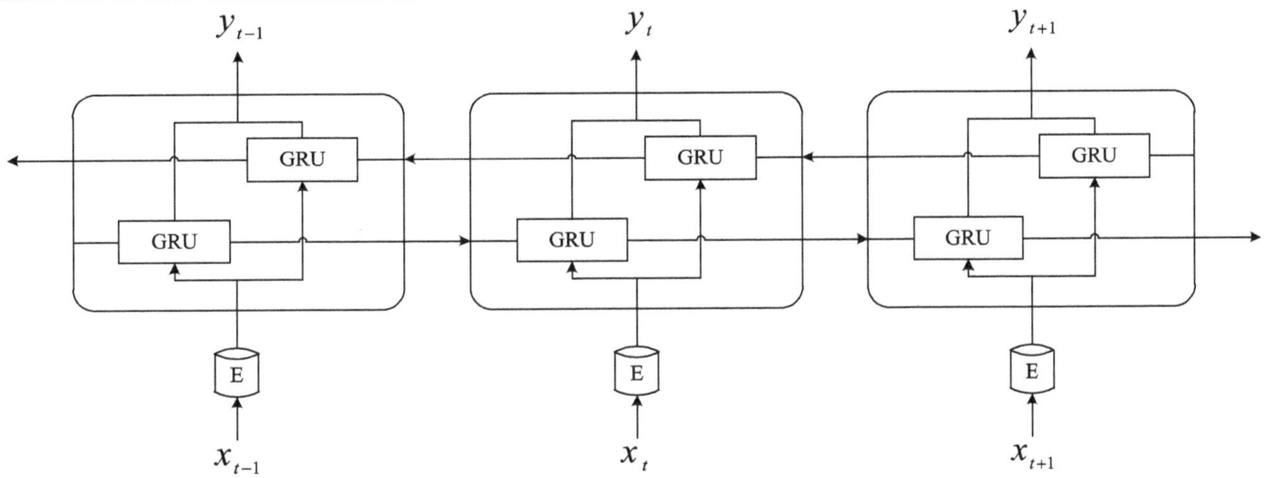

Fig. 2 The RNN model for de-identification

information over long periods of time. Cho et al. proposed Gated Recurrent Unit (GRU) [21] which is a simplification of the LSTM architecture. Cho and his colleagues used neither peephole connections nor output activation functions, but they combined the forget gate and the input gate into a single update gate. They also merged the cell state with hidden state, thus the final model is simpler than standard LSTM models. The GRU architecture can be precisely specified as following equations:

$$r_t = \sigma(W_r \cdot [h_{t-1}, x_t]), \quad (1)$$

$$z_t = \sigma(W_z \cdot [h_{t-1}, x_t]), \quad (2)$$

$$h_t = (1-z_t) * h_{t-1} + z_t * tanh(W \cdot [r_t * h_{t-1}, x_t]), \quad (3)$$

where functions $\boldsymbol{\sigma}$ and $\boldsymbol{tanh}$ are non-linear activation functions. $\boldsymbol{r_t}$ is reset gate, $\boldsymbol{z_t}$ is update gate, and $\boldsymbol{W}$ represent weights.

A bidirectional GRU consists of a forward GRU that moves forward through time beginning from the start of the sequence with another GRU that moves backward through time beginning from the end of the sequence. This structure can provide the output layer with whole past and future context for each point in the input sequence.

The RNN model for de-identification uses the bidirectional GRU, as shown in Fig. 2. x_t is a word of the medical record, E is mapping from words to word embeddings, y_t is the predicted label of the i-th word.

Text skeleton

Compared with normal articles or records, there are a mass of short sentences and abbreviations in EMRs. In addition, there are a great number of table-like texts and special writing formats. Therefore, EMRs are a kind of semi-structured text and the efforts to solve the problem of de-identification can also focus on the text structure of the records.

Because the forms of EMRs are different from normal traditional text, the skeleton of a record, which helps to privacy information recognition. A statistical approach, proposed by us, extracts the skeletons of records, which reveal the different format and punctuation usage between corpora. Especially, only words that appear more than t times during training will be retained and the rest of the words are marked as <UNK> (words in both training set and test set). It should be clearly noted that not only named entities retain but also other words, such as stop words. A text skeleton sample shows in Fig. 3.

We can get various amount of information different skeletons by tuning t. In fact, the scope of t cannot be easily estimated. Therefore, we propose a method to determine the value of t as in Eq. (4). Here *vocabSize* is the vocabulary size of the dataset, f_i is the number of words whose frequency equal to i, maxFreq is the maximum

Original: Mr. HESS was seen by me in BCH with Dr. Whittaker …

Skeleton: Mr. <UNK> was seen by me in <UNK> with Dr.

Fig. 3 A sample of the text skeleton

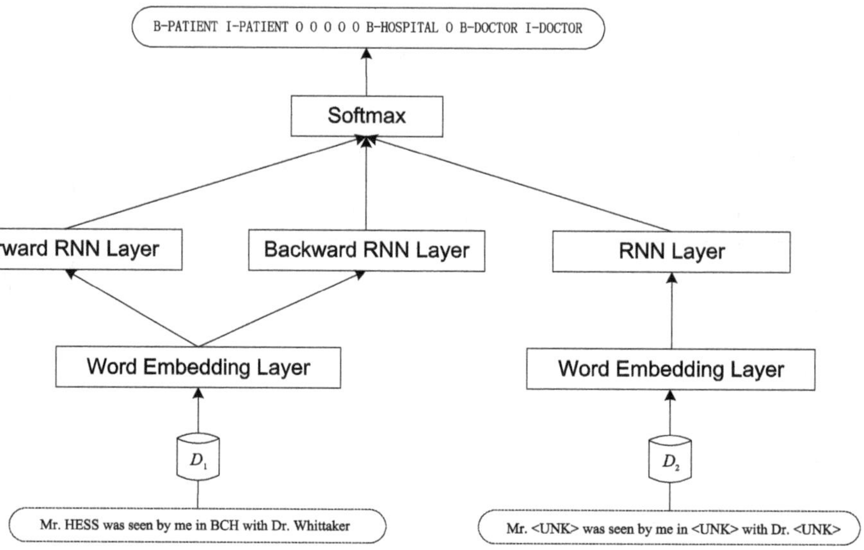

Fig. 4 The structure of TS-RNN model

frequency. *r*, a factor which value of is between 0 and 1, which determines the vocabulary size of the skeleton approximately. Thus, appropriate value of *t* can be obtained by tuning *r*.

$$t = \arg\min_{n} \left| \sum_{i=t}^{n} f_i - r * vocabSize \right|, \tag{4}$$

$$s.\ t.\ 0 < n < \max Freq,$$

$$0 < r < 1,$$

This approach avoids searching in a large range: by adopting (4) the appropriate *t* often falls in a small range. In different datasets, the best *t* can be smaller than 15 or larger than 100 but the corresponding *r* frequently falls between 0.1 and 0.3.

Sentence is the processed unit, within which the named entities are searched for by many existing systems. If we use the sentence context for the EMRs de-identification, there will be one problem is that there is only one or two words in many sentences. Especially in some extreme cases, a PHI instance is the whole sentence. In order to solve this problem, we concatenate all sentences which come from a record to a unique string, and add a "#RETURN" symbol between every two sentences. Digits whether from training data or from test data are converted into the string DIGIT. For example, "a 46 year old male" we mentioned above will be converted to "a DIGITDIGIT year old male".

Combine RNN and text skeleton

We propose TS-RNN (Text Skeleton- Recurrent Neural Network) by combining RNN with text skeleton. The TS-RNN model is summarized in Fig. 4. There are two branches at the input layer of TS-RNN, which receive original medical record and the text skeleton respectively. Each branch has its own word embedding layer and RNN layer. Through the Softmax layer, each word of the medical record generates a corresponding label. Since the output of the labels are mutually exclusive, we apply Softmax regression after the RNN layer. A label dictionary, which generative process can be combined with the automatic generation of word dictionary, is considered as a necessary condition for determining the Softmax output dimension.

Once the word embeddings have been learned in an unsupervised fashion [22], fine-tuning them during supervised training on the task of interest is possible and has some advantages [23]. Note that there are two dictionaries D_1 and D_2, which are used to map words to the index. Therefore, the two embedding layers are also different. In Fig. 4, the left input branch receives the original text of medical records, and the right branch receives the text skeleton we have introduced. The output labels use BIO tagging scheme to identify PHIs.

A context window is essential for scanning the record, as a record is too long for RNNs. The size of the context window should be selected carefully: a small window size cannot contain enough context information while a large window goes against the learning of model.

Table 2 Comparison with the i2b2 shared task submissions

	2006 i2b2		2014 i2b2	
	Entity-level	Token-level	Entity-level	Token-level
Submissions	**0.76–0.96**	**0.80–0.97**	0.44–0.93	0.58–0.96
TS-GRU	0.9452	0.9540	0.9344	0.9401

Table 3 Comparison between the state-of-the-art methods and our framework

Model	2006 i2b2			2014 i2b2			Chinese		
	Precision	Recall	F1-score	Precision	Recall	F1-score	Precision	Recall	F1-score
Wellner	0.9870	0.9750	0.9810	–	–	–	–	–	–
Nottingham	–	–	–	0.9900	0.9640	0.9768	–	–	–
MIST	–	–	–	0.9529	0.7569	0.84367	–	–	–
CRF	0.9640	0.9371	0.9504	0.9842	0.9663	0.9752	0.9863	0.9705	0.9783
CRF + ANN	–	–	–	0.9792	0.9784	0.9788	–	–	–
Bi-LSTM	0.9723	0.9656	0.9689	0.9878	0.9389	0.9627	0.9908	0.9584	0.9743
Bi-GRU	0.9871	0.9664	0.9766	0.9750	0.9704	0.9727	0.9898	0.9624	0.9759
TS-GRU	0.9903	0.9855	0.9879	0.9889	0.9723	0.9805	0.9875	0.9719	0.9797

Parameters of the model

Through training subsets of i2b2 datasets, we acquired optimized parameters of the TS-RNN model. The model is trained using Keras [24] with the RMSprop optimizer. Dropout is applied before Softmax for regularization. We used the early-stopping to choice suitable hyperparameters of model on validation set (20% of the training data).

Here are some optimized parameters:

- Dropout: 0.5
- RNN architecture: GRU
- Hidden dimension: 150
- Embedding dimension: 150
- Early-stopping epoch: 8
- Window size: 7
- r: 0.25 (0.1 for 2014 i2b2 dataset and 0.14 for Chinese dataset)

Results

PHI identification results on token-level and entity-level

The i2b2 de-identification challenge evaluated at token-level and entity-level, and we used the same way to evaluate our model [7, 14]. Meantime, it is significant to evaluate at binary token-level (PHI token versus non-PHI token). Obviously, the EMRs can be displayed for its completeness. The comparison result is shown in Table 2. Table 2 presents the comparison of F1-scores at entity-level and token-level between the i2b2 submissions and the TS-GRU model. Our goal is to retain non-PHI and to use the complete de-identified EMRs for further medical research.

PHI identification results on different datasets

Here are some the novel models and frameworks for PHI identification. We compare them with our framework, and the results, including the binary token-based precisions, recalls and F1-scores, are shown in Table 3. In the i2b2 2006 de-identification challenge, Wellner et al. [9] achieved the best results, there is no results on the 2014 i2b2 dataset. The Nottingham system [17] was the best system in i2b2 2014 de-identification challenge. Because it's not publicly available, the system has no results on 2006 i2b2 dataset. MIST [25] is an off-the-shelf program for de-identification and CRF + ANN was proposed by Dernoncourt et al. [19]. CRF is the model based on Conditional Random Field, Bi-LSTM (Bidirectional Long Short-Term Memory) and Bi-GRU (Bidirectional Gated Recurrent Unit) are classic bidirectional RNN models. TS-GRU is the model we proposed in this work.

From the binary token-based results we can conclude that the TS-GRU model outperform classical models and previous RNN-based models. Moreover, the TS-GRU model is also competitive at token-level and entity-level. There is an interesting phenomenon: precision of machine learning methods is generally higher than the corresponding recall value but handmade rules can achieve a better recall. Most of medical records are edited on templates, therefore they are semi-structured text. An elaborated regular expression set can work effectively, but these over-complicated rules can match many non-PHIs by mistake.

Influence on the results by using different factor *r* value

Figure 5 shows the impact of the factor *r* on the performance of our model on the 2006 i2b2 dataset. When

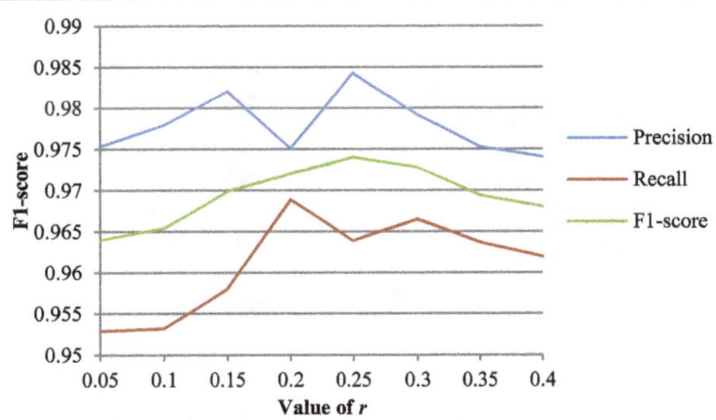

Fig. 5 Impact of the value of *r*

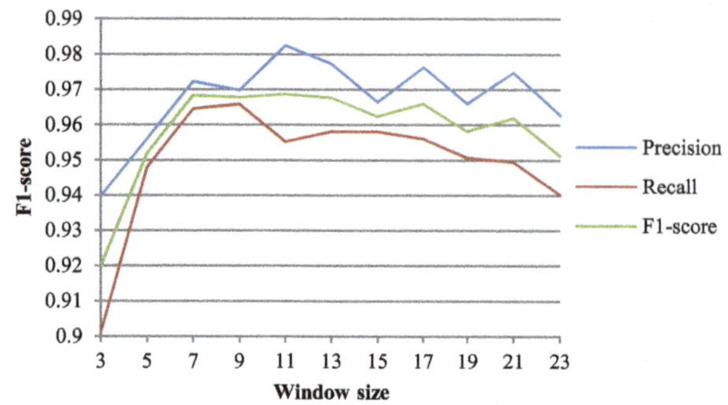

Fig. 6 The performance under different window sizes

Table 4 Performance at entity-level and token-level

Model	Entity-level			Token-level		
	Precision	Recall	F1-score	Precision	Recall	F1-score
Rule-based	0.8747	0.9276	0.9003	0.8802	**0.9478**	0.9128
CRF	**0.9815**	0.8972	0.9375	0.9669	0.9236	0.9448
Bi-LSTM	0.9701	0.9235	0.9462	0.9545	0.9027	0.9279
Bi-GRU	0.9665	0.9470	0.9567	0.9592	0.9270	0.9428
TS-GRU	0.9778	**0.9502**	**0.9638**	**0.9777**	0.9447	**0.9609**

r is between 0.15 and 0.35, the model performs better. If r is very small (0.05 or smaller), the dictionary of the skeleton would be small and then the remaining words of a medical record could not reveal the structure of this record. On the other hand, if r is very big (bigger than 0.3), the text skeleton will degrade into the original text. The maximum value of r in this experiment is 0.4, as the corresponding t equals to 2 when r is larger than 0.4.

Influence on the result by setting different window size

Figure 6 shows the impact of the size of context window on the performance. With the increasing of the window size, precision, recall and F1-measure increase as well. Yet after 7, F1-score begins to fluctuate slightly around a fixed value.

Discussion

Figure 7 shows the token-level F1-scores for all PHI categories on the 2006 i2b2 challenge dataset. Due to the relatively small number of i2b2 datasets in 2006 (the percentages 1% and 0.1% respectively), the LOCATION and AGE categories performed significantly lower than the other categories. Compared with the recall, the precision is higher on most categories except ID. On the category of ID, the recall is about 0.4 higher than the precision. This is due to the fact that all numbers were replaced with the string DIGIT, so the ID numbers can be recognized more easily. In Figs. 6 and 7, the results on the 2014 i2b2 dataset and the Chinese dataset also show that recall is higher than precision on the ID category, which highlights the point.

Table 4 presents the results on the Chinese dataset at entity-level and token-level. In the early stage of our work, the system, based on rule, was established by dictionaries and regular expressions.

Figure 8 shows the token-level F1-scores for all PHI categories on the 2014 i2b2 challenge dataset. The performance of HOSPITAL, CITY and STATE are lower than others because these three categories are quite similar. Sometimes, it's also hard for humans to classify these words. The performance of AGE is remarkable higher than that in 2006 i2b2 dataset. And because LOCATION is divide into CITY, STATE and so on, the performance of these location names are also superior.

Figure 9 shows the token-level F1-scores for all PHI categories on our own dataset. Compared with recall obtained for other categories, the recall of the PATIENT category is clearly lower. Due to China's cultural habits, there is no contextual explanation that the patient's name information does not appear on the record with a uniform format. A more serious problem is that most of the names only appear once in the dataset, and <UNK> information is an important factor in reducing the size of the dictionary. Perhaps it is another reason the names are hard to recognize.

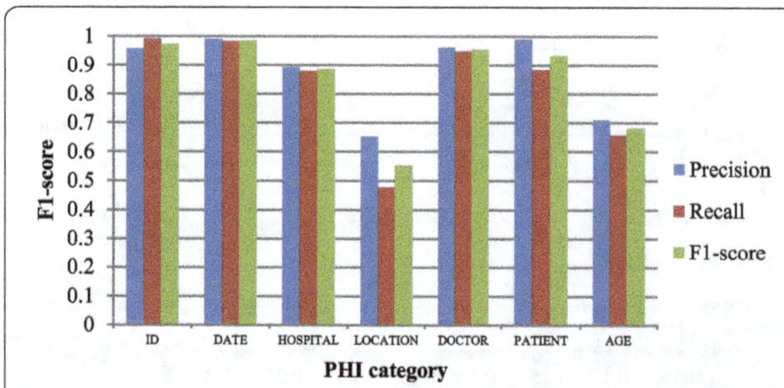

Fig. 7 Token-level F1-scores for each PHI category on 2006 i2b2 dataset

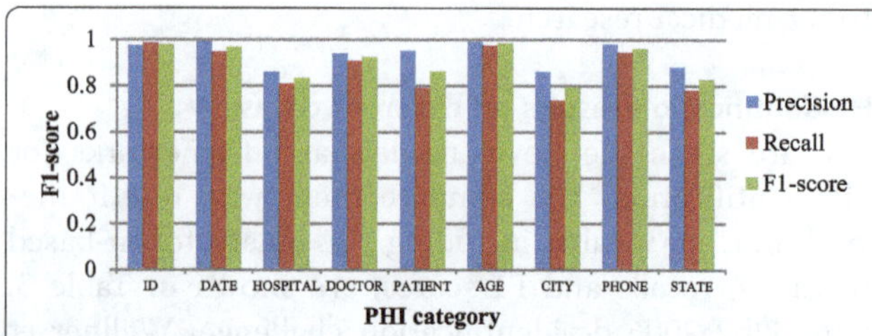

Fig. 8 Token-level F1-scores for each PHI category on 2014 i2b2 dataset

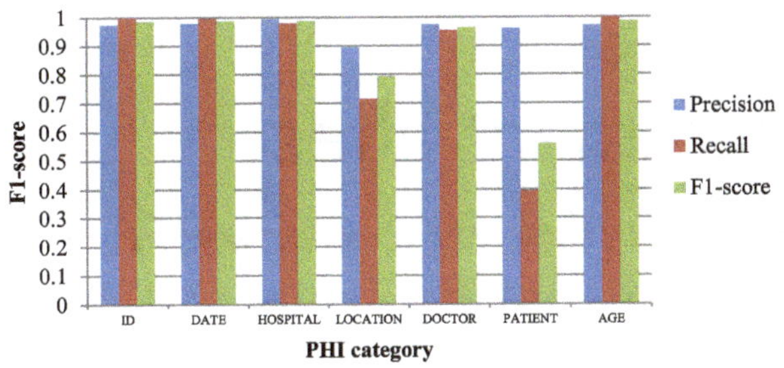

Fig. 9 Token-level F1-scores for each PHI category on Chinese dataset

Conclusions

We proposed a novel de-identification system based on text skeleton and recurrent neural network. Without any structure transform, our method performs well on three datasets mentioned above (two English datasets and a Chinese dataset) at entity-level, token-level and binary token-level. Especially, the results on i2b2 datasets show that the TS-GRU model outperforms classic systems at binary token-level.

Further analysis indicates our method better incorporates the special context in EMRs and is more flexible to different languages than previous systems. Therefore, future research base on TS-RNN will focus on the usage of context and the generation of text skeleton.

Abbreviations

ANN: Artificial Neural Network; Bi-GRU: Bidirectional Gated Recurrent Unit; Bi-LSTM: Bidirectional Long Short-Term Memory; CRFs: Conditional Random Fields; EMR: Electronic Medical Record; GRU: Gated Recurrent Unit; HIPAA: Health Insurance Portability and Accountability Act; HMM: Hidden Markov Models; LSTM: Long Short-Term Memory; PHI: Protected Health Information; RNN: Recurrent Neural Network; SVM: Support Vector Machines; TS: Text Skeleton; TS-RNN: Text Skeleton- Recurrent Neural Network

Funding

Publication of this article was funded by the National Natural Science Foundation of China (No.61402419) and the science and technology project of Science and Technology Department of Henan Province (No. 172102210478).

Authors' contributions

YSZ was involved in data collection and annotation, literature review, statistical analysis and the sections Background and Discussion writing. KLZ designed algorithms and experiments and wrote the rest of the article. HCM and KL implemented the algorithms and performed the calculation. All authors have read and approved the final manuscript.

Competing interests

The authors declare that they have no competing interests.

Author details

[1]The Third Affiliated Hospital of Zhengzhou University, Kangfu Road, Zhengzhou, Henan 450072, China. [2]School of Information Engineering, Zhengzhou University, Science Avenue, Zhengzhou, Henan 450001, China.

References

1. Dorr DA, Phillips WF, Phansalkar S, et al. Assessing the difficulty and time cost of de-identification in clinical narratives. Methods Inf Med. 2006;45:246–52.
2. Sweeney L. Replacing personally-identifying information in medical records, the Scrub system. Proceedings of the AMIA annual fall symposium. J Am Med Inform Assoc. 1996:333.
3. Ruch P, Baud RH, Rassinoux AM, et al. Medical document anonymization with a semantic lexicon. Proceedings of the AMIA Symposium. J Am Med Inform Assoc. 2000:729.
4. Fielstein EM, Brown SH, Speroff T. Algorithmic de-identification of VA medical exam text for HIPAA privacy compliance: preliminary findings. Medinfo. 2004;1590
5. Gupta D, Saul M, Gilbertson J. Evaluation of a deidentification (de-id) software engine to share pathology reports and clinical documents for research. Am J Clin Pathol. 2004;121:176–86.
6. Beckwith BA, Mahaadevan R, Balis UJ, et al. Development and evaluation of an open source software tool for deidentification of pathology reports. BMC Medical Informatics and Decision Making. 2006;6:12–21.
7. Uzuner Ö, Luo Y, Szolovits P. Evaluating the state-of-the-art in automatic de-identification. J Am Med Inform Assoc. 2007;14:550–63.
8. Ishna N, Douglass MM, Lehman LH, et al. Automated de-identification of free-text medical records. BMC Medical Informatics & Decision Making. 2008; 8(1):1–17.
9. Wellner B, Huyck M, Mardis S, et al. Rapidly retargetable approaches to de-identification in medical records. J Am Med Inform Assoc. 2007;14:564–73.
10. Hara K. Applying a SVM based Chunker and a Text Classifier to the Deid Challenge . I2B2 Workshop on Challenges in Natural Language Processing for Clinical Data 2006. Available as a JAMIA on-line data supplement to the current overview article, at www.jamia.org.
11. Szarvas G, Farkas R, Busa-Fekete R. State-of-the-art anonymization of medical records using an iterative machine learning framework. J Am Med Inform Assoc. 2007;14:574–80.
12. Sweeney L. Uniqueness of simple demographics in the US population. Technical Report: Carnegie Mellon University; 2000.
13. Stubbs A, Kotfila C, Uzuner Ö. Automated Systems for the de-Identification of longitudinal clinical narratives: overview of 2014 i2b2/UTHealth shared task track 1. J Biomed Inform. 2015;58:S11–9.
14. Stubbs A, Uzuner Ö. Annotating longitudinal clinical narratives for de-identification: the 2014 i2b2/UTHealth corpus. J Biomed Inform. 2015;58:S20–9.
15. Dehghan A, Kovacevic A, Karystianis G, et al. Combining knowledge and data-driven methods for de-identification of clinical narratives. J Biomed Inform. 2015;58:S53–9.
16. Liu Z, Chen Y, Tang B, et al. Automatic de-identification of electronic medical records using token-level and character-level conditional random fields. J Biomed Inform. 2015;58:S47–52.
17. Yang H, Garibaldi JM. Automatic detection of protected health information from clinic narratives. J Biomed Inform. 2015;58:S30–8.
18. Li M, Carrell D, Aberdeen J, et al. Optimizing annotation resources for natural language de-identification via a game theoretic framework. J Biomed Inform. 2016;61:97–109.
19. Dernoncourt F, Lee JY, Uzuner O, et al. De-identification of patient notes with recurrent neural networks. Journal of the American Medical Informatics Association Jamia. 2016;24(3):596–81.
20. Graves A: Supervised sequence labelling with Recurrent Neural Networks Springer Berlin Heidelberg, 2012.
21. Hochreiter S, Schmidhuber J. Long short-term memory. Neural Comput. 1997;9:1735–80.
22. Cho K, Van Merriënboer B, Gulcehre C, et al. Learning Phrase Representations Using RNN Encoder-decoder for Statistical Machine Translation. Proceedings of the 2014 Conference on Empirical Methods in Natural Language Processing. 2014:1724–34.
23. Collobert R, Weston J: A Unified Architecture for Natural Language Processing: Deep Neural Networks with Multitask Learning. Proceedings of the 25th International Conference on Machine Learning. ACM, 2008: 160–167.
24. Mesnil G, He X, Deng L, et al. Investigation of recurrent-neural-network architectures and learning methods for spoken language understanding. Interspeech. 2013:3771–5.
25. Chollet F. Keras. GitHub repository: https://github.com/fchollet/keras, 2015.

12

Length of time periods in treatment effect descriptions and willingness to initiate preventive therapy

Erik Berglund[1*], Ragnar Westerling[1], Johan Sundström[2] and Per Lytsy[1]

Abstract

Background: Common measures used to describe preventive treatment effects today are proportional, i.e. they compare the proportions of events in relative or absolute terms, however they are not easily interpreted from the patient's perspective and different magnitudes do not seem to clearly discriminate between levels of effect presented to people.

Methods: In this randomised cross-sectional survey experiment, performed in a Swedish population-based sample ($n = 1041$, response rate 58.6%), the respondents, aged between 40 and 75 years were given information on a hypothetical preventive cardiovascular treatment. Respondents were randomised into groups in which the treatment was described as having the effect of delaying a heart attack for different periods of time (Delay of Event, DoE): 1 month, 6 months or 18 months. Respondents were thereafter asked about their willingness to initiate such therapy, as well as questions about how they valued the proposed therapy.

Results: Longer DoE:s were associated with comparatively greater willingness to initiate treatment. The proportions accepting treatment were 81, 71 and 46% when postponement was 18 months, 6 months and 1 month respectively. In adjusted binary logistic regression models the odds ratio for being willing to take therapy was 4.45 (95% CI 2.72–7.30) for a DoE of 6 months, and 6.08 (95% CI 3.61–10.23) for a DoE of 18 months compared with a DoE of 1 month. Greater belief in the necessity of medical treatment increased the odds of being willing to initiate therapy.

Conclusions: Lay people's willingness to initiate preventive therapy was sensitive to the magnitude of the effect presented as DoE. The results indicate that DoE is a comprehensible effect measure, of potential value in shared clinical decision-making.

Keywords: Medical decision-making, Risk communication, Risk perception, Necessity-concern framework

Background

Insufficient adherence to cardiovascular treatments is considered an important factor in treatment failure [1], and insufficient adherence may increase cardiovascular morbidity [2, 3]. Several studies link patient/person-centred care (PCC) to adherence, as part of a successful preventive medical treatment strategy [4, 5]. To enable optimal adherence, using a patient-centred approach and informed decision-making, patients need to receive treatment information that is both correct and easy to understand. Statistical effect measures from clinical trials are known to influence patients' views and understandings of a treatment, and it has been shown that the format of the effect measure communicated influences decisions by both physicians and patients [6–9]. The most common measures used to describe a preventive treatment effect include relative risk reductions (RRR) and absolute measures such as absolute risk reductions

* Correspondence: Erik.Berglund@pubcare.uu.se
[1]Department of Public Health and Caring Sciences, Uppsala University, Box 564, SE-751 22 UPPSALA, Sweden
Full list of author information is available at the end of the article

(ARR) and numbers-needed-to-treat (NNT) [10]. These measures are proportional, i.e. they compare the proportions of events in relative or absolute terms. RRRs have, compared to ARRs and NNTs been shown to score more favourably in evaluations of treatments [10, 11]. RRRs, however, does not account for of the baseline risk and are, thus, alone not sufficient to distinguish a treatment effect that is clinically valuable from one that is not. Furthermore, different magnitudes of RRRs do not seem to clearly discriminate between levels of effect presented to lay people [12]. It has been argued that the amplification effect, following a RRR effect description, biases or misleads patients towards accepting interventions in a way that is not consistent with their own values [13, 14]. For that reason, RRRs are not alone recommended in shared decision making. In a search for effect measures that are appropriate for communication of risk and treatment effect in the preventive setting, different measures depicting postponement of events, time-to-event or prolongation of life have been suggested [15–18]. A gain in disease free time or a gain in life expectancy estimates treatment effect in a way that might be of intuitive value to patients. Lay people seems to have the capacity to determine and choose between different levels of treatment effect in settings such as hip fracture [17] and heart attack [18], when the treatment effect is explained as postponements of time to events. Such time estimations studies have, hitherto, used hypothesised or extrapolated data, which proves the concept of time-based measures, but provides little value for risk and effect communication in clinical practice. A set of complementary measures that go beyond the proportional measures has recently been proposed, that involve assessing between-group differences in percentiles of the survival function [19–21]. By the use of Laplace regression modelling [22], it is possible to assess a treatment effect as the time an event is delayed due to treatment, which can be expressed as the Delay of Event (DoE) measure [19]. The DoE measure evaluates the time difference between two treatment arms at equal event rates. Over the follow-up period, it presents a curve of how the treatment effect develops over time, which has been exemplified using data from clinical studies [19, 21]. The DoE is an absolute measure and conditional on the event. This means that for a study participant who would have an event during the follow-up without treatment, the DoE depicts the time of the delay when treated. A person who does *not* experience the event of interest during a follow-up cannot benefit from treatment during this period. The DoE is a complimentary effect measure, and recent results suggest that the DoE compares well to RRR and better than ARR when measuring laymen's willingness to initiate a hypothetical preventive treatment [20].

The objective of this study was to investigate if the length of time in the DoE measure influences lay people's willingness to initiate a preventive treatment against cardiovascular disease (CVD). Secondary objectives were to investigate how the different magnitudes of DoE treatment effects affect individuals' understanding and confidence in the medication and their willingness to pay for treatment (WTP). We hypothesised that people's preference for a preventive therapy is positively influenced by the length of the delayed disease when it is expressed in terms of DoE.

Methods

Design and sample

This is a cross-sectional randomised survey experiment [23, 24], in a population-based sample, aged 45–75 years. Eighteen hundred (1800) randomly selected persons from the Swedish national population registry were randomly allocated into three equally sized groups. The groups received information about a hypothetical treatment's effect as three different delayed event times of heart attack: 1 month, 6 months or 18 months and were then asked different follow-up questions. The questionnaire was returned by 1041 individuals; 23 persons could not be reached or declined to participate, and 736 did not answer, making the response rate of the distributed questionnaires 58.6% (1041/1777). The response rate in the three groups varied from 56.8 to 59.8%. Data were collected from November 2013 to February 2014. A previous study compared the 18 months DoE arm to proportional effect measures [20].

Background questions

Background data were assessed using questions about the respondent's gender (dichotomous variable), age (continuous variable), and educational level (categorised in three groups).

History of cardiovascular disease

Data were collected using questions about history of CVD (dichotomised to having had myocardial infarction and/or angina, or not); these questions have been used in previous studies [25, 26].

Beliefs about medicines

Patients beliefs was assessed using the Necessity-Concern Framework (NCF) which was developed specifically to address views of drug treatments [27]. According to the NCF, a patient's decision regarding approving and adhering to a treatment is the result of a trade-off between the patient's perceived need for a prescribed treatment (necessity) and their worries about potential adverse effects as a result of the treatment (concern). NCF has been used in a broad range of different quantitative studies exploring drug treatment adherence [28–31], including cardiovascular diseases [32–35]. NCF was assessed by using the

Beliefs about Medicines Questionnaire (BMQ) in specific version [27]. The BMQ questionnaire has been translated into Swedish and has been used previously in Sweden [26, 36–39].

Hypothetic scenario and treatment effect information

The study was conducted as an information intervention with randomised groups in a survey experiment. Respondents were asked to imagine a scenario where they had an increased risk of CVD, and that their physician suggested a preventive cardiovascular drug treatment (comparable to statin treatments). The text was outlined: "Imagine that in the next five years you will have an increased risk of having a heart attack. Your physician offers you a treatment with rare and mild side effects, to be taken in pill form once a day. The usefulness of the treatment has been evaluated in scientific studies, and the effect can be described as follows: If you would have a heart attack in the next 5 years it will be delayed for up to [1 month] if you take the treatment." The text describing the effect measure, in square brackets above, expressed different magnitudes of the Delay of Event measure. The first group received a treatment effect described as 1 month DoE, the second group 6 months DoE, and the third group 18 months DoE.

Outcome variables

Information about willingness to initiate treatment, the dependent variable in the analyses, was assessed using the question: "If you were in the same situation as the person in this case would you take the treatment?". Response alternatives were yes or no. Other questions that were used to evaluate the views of the treatment were: "How much benefit do you assess that the drug would have?"; "Would you feel safe to take the drug?"; "Would you, based on the description, be motivated to take the medication on a daily basis?"; "How important is it to adhere to the treatment prescription?" and "To what extent does the description help you make a medical decision?". The answers to these questions were assessed on seven-point Likert scales ranging from: 1 (not at all) to 7 (very much). Little is known about the monetary value that individuals assign in relation to the proposed medication. Willingness to pay (WTP) is an assessment of the highest price an individual will pay for a good or service [40]. WTP was assessed with an open-ended question: "What is the maximum amount of money that you would pay per month during a five-year period to receive the treatment?". WTP was measured in Swedish currency (SEK), and for the purpose of this study was converted to Euros (€) at an exchange rate of 0.10.

Statistical analysis

Chi-square analyses and multivariate logistic regression analyses were used to investigate associations between willingness to initiate therapy and the presented DoE magnitudes. Associations between lay people's views of the treatment descriptions, WTP and presented DoE magnitudes were tested with Kruskal-Wallis H tests. Consent to initiate preventive therapy was tested in multivariate binary logistic regression models. A stepwise approach was performed to build these models. Model 1 included length of time delay and demographics. Model 2 included model 1, history of cardiovascular diseases and NCF. In order to examine the interaction effects of DoE and age group (categorised as over/under 60 years of age), multiplicative interaction terms of length of time delay × age group were included in model 3. Statistical Package for the Social Sciences (SPSS)® version 22 (IBM SPSS Statistics for Windows, Armonk, NY: IBM Corp Chicago, IL, U.S.A.) was used for descriptive statistics and statistical tests. A p-value ≤0.05 was considered statistically significant.

Results

The study population was on average 61.8 years old and consisted of slightly more women than men. College or university was the most common completed education level. A distribution of demographic variables, overall and according to group allocation, is shown in Table 1. In the study population the prevalence of a history of cardiovascular disease (heart attack and/or angina) was 5.8%. Overall the three groups were well balanced in baseline characteristics.

Decision to initiate treatment and views of treatment

Overall, 65.4% of the respondents were willing to take the suggested medication. The proportions accepting the treatment were 80.5, 70.6 and 45.5%, for a DoE of 18 months, 6 months and 1 month, respectively. The difference was statistically significant between the three groups (Table 2).

There were statistically significant differences between the three groups due to the presented DoE regarding respondents' views of the benefit from treatment, feeling safe to take the drug, motivation to take treatment, views on importance of adhering to prescription, and WTP. The longer time periods presented as DoE, the more favourable did the respondents consider the drug. The median WTP for the three different treatment descriptions ranged from €13.4 for DoE of 1 month, €23.2 for DoE of 6 months, to €25.7 for DoE of 18 months ($P < 0.001$). There was no difference in use of information from prescriptions (Table 2).

Logistic regressions

The willingness to initiate therapy was further explored in logistic regression models (Table 3). The odds of being willing to initiate treatment increased with a longer

Table 1 Distribution of characteristics among participants

Category	Subcategory	Delay of Events 1 month	6 months	18 months	Overall
Gender	Men, % (n)	48.6 (169)	40.2 (141)	44.3 (148)	44.3 (458)
	Women, % (n)	51.4 (179)	59.8 (210)	55.7 (186)	55.7 (575)
Age	Mean (SD)	61.7 (8.5)	61.8 (8.7)	61.8 (8.6)	61.8 (8.6)
Education level	Compulsory school, % (n)	27.2 (94)	29.0 (101)	27.5 (92)	27.9 (287)
	Secondary school, % (n)	35.9 (124)	35.3 (123)	35.8 (120)	35.7 (367)
	College or university, % (n)	36.8 (127)	35.6 (124)	36.7 (123)	36.4 (374)
History of cardiovascular disease	Have had heart attack or angina, % (n)	7.4 (25)	5.5 (19)	4.5 (15)	5.8 (59)
	No history of heart attack or angina, % (n)	92.6 (315)	94.5 (327)	95.5 (315)	94.2 (957)
Necessity-concern Framework	Necessity, median[a] (mean)	12 (12.1)	11 (11.0)	12 (12.6)	12 (11.6)
	Concern, median[a] (mean)	4 (4.8)	3 (4.4)	4 (5.1)	4 (4.8)

Figures as percentages and numbers (n) if not stated otherwise. Mean values are presented with standard deviation (SD)
[a]Necessity and concern was used in index form, ranging from 0 to 20

DoE, in adjusted models: odds ratio (OR) 4.45 (95% confidence interval (CI) 2.72–7.30) for a DoE of 6 months, OR 6.08 (95% CI 3.61–10.23) for a DoE of 18 month compared with a DoE of 1 month (reference category). The results were similar also when interaction terms were included in the model: OR 5.51 (95% CI 2.47–12.30) for a DoE of 6 months and OR 5.69 (95% CI 2.44–13.27) for a DoE of 18 months. A higher perceived necessity of medication in medical treatments in the NCF slightly increased the odds (OR 1.07, CI 1.03–1.11) for being willing to initiate therapy. Having a history of cardiovascular disease (heart attack and/or angina) was significantly associated with having a higher willingness to initiate treatment in the crude and adjusted models. No statistically significant interaction effect was found between length of time delay and age group.

Discussion

This study had the objective of investigating whether the length of time in the Delay of Event measure affected lay peoples' willingness to accept a proposed treatment. This study also aimed to investigate how the different time periods of delay affect individuals' evaluation and confidence in a proposed treatment as well as their willingness to pay for a therapy with a certain stated effect.

A higher proportion of individuals were willing to accept the treatment when the effect was presented with a greater time period in DoE. These findings are in agreement with similar studies that have demonstrated that lay people's choices are sensitive to length of time periods of a treatment effect when it is expressed as postponements in time [17, 18]. Time-based measures, such as DoE, are considered to be easier to comprehend than proportional measures [18]. The results in the present study suggest that time-based measures of treatment effects enable lay people to evaluate and choose between different magnitudes of delay, in contrast to RRR measures which do not help lay people to a sufficient extent [12].

Relative measures of risk reductions depict a perspective that is relevant to individual patients. Relative risk reductions are usually relatively stable over the follow-up time

Table 2 Treatment decision and evaluation of descriptions

Outcome	Delay of Events 1 month	6 months	18 months	Overall	CHI-Square	*P*-value
Willingness to initiate treatment, % (n)	45.5 (156)	70.6 (243)	80.5 (268)	65.4 (667)	98.71[a]	< 0.001
Benefit from medication, md (q1, q3), m	3 (2,5), 3.18	4 (2,5), 3.99	5 (4,6), 4.58	4 (2,5), 3.91	96.20[b]	< 0.001
Feel safe with medication, md (q1, q3), m	3 (2,5), 3.45	4 (2,5), 3.95	4 (3,6), 4.25	4 (2,5), 3.88	30.35[b]	< 0.001
Be motivated to take medication, md (q1, q3), m	2 (1,5), 3.17	4 (2,6), 4.09	5 (3,6), 4.66	4 (2,6), 3.97	79.64[b]	< 0.001
Importance to adhere, md, (q1, q3), m	5 (2,7), 4.47	6 (4,7), 5.27	5 (5,7), 5.67	6 (4,7), 5.13	41.91[b]	< 0.001
Willingness to pay (Euro), md (q1, q3), m[c]	5 (0, 16), 13.4	10 (5, 30), 23.2	20 (10,30), 25.7	10 (0, 30), 20.8	65.10[b]	< 0.001
Use of information, md (q1, q3), m	5 (3,6), 4.63	5 (4,6), 4.65	5 (4,6), 4.91	5 (4,6), 4.72	3.25[b]	0.20

[a]Pearson Chi-Square
[b]Kruskal-Wallis H test
[c]Willingness to pay was measured in Swedish krona (SEK) 1SEK/0.10 Euro (€)

Table 3 Multivariate models of the odds of consenting to therapy

		Crude OR 95% CI	Model 1 OR 95% CI	Model 2 OR 95% CI	Model 3 OR 95% CI
Delay of Events (DoE)	Length of time delay				
	1 month (ref. cat.)	1	1	1	1
	6 month	2.88** (2.11 to 3.95)	3.01** (2.17 to 4.16)	4.45** (2.72 to 7.30)	5.51** (2.47 to 12.30)
	18 month	4.94** (3.50 to 6.97)	5.15** (3.62 to 7.33)	6.08** (3.61 to 10.23)	5.69** (2.44 to 13.27)
Demographic	Gender				
	Male (ref. cat.)	1	1	1	1
	Female	1.11 (0.85 to 1.43)	1.02 (0.77 to 1.35)	0.87 (0.56 to 1.33)	0.87 (0.57 to 1.32)
	Age group				
	under 60 years of age (ref. cat.)	1	1	1	1
	60 years of age or older	1.80** (1.35 to 1.28)	1.64** (1.12 to 2.20)	1.34 (0.87 to 2.07)	1.45 (0.76 to 2.70)
	Education level				
	University (ref. cat.)	1	1	1	1
	Secondary school or equal	1.43* (1.06 to 1.93)	1.54** (1.12 to 2.12)	1.13 (0.70 to 1.83)	1.12 (0.69 to 1.81)
	Compulsory school	2.28** (1.62 to 3.20)	2.19** (1.51 to 3.17)	1.87* (1.11 to 3.16)	1.89* (1.12 to 3.19)
History of cardiovascular diseases	History of heart attack or angina				
	No (ref. cat.)	1		1	1
	Had heart attack and/or angina	3.47** (1.62 to 7.41)		2.89* (1.13 to 7.41)	2.86* (1.11 to 7.36)
Necessity concerns framework[a]	Beliefs about medicine				
	Necessity	1.06** (1.03 to 1.10)		1.07** (1.03 to 1.11)	1.07** (1.03 to 1.11)
	Concern	1.03 (0.99 to 1.07)		1.00 (0.95 to 1.05)	1.00 (0.95 to 1.05)
Interaction effect[b]	DoE 6 month × 60 years of age or older	0.98 (0.52 to 1.87)			0.71 (0.26 to 1.92)
	DoE 18 month × 60 years of age or older	1.18 (0.58 to 2.39)			1.11 (0.38 to 3.22)

Odds ratio (OR), significance level and confidence interval (CI) for willing to initiate therapy (0 = "no", 1 = "yes")
[a]Necessity and concern was used in index form, ranging from 0 to 20
[b]Interaction effects was adjusted for variables included in the interaction term
* $P \leq 0.05$, ** $P \leq 0.01$ Model 1 = Length of time delay+demographics, Model 2 = Model 1 + History of cardiovascular diseases+Necessity concerns framework, Model 3 = Model 2+ interaction effect

and across different risk groups, but they are not easily interpreted from the patient's perspective. This may be because RRRs do not consider the time perspective, which is of profound meaning for patients. RRRs do not apply to the patients' long-term perspective for events that eventually will occur, such as death or other major adverse events of which absolute risk increases with time. This is linked to the fact that RRRs does not account for the underlying absolute risk at baseline. On the other hand, absolute numbers, such as risk differences, are easy to grasp and emphasise the fraction of treated patients that do experience a benefit. Such an interpretation - that only some benefit - is, however, likely to be an underestimation of the effect, as ARRs and NNTs only consider treatment benefit that will persist over the time point of evaluation [41]. Absolute effect measures are further sensitive to the time period of evaluation as well as to the baseline risk of the study population, and is thus of unclear relevance for patients who are likely to be taking the medication on a different timescale than the study population. Time-based non-parametric measures such as the DoE can be favourably expressed as curves, which depict the development of the effect over time and may support well-informed treatment decisions.

The DoE measure is not an average that applies to everyone which is a potentially difficult aspect in a clinical situation. Rather it is an estimation of the time an event is delayed due to treatment for people who would have developed the event, if untreated. To assume that one will have the event might be a cognitive challenge, and there is a risk such an assumption will tend to inflate patients' perceived necessity and concerns of the treatment. If so, it might bias treatment decisions in favour of taking the treatment. On the other hand, if a DoE effect is perceived as short, it might do the opposite. Clinical use of the DoE measure will provide patients and physicians an opportunity to reflect on several important aspects, such as the patient's medical status, risk and the benefits from treatment, which is one of the suggested routines to achieve shared decision making within patient-centred care [42, 43]. It cannot be taken for granted that different populations will assess the DoE measure in equal ways. The absolute risk of having an event, as well as the perceived severity and consequences of having that event, might vary for different conditions over different populations. For instance, the risk of having an event following a chronic disease usually increases with age. At the same time older age might go with declining quality of life, which may affect the perceived importance of delaying (or avoiding) events. Hence, there is a need to investigate the appropriateness of present treatment effect as DoE, for different conditions and populations.

Our observations suggest that the length of the DoE affects several aspects of lay people's view of the proposed treatment, including their degree of motivation for taking it. The magnitude of the DoE showed no influence on the perceived usefulness of the information provided; consequently the quality of information and the ability to be informed was not dependent on the presented effect. This indicates that the data and their presentation were useful for decision and evaluation of effect, regardless of the presented DoE magnitude. Respondents' willingness to pay for the treatment was higher for longer time periods of DoE. However, the relationship seems to level off in a way sometimes referred to as "the law of diminishing marginal utility", which means that the first unit of consumption of a goods or service yields more utility than the second and subsequent units. In this case lay people tended to have higher WTP for a month in a shorter total time period than for a month in a longer time period. Previous research has discussed diminishing marginal utility in relation to gain of future life-years compared to those at present age. People tend to value life-years in the future less than those at present not because of the timing of these life-years, but simply because a life-year in the distant future implies a long life, which may stand for a satiation effect [44].

No statistically significant interaction effect was found between length of time delay and age group, which suggests that there are no multiplicative effects. However, it is possible that such an interaction exists in other populations, where the events and treatment effects are more closely related to the age.

High belief in treatment necessity in the NCF are known to be associated with adherence and behaviour related to treatment [26]. In this study, greater belief of necessity was associated with increased willingness to initiate therapy; however, adjusting for necessity and concerns did not abolish the effect of an increased DoE effect. The NCF was developed to explore patients' views on drugs in general and not specifically preventive drugs; consequently the measure is not optimal for use in a study with lay people and a hypothetical scenario. The reason for including the NCF in this study was to capture a general attitude to drugs rather than specific benefits/concerns about the treatment presented in the scenario.

To summarise: the results in this study imply that time magnitudes described as DoE are useful for lay people in decision-making regarding medical treatments. The DoE measure might be an adequate alternative, and/or a complement to other treatment descriptions and a useful tool in shared clinical decision-making. This was the first study of differences in magnitudes for DoE and therefore relatively large differences in the time periods were chosen to explore the concept. Future studies should investigate if patients also are sensitive to minor differences in DoE, and if patient groups with different baseline risks and conditions also are sensitive to minor differences in DoE. This study does not compare variations in DoE magnitudes with variations in other measure such as RRRs or ARRs, therefore no conclusion can be drawn on these matters. It is suggested that future studies address the question on how variations of magnitude of different effect measures relates to each other as well as decision-making in different situations. There is a need to further investigate if time-based measures, such as DoE, may have an advantageous role in clinical decision making for specific patient groups and treatments, especially if they may improve long-term adherence.

Strengths and limitations

The strengths of this study include the community setting and the randomised approach. This study also has some limitations worth noting. The study used a hypothetical scenario and the study population mainly consisted of lay people (without previous heart disease); thus, the study population were different than typical patient groups. The response rate is reasonable according to that anticipated from mailed questionnaire-based studies, but unfortunately there is no information about non-responders. Further, reporting bias may exist due to the nature of self-reported data.

Conclusion

Lay people's willingness to initiate preventive therapy was sensitive to the length of time periods when treatment effect was presented as the time-based measure Delay of Event. The results indicate that Delay of Event is a comprehensible measure of effect, which holds potential value for communicating treatment benefit and shared clinical decision-making.

Abbreviations

€: Euros; ARR: Absolute risk reductions; BMQ: Beliefs about Medicines Questionnaire; CI: Confidence interval; CVD: Cardiovascular disease; CVM: Contingent valuation method; DoE: Delay of Event; NCF: Necessity-Concern Framework; NNT: Numbers-needed-to-treat OROdds ratio; PCC: Patient/person-centred care; RRR: Relative risk reductions; SEK: Swedish currency; SPSS: Statistical Package for the Social Sciences; WTP: Willingness to pay

Acknowledgments

We are grateful to all of the responders who gave up their time to contribute to this research.

Funding

The study was financially supported by grants from Uppsala University and The Swedish Society of Medicine. The funders had no role in the study design, collection and analysis of the data or in preparation of the manuscript.

Authors' contributions

EB designed the study, undertook the statistical modelling and led the writing. PL, RW and JS designed the study, contributed to data interpretation, and commented on successive drafts of the manuscript and handling of data. All authors read and approved the final manuscript.

Competing interests

All the authors declare that there is no potential competing interest.

Author details

[1]Department of Public Health and Caring Sciences, Uppsala University, Box 564, SE-751 22 UPPSALA, Sweden. [2]Department of Medical Sciences, Uppsala University, Uppsala, Sweden.

References

1. Cheng CW, Woo KS, Chan JC, Tomlinson B, You JH. Association between adherence to statin therapy and lipid control in Hong Kong Chinese patients at high risk of coronary heart disease. Br J Clin Pharmacol. 2004; 58(5):528–35. https://doi.org/10.1111/j.1365-2125.2004.02202.x.
2. Blackburn DF, Dobson RT, Blackburn JL, Wilson TW. Cardiovascular morbidity associated with nonadherence to statin therapy. Pharmacotherapy. 2005; 25(8):1035–43. https://doi.org/10.1592/phco.2005.25.8.1035.
3. Wei L, Wang J, Thompson P, Wong S, Struthers AD, MacDonald TM. Adherence to statin treatment and readmission of patients after myocardial infarction: a six year follow up study. Heart. 2002;88(3):229–33.
4. Robinson JH, Callister LC, Berry JA, Dearing KA. Patient-centered care and adherence: definitions and applications to improve outcomes. J Am Acad Nurse Pract. 2008;20(12):600–7. https://doi.org/10.1111/j.1745-7599.2008.00360.x.
5. WHO. Adherence to Long-term Therapies: Evidence for action. Geneva: World Health Organization; 2003.
6. Hux JE, Naylor CD. Communicating the benefits of chronic preventive therapy: does the format of efficacy data determine patients' acceptance of treatment? Med Decis Mak. 1995;15(2):152–7.
7. Morris JN, Heady JA, Raffle PA, Roberts CG, Parks JW. Coronary heart-disease and physical activity of work. Lancet. 1953;265(6796):1111–20; concl.
8. Edwards A, Elwyn G, Stott N. Communicating risk reductions. Researchers should present results with both relative and absolute risks. BMJ. 1999; 318(7183):603 author reply –4.
9. Nexoe J, Gyrd-Hansen D, Kragstrup J, Kristiansen IS, Nielsen JB. Danish GPs' perception of disease risk and benefit of prevention. Fam Pract. 2002;19(1):3–6.
10. Covey J. A meta-analysis of the effects of presenting treatment benefits in different formats. Med Decis Mak. 2007;27(5):638–54. https://doi.org/10.1177/0272989X07306783.
11. Misselbrook D, Armstrong D. Patients' responses to risk information about the benefits of treating hypertension. Br J Gen Pract. 2001; 51(465):276–9.
12. Sorensen L, Gyrd-Hansen D, Kristiansen IS, Nexoe J, Nielsen JB. Laypersons' understanding of relative risk reductions: randomised cross-sectional study. BMC Med Inform Decis Mak. 2008;8:31. https://doi.org/10.1186/1472-6947-8-31.
13. Akl EA, Oxman AD, Herrin J, Vist GE, Terrenato I, Sperati F, et al. Using alternative statistical formats for presenting risks and risk reductions. Cochrane Database Syst Rev. 2011;(3):Cd006776. https://doi.org/10.1002/14651858.CD006776.pub2.
14. Fagerlin A, Zikmund-Fisher BJ, Ubel PA. Helping patients decide: ten steps to better risk communication. J Natl Cancer Inst. 2011;103(19):1436–43. https://doi.org/10.1093/jnci/djr318.
15. Christensen PM, Brosen K, Brixen K, Kristiansen IS. Expressing effects of osteoporosis interventions in terms of postponing of fractures. Eur J Clin Pharmacol. 2002;58(9):629–33. https://doi.org/10.1007/s00228-002-0526-6.
16. Halvorsen PA, Selmer R, Kristiansen IS. Different ways to describe the benefits of risk-reducing treatments: a randomized trial. Ann Intern Med. 2007;146(12):848–56.
17. Christensen PM, Brosen K, Brixen K, Andersen M, Kristiansen IS. A randomized trial of laypersons' perception of the benefit of osteoporosis therapy: number needed to treat versus postponement of hip fracture. Clin Ther. 2003;25(10):2575–85.
18. Dahl R, Gyrd-Hansen D, Kristiansen IS, Nexoe J, Bo Nielsen J. Can postponement of an adverse outcome be used to present risk reductions to a lay audience? A population survey. BMC Med Inform Decis Mak. 2007;7:8. https://doi.org/10.1186/1472-6947-7-8.
19. Lytsy P, Berglund L, Sundstrom J. A proposal for an additional clinical trial outcome measure assessing preventive effect as delay of events. Eur J Epidemiol. 2012;27(12):903–9. https://doi.org/10.1007/s10654-012-9752-0.
20. Berglund E, Westerling R, Sundstrom J, Lytsy P. Treatment effect expressed as the novel delay of event measure is associated with high willingness to initiate preventive treatment - a randomized survey experiment comparing effect measures. Patient Educ Couns. 2016. https://doi.org/10.1016/j.pec.2016.07.028.
21. Bellavia A, Wallentin L, Orsini N, James SK, Cannon CP, Himmelmann A, et al. Time-based measures of treatment effect: reassessment of ticagrelor and clopidogrel from the PLATO trial. Open Heart. 2017;4(2):e000557. https://doi.org/10.1136/openhrt-2016-000557.
22. Bottai M, Zhang J. Laplace regression with censored data. Biom J. 2010; 52(4):487–503. https://doi.org/10.1002/bimj.200900310.
23. Sniderman PM, Grob DB. Innovations in experimental Design in Attitude Surveys. Annu Rev Sociol. 1996;22:377–99.
24. Gaines BJ, Kuklinski JH, Quirk PJ. The logic of the survey experiment reexamined. Polit Anal. 2007;15:1):1–20. https://doi.org/10.1093/pan/mpl008.
25. Lytsy P, Westerling R. Patient expectations on lipid-lowering drugs. Patient Educ Couns. 2007;67(1–2):143–50. https://doi.org/10.1016/j.pec.2007.03.004.
26. Berglund E, Lytsy P, Westerling R. Adherence to and beliefs in lipid-lowering medical treatments: a structural equation modeling approach including the necessity-concern framework. Patient Educ Couns. 2012. https://doi.org/10.1016/j.pec.2012.11.001.
27. Horne R, Weinman J, Hankins M. The beliefs about medicines questionnaire: the development and evaluation of a new method for assessing the cognitive representation of medication. Psychol Health. 1999;14:1–24.

28. Aikens JE, Nease DE Jr, Nau DP, Klinkman MS, Schwenk TL. Adherence to maintenance-phase antidepressant medication as a function of patient beliefs about medication. Ann Fam Med. 2005;3(1):23–30. https://doi.org/10.1370/afm.238.
29. Horne R, Weinman J. Self-regulation and self-management in asthma: exploring the role of illness perceptions and treatment beliefs in explaining non-adherence to preventer medication. Psychol Health. 2002;17(1):17–32. https://doi.org/10.1080/08870440290001502.
30. Llewellyn CD, Miners AH, Lee CA, Harrington C, Weinman J. The illness perceptions and treatment beliefs of individuals with severe Haemophilia and their role in adherence to home treatment. Psychol Health. 2003;18(2): 185–200. https://doi.org/10.1080/0887044031000098198.
31. Neame R, Hammond A. Beliefs about medications: a questionnaire survey of people with rheumatoid arthritis. Rheumatology. 2005;44(6):762–7. https://doi.org/10.1093/rheumatology/keh587.
32. Allen LaPointe NM, Ou FS, Calvert SB, Melloni C, Stafford JA, Harding T, et al. Association between patient beliefs and medication adherence following hospitalization for acute coronary syndrome. Am Heart J. 2011;161(5):855–63. https://doi.org/10.1016/j.ahj.2011.02.009.
33. Allen LaPointe NM, Ou FS, Calvert SB, Melloni C, Stafford JA, Harding T, et al. Changes in beliefs about medications during long-term care for ischemic heart disease. Am Heart J. 2010;159(4):561–9. https://doi.org/10.1016/j.ahj.2009.12.025.
34. Magadza C, Radloff SE, Srinivas SC. The effect of an educational intervention on patients' knowledge about hypertension, beliefs about medicines, and adherence. Res Social Adm Pharm. 2009;5(4):363–75. https://doi.org/10.1016/j.sapharm.2009.01.004.
35. Sud A, Kline-Rogers EM, Eagle KA, Fang J, Armstrong DF, Rangarajan K, et al. Adherence to medications by patients after acute coronary syndromes. Ann Pharmacother. 2005;39(11):1792–7. https://doi.org/10.1345/aph.1G249.
36. Jorgensen TM, Andersson KA, Mardby AC. Beliefs about medicines among Swedish pharmacy employees. Pharm World Sci. 2006;28(4):233–8. https://doi.org/10.1007/s11096-005-2907-2.
37. Mardby AC, Akerlind I, Jorgensen T. Beliefs about medicines and self-reported adherence among pharmacy clients. Patient Educ Couns. 2007; 69(1–3):158–64. https://doi.org/10.1016/j.pec.2007.08.011.
38. Mardby AC, Akerlind I, Hedenrud T. Different development of general beliefs about medicines during undergraduate studies in medicine, nursing and pharmacy. Patient Educ Couns. 2009;75(2):283–9. https://doi.org/10.1016/j.pec.2008.10.012.
39. Mardby AC, Akerlind I, Hedenrud T. General beliefs about medicines among doctors and nurses in out-patient care: a cross-sectional study. BMC Fam Pract. 2009;10:35. https://doi.org/10.1186/1471-2296-10-35.
40. Kopits IM, Chen C, Roberts JS, Uhlmann W, Green RC. Willingness to pay for genetic testing for Alzheimer's disease: a measure of personal utility. Genet Test Mol Biomarkers. 2011;15(12):871–5. https://doi.org/10.1089/gtmb.2011.0028.
41. Kristiansen IS, Gyrd-Hansen D, Nexoe J, Nielsen JB. Number needed to treat: easily understood and intuitively meaningful? Theoretical considerations and a randomized trial. J Clin Epidemiol. 2002;55(9):888–92.
42. Barry MJ, Edgman-Levitan S. Shared decision making--pinnacle of patient-centered care. N Engl J Med. 2012;366(9):780–1. https://doi.org/10.1056/NEJMp1109283.
43. Ekman I, Swedberg K, Taft C, Lindseth A, Norberg A, Brink E, et al. Person-centered care--ready for prime time. Eur J Cardiov Nursing. 2011;10(4):248–51. https://doi.org/10.1016/j.ejcnurse.2011.06.008.
44. Dorte G-H, Jes S. Discounting life-years: whither time preference? Health Economics. 1998;7(2):121–7. https://doi.org/10.1002/(SICI)1099-1050(199803)7:2<121::AID-HEC318>3.0.CO;2-H.

13

Extracting psychiatric stressors for suicide from social media using deep learning

Jingcheng Du[1†], Yaoyun Zhang[1†], Jianhong Luo[1,2], Yuxi Jia[1,3], Qiang Wei[1], Cui Tao[1] and Hua Xu[1*]

Abstract

Background: Suicide has been one of the leading causes of deaths in the United States. One major cause of suicide is psychiatric stressors. The detection of psychiatric stressors in an at risk population will facilitate the early prevention of suicidal behaviors and suicide. In recent years, the widespread popularity and real-time information sharing flow of social media allow potential early intervention in a large-scale population. However, few automated approaches have been proposed to extract psychiatric stressors from Twitter. The goal of this study was to investigate techniques for recognizing suicide related psychiatric stressors from Twitter using deep learning based methods and transfer learning strategy which leverages an existing annotation dataset from clinical text.

Methods: First, a dataset of suicide-related tweets was collected from Twitter streaming data with a multiple-step pipeline including keyword-based retrieving, filtering and further refining using an automated binary classifier. Specifically, a convolutional neural networks (CNN) based algorithm was used to build the binary classifier. Next, psychiatric stressors were annotated in the suicide-related tweets. The stressor recognition problem is conceptualized as a typical named entity recognition (NER) task and tackled using recurrent neural networks (RNN) based methods. Moreover, to reduce the annotation cost and improve the performance, transfer learning strategy was adopted by leveraging existing annotation from clinical text.

Results & conclusions: To our best knowledge, this is the first effort to extract psychiatric stressors from Twitter data using deep learning based approaches. Comparison to traditional machine learning algorithms shows the superiority of deep learning based approaches. CNN is leading the performance at identifying suicide-related tweets with a precision of 78% and an F-1 measure of 83%, outperforming Support Vector Machine (SVM), Extra Trees (ET), etc. RNN based psychiatric stressors recognition obtains the best F-1 measure of 53.25% by exact match and 67.94% by inexact match, outperforming Conditional Random Fields (CRF). Moreover, transfer learning from clinical notes for the Twitter corpus outperforms the training with Twitter corpus only with an F-1 measure of 54.9% by exact match. The results indicate the advantages of deep learning based methods for the automated stressors recognition from social media.

Keywords: Suicide, Mental health, Psychiatric stressors, Social media, Deep learning, Named entity recognition

* Correspondence: hua.xu@uth.tmc.edu
†Jingcheng Du and Yaoyun Zhang contributed equally to this work.
[1]The University of Texas School of Biomedical Informatics, 7000 Fannin St Suite 600, Houston, TX 77030, USA
Full list of author information is available at the end of the article

Background

Suicide has been one of the leading causes of deaths in the United States [1]. An average of 44,965 Americans die by suicides each year [2]. The national cost of suicides and suicidal behavior in the United States was $93.5 billion in 2013 after adjustment for under-reporting [3]. According to the National Institute of Mental Health, the total suicide rate has increased 24% over the past 15 years [4]. Suicide and suicidal behaviors not only cause unbearable impacts on the specific individuals and surviving family and friends, but also create long lasting effects on whole communities [5].

One of the first steps toward suicide prevention is the identification of risk factors and causes associated with suicide [6].The multiple causes of suicide and suicidal behaviors can be broadly divided into stressors or triggers and predisposition [7]. As one of the major causes to suicide, psychiatric stressors are psychosocial or environmental factors that can profoundly impact cognition, emotion, and behavior of people [8]. The causes of suicide and suicidal behaviors can be complex and vary greatly from individual to individual. The identification of psychiatric stressors is critical to understanding the causes of potential suicide and suicidal behaviors for a specific individual, which is critical to provide a tailored and precise intervention strategy. For example, if the primary stressor for an individual is identified as school bullying, we can offer intensive individual interventions that provide the victim with individual support through meetings with students and parents, counseling, and sustained child and family support [9].

Mentions of stressors are often embedded in narratives such as clinical text or social media posts, and thus need to be recognized first for further investigation. Fortunately, the advances in machine learning and natural language processing (NLP) provide great opportunities to access mental health issues from large-scale narrative data. For example, Zhang et al. mined Electronic Health Records (EHR) to extract psychiatric stressors and symptoms from clinical text [8, 10]. In recent years, social media has shown significant value for many public health related issues [11], as well as the influence on mental health and suicide-related behaviors [12, 13]. The wide popularity of social media provides unprecedented opportunities to access mental health and suicide risk from a large-scale population. The real-time information sharing flow on social media allows potential early detection and intervention for at-risk users.

Most previous studies focused on analyzing the association between suicidal ideation and the linguistic features of the contents (i.e. lexical analysis [14–18]) or posting behaviors (i.e. posting frequency [5, 19]) on social media platforms. Some recent efforts attempted to classify tweets by levels of distress [6], concerns [20, 21] or types of suicidal communication [22] using machine learning or rule based approaches. However, few studies have been done mining the risk factors from social media. Jashinsky et al. tracked suicide risk factors from Twitter using keywords-based approaches [5]. We explored the association between psychiatric stressors and symptoms in tweets based on domain terminologies using Elasticsearch in the paper published in BIBM SEPDA 2017 workshop [23]. However, the keywords-based approaches often retrieve many irrelevant tweets, which introduce much noise into the further analyses.

As an extension to the conference paper, we narrowed down the focus of this paper to automatic identification of suicide related psychiatric stressors and propose a complete deep learning based pipeline to extract psychiatric stressors for suicide from Twitter data. This pipeline first collected and filtered suicide related tweets using keywords. Then, a convolutional neural network (CNN) based classifier removed more noise by further filtering out irrelevant tweets. After that, we applied a recurrent neural network (RNN) based algorithm to extract the mentions of stressors from texts of the suicide related tweets. Furthermore, given that it is time-consuming and costly to build an annotation dataset of stressors in tweets, we also examined the impact of transfer learning based approaches by leveraging pre-trained neural network layers training on clinical notes. To the best of our knowledge, it is the first effort to use systematic machine learning based approaches to extract psychiatric stressor from social media. It could have significant impacts on how people identify those in need of mental health services such as suicide prevention.

Methods

System overview

As illustrated in Fig. 1, the pipeline of the psychiatric stressor recognition from Twitter consisted of four steps. First, we retrieved a coarse set of suicide-related tweets using suicide-related keywords. Here we define the suicide related tweets as the tweets that contain the potential suicidal ideations, suicide history or plan etc. for the Twitter users. Second, we generated a refined candidate set of suicide related tweets by filtering tweets with the obvious stop words collected manually. Third, considering that keywords based tweets collection will introduce much noise, we employed a deep learning based classification model to further select out the precise suicide related tweets. Specifically, the CNN based approach was employed in this step. Finally, we detected the mentions of psychiatric stressors from the suicide-related tweets generated from the previous step. This problem was conceptualized as a named entity recognition (NER) task and we leveraged a state-of-art RNN based framework for this step. In addition, we further investigated transfer

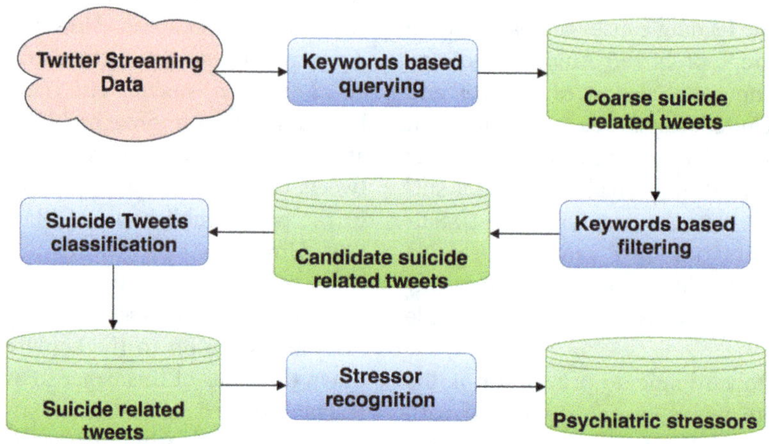

Fig. 1 Pipeline of suicides related psychiatric stressor recognition from Twitter

learning strategy to improve the performance of stressor extraction.

Tweets collection and filtering

We manually curated a suicide related keywords/phrases list to collect public suicide related tweets from June 26th, 2017 to Oct. 19th, 2017 through Twitter streaming API. The keywords/phrases list contains 21 keywords/phrases, such as "suicide", "kill myself", "want death", etc. While manually reviewing the collected tweets, we found most of the tweets were discussing news or advertisements instead of personal ideation or experience. It would have created higher annotation burden and would have deteriorated the performance of the machine learning system if we used the collected tweets directly. To create a refined candidate set of more precise suicide related tweets, we removed all the tweets that contained an URL or keywords such as "hotline", "suicide bomb", "suicide attack", etc. during the collection period. We inductively generated the stop words list to filter the tweets. By doing so, we observed a strong increase in the relevant tweets, which is beneficial for the training and evaluation of the deep learning system. The full list of keywords and stop keywords can be seen in Table 1. After filtering, 1,962,766 tweets were collected during this time period.

Tweets annotation

To identify tweets related to suicide and recognize the psychiatric stressors from tweets, two types of information were annotated. The first type of information is the label of the tweets. We annotated true suicide related tweets by choosing the label from *Positive/Negative*. *Positive* means the tweet is related to suicide or suicide ideation of the Twitter user (personal experience or feeling); tweets with the *Negative* label can be further categorized as 1) not related to suicide or suicide ideation, 2) the negation of suicide or suicide ideation (e.g. I don't want suicide), 3) the discussion of suicide or suicide ideation of other people, 4) the news or reports, 5) other non-positive tweets. Sample tweets with positive and negative labels are illustrated in Table 2.

The second type of information is the mention of psychiatric stressors in tweets text. For the tweets annotated with label *Positive* (i.e., suicide-related), we further annotated the mentions of psychiatric stressors. Some examples of stressors are listed in Table 3.

Here we divided this annotation process into two rounds: we first assigned *Positive/Negative* labels to 3263 tweets. We then trained a binary deep learning based classifier. We will introduce the classifier in the next section. We used this classifier to further select 3000 additional suicide related tweets with *Positive* labels that were relatively more precise than the original set. In the second round of annotation, we annotated the *Positive/Negative* labels as well as the mentions of psychiatric stressors on the new 3000 tweets. We leveraged the Clinical Language Annotation, Modeling, and Processing Toolkit (CLAMP) for the annotation process [24].

CNN based binary classification to recognize suicide related tweets

As one deep learning based algorithm commonly used in various computer vision tasks [25], CNN also demonstrated excellent performance in many NLP tasks, including various text classification tasks [26–29]. We leveraged a classic CNN model for short text classification proposed by Kim et al. [26] to build the tweets binary classifier. We cleaned the tweets using the script from Stanford [30]. Then, we converted the tokens in each tweet to one-hot vectors and mapped the one-hot vectors to pre-trained GloVe Twitter embedding. The mapped embedding was used as the initial input feature to the CNN model. For the CNN model training, various filters were applied to generate the convolutional layers.

Table 1 Examples of suicide-related keywords as queries for tweets retrieval and stop keywords used for irrelevant tweets filtering

Keywords	Stop Keywords
"suicide", "suicidal", "suic", "self-harm", "self-injury", "self harm", "self injury", "hang myself", "hung myself", "kill myself", "kills myself", "killed myself", "take my life", "takes my life", "want to die", "wanted to die", "wants to die", "want death", "wants death", "wanted death", "to be dead"	"bomb", "suicide attack", "suicide attacks", "car attack", "car attacks", "suicide hotline", "https://", "http://"

We applied the max pooling strategy on the feature maps generated by different filters. We added dropout on the pooling layer to avoid overfitting. The pooling layer was connected to a fully connected layer with softmax output. The architecture of the CNN framework is shown in Fig. 2.

RNN-based named entity recognition for stressors

We conceptualized the stressor recognition as a NER task and leveraged a state-of-art RNN framework proposed by Dernoncourt el al [31, 32] to extract the mentions of stressors. The architecture of the framework is shown in Fig. 3. The token embedding mapped each token in the tweets text to a token vector. The character embedding mapped the characters in each token to character vectors. The character Bi-LSTM took the character embedding at each time step as the input and outputs the summary of each character for each token. The token embedding was concatenated with the character LSTM output and then fed to the token Bi-LSTM layer together. On top of token Bi-LSTM, we applied a sequential CRF to jointly decode labels for the whole tweet.

Table 2 Examples of tweets labeled with *Positive* or *Negative* in terms of relatedness to suicide

Positive	i don't know why my dad always comments on how much i'm eating because it makes me want to die
	i'm tired of losing friends and people close to me cause of being suicidal
	i want to kill my self
	i'm in pain, wanna put ten shots in my brain i've been tripped by some things i can't change suicidal
Negative	in the uk the biggest killer for men is suicide. Good job feminists ignoring their issues
	a dear friend of mine committed suicide with a shotgun two years ago
	i don't say this lightly - hemingway's life ended by suicide. His life was actually a loss
	these r not ur problems dear!! these r ur x bf's commitng suicide

Transfer learning-based stressor recognition from tweets

Transfer learning has proven to be an effective technique to improve the performance on a target task with limited annotation data, by using some knowledge learned from a source task [33, 34]. Instead of training the model for a target task from a completely blank network, transfer learning can re-use all or some of the parameters trained from a source task. In our previous studies on extraction of stressors from clinical notes [8, 10], we created a dataset with stressors annotations from the psychiatric notes provided by the CEGS N-GRID 2016 challenge organizers [35]. The annotated dataset contained 946 sentences with stressors annotation. For the transfer learning based approach, clinical notes were used as the source domain to transfer stressor related knowledge to the target domain: Twitter.

Experiment configuration

The core of the deep learning based framework in this study had two modules: a CNN based binary classifier to select suicide related tweets and a RNN based NER system to extract the mentions of stressors. The following experiments were performed for these two modules separately.

For the binary classifier, we trained the CNN model in two steps using two rounds of annotations, respectively. We first trained a CNN model on the first round of annotations with *Positive/Negative* labels. To improve the classifier performance on the unbalanced class distribution (623 *Positives*/3263 tweets), especially on the *Positive* class (suicide related), the training corpus was built with equal sample sizes of the *Positive* class and the *Negative* class (*Positive*: 498 tweets, *Negative*: 498 tweets); the evaluation corpus was built using the same distribution of origin tweets class (*Positive*: 125 tweets, *Negative*: 652 tweets). We further used the best classifier on the evaluation corpus to select another 3000 candidate suicide related tweets that potentially have a high proportion of *Positive* labels for the second round of annotation. The labeled tweets in the later 3000 candidate tweets were divided into training, validation and testing sets with a proportion of 7: 1: 2.

Table 3 Examples of psychiatric stressors annotation from the suicide-related tweets. **Bold** refers to the annotated stressors

job hunting makes me want to commit suicide lmao
honestly every time i think about me **getting pregnant** i wanna kill myself
i just realized that i was completely **sexually assaulted** by some disgusting photographer and i want to fucking kill myself
well i guess it's too bad that i'm just **young adult without a degree** about to lose my **job** and probably planning my suicide afterwards
school and **work** make me want to die everyday

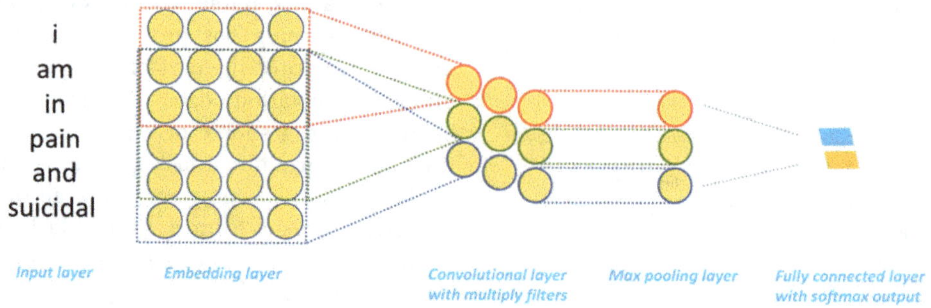

Fig. 2 The architecture of CNN based binary classifier for suicide related labels prediction

The CNN based classifier was trained and evaluated based on the three sets. We used the GloVe Twitter embedding to initialize the embedding layer of CNN and compare the performance using dimensions at 50, 100, and 200 respectively. In order to confirm the superiority of the CNN model, we also evaluated several traditional machine learning algorithms, including Extra Trees (ET), Random Forest (RF), Logistics Regression (LR) and Support Vector Machine (SVM) with Radial Basis Function (RBF) as the kernel, as well as a Bidirectional Long Short-Term Memory (Bi-LSTM) classifier. All the algorithms use GloVe Twitter embedding (dimension 50) as the input. The traditional classification algorithms take the average of the word vectors of the tweet text as the input feature. We evaluated the performance of the classifiers using standard metrics, including precision, recall and F-measure.

For the RNN based NER, we performed the following experiments:

1. To demonstrate the superiority of the RNN model, we used classic Conditional Random Fields (CRF) as the baseline model. We leveraged CLAMP for implementation [24]. Typical features for named entity recognition in CLAMP were employed including lexical features (e.g., bag-of-word, cases, prefix/suffix/stem patterns), syntactic features (e.g. Part of Speech tags), context features (e.g., n-grams), distributional representation of words (e.g., brown clustering, word embedding), and domain knowledge features (e.g., semantic types in UMLS), etc.
2. Performance comparison of different GloVe Twitter embedding dimensions at 50, 100, and 200 on stressor recognition tasks. Performance of different embedding dimensions were evaluated and reported using standard metrics, including precision, recall and F-measure, based on exact match (same entity boundary) and inexact match (overlap in entity boundary) respectively.
3. Performance comparison between using transfer learning strategy and training on Twitter data only for stressor recognition. For the transfer learning approach, clinical notes were used as the source domain to transfer stressor related knowledge to the target Twitter domain. The tweets with *Positive* label in the second round of annotation were divided into training, validation and testing set with

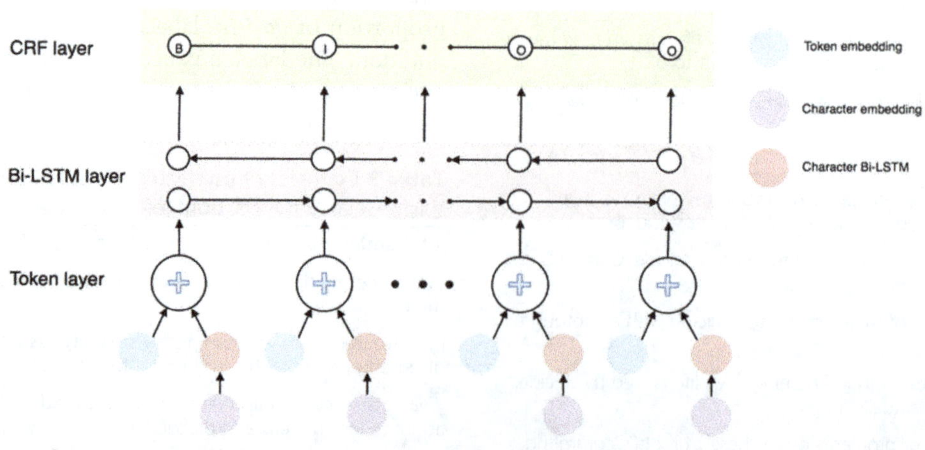

Fig. 3 The architecture of the RNN framework for NER

a proportion of 6: 2: 2. Specifically, the following experiments were conducted:

a. Performance comparison using different sizes of annotated tweets for training in the transfer learning strategy and training on Twitter data only. We evaluated the performance of using different training data sizes from 5, 10, 20, 30, 40, 50 to 60% (all training data) respectively. The validation and testing datasets were kept with the same configuration consistently. We reported the standard metrics, including precision, recall and F-measure, based on exact match and inexact match respectively.
b. Performance comparison of transferring pre-trained parameters up to different layers of the RNN framework, from token embedding layer, character embedding layer, character LSTM layer, token LSTM layer, to fully connected layer to the final CRF layer.

Results

Annotation of suicide related tweets and psychiatric stressors

In the first round of annotation, we assigned the *Positive/Negative* labels to 3263 tweets. Among these tweets, only 623 tweets were annotated as *Positive* (suicide related). We trained the binary classifier (P: 0.66, R: 0.79, F: 0.72) on this annotated dataset and further selected 3000 tweets for the second round of annotation. Among these 3000 tweets, 1985 tweets were annotated as *Positive*, and 2162 stressor entitles were annotated in the *Positive* tweets.

Suicide-related tweet classification

Table 4 lists the performance of suicide-related tweets classification, using the CNN based algorithm and GolVe Twitter embedding features of different dimensions. As shown, the *Positive* type had a high recall (0.90 as the optimal). It also achieved an overall F-measure sufficient (0.83 as the optimal) for practical applications.

Table 5 lists the comparison of the CNN based algorithm with traditional machine learning algorithms as well as the Bi-LSTM model, using GloVe Twitter embedding (dimension 50) as the input. As shown, the CNN model led the performance in *Positive* type, *Negative* type and the overall accuracy. Bi-LSTM was second to the CNN model.

Table 4 Experimental performance of suicide-related tweets classification, using the CNN based algorithm and word embedding features of different dimensions. **Bold** number denotes the largest number in that row

		D = 50	D = 100	D = 200
Precision	Positive	0.78	0.76	**0.79**
	Negative	0.69	**0.70**	0.65
Recall	Positive	0.88	**0.90**	0.84
	Negative	0.51	0.45	**0.56**
F-1 measure	Positive	**0.83**	0.82	0.81
	Negative	0.59	0.55	**0.60**

Psychiatric stressor extraction

Performance of RNN-based stressor recognition

In our pilot work, we evaluated the impact of different types of word embedding for stressors recognition. We first set embedding dimension at 100 and compared GloVe Twitter embedding, GloVe embedding and MIMIC embedding. GloVe Twitter embedding achieved best exact match and inexact match F-measure at 53.25 and 65.46% respectively. As a result, we chose GloVe Twitter embedding for further analysis. We further evaluated the impact of dimensions of the word embedding. The dimension at 100 achieves best exact match F-1 measure (53.25%), while the dimension at 50 achieves best inexact match F-1 measure (67.94%). Although the CRF baseline model led the precision of stressor recognition, however, as we can observe, the RNN based models greatly improved the recall, thus achieving better F-1 measure. The details of metric scores are in Table 6.

Performance of transfer learning -based stressor recognition

Initialized with GloVe Twitter embedding with dimensions of 100, the best model trained on clinical notes achieved precision of 53.08%, recall of 47.51% and F-1 measure of 50.14% on the clinical notes validation set. We transferred parameters up to different layers from this model to initialize the RNN model training on Twitter dataset.

We first investigated the impact of varying training set sizes of the Twitter dataset (see Fig. 4). For both learning strategies, F-measure improved as more training samples were used. Transfer learning improved the F-measure

Table 5 Performance comparison of the CNN model with other algorithms. SVM: Support Vector Machine; ET: Extra Trees; RF: Random Forest; LR: Logistics Regression; Bi-LSTM: Bi-directional Long Short-Term Memory. **Bold** number denotes the largest number in that row

		CNN	SVM	ET	RF	LR	Bi-LSTM
Precision	Positive	**0.78**	0.7	0.69	0.69	0.7	0.73
	Negative	0.69	**0.72**	0.58	0.5	0.67	0.65
Recall	Positive	0.88	**0.96**	0.94	0.88	0.94	0.9
	Negative	**0.51**	0.21	0.17	0.24	0.23	0.37
F-1 measure	Positive	**0.83**	0.81	0.79	0.77	0.8	0.81
	Negative	**0.59**	0.33	0.27	0.33	0.34	0.47
Accuracy		**0.74**	0.703	0.689	0.665	0.697	0.72

Table 6 Experimental performance metric of stressors recognition on different types of word embedding for both exact and inexact match. CRF: Conditional Random Fields. **Bold** number denotes the largest number in that column

	Precision		Recall		F-1 measure	
	exact	inexact	exact	inexact	exact	inexact
GloVe Twitter 50	0.4868	0.6843	0.4765	**0.6745**	0.4816	**0.6794**
GloVe Twitter 100	0.5822	0.7123	0.4906	0.6057	**0.5325**	0.6546
GloVe Twitter 200	0.5248	0.6808	**0.4977**	0.6484	0.5108	0.6642
CRF	**0.600**	**0.784**	0.398	0.572	0.478	0.661

over training with Twitter data only, though the improvement diminished as more training samples were used. This phenomena is consistent with transfer learning on other NER tasks [34]. Compared to training with Twitter data only, transfer learning strategy can save on the number of annotations to achieve the same level of performance. For example, as shown in Fig. 4, transfer learning using 30% of the Twitter training data can achieved a higher F-measure than the baseline strategy where 40% of the training data was used.

Figures 5 and 6 show the impact of transferring the parameters up to each layer of the RNN model measured by exact match and inexact match respectively. For exact match, transferring the layers up to character LSTM achieved best F-measure at 54.9% (see Fig. 7), compared with 53.25% achieved by the model without transfer learning. Transferring all layers could also increase the F-measure, but not as much as transferring some lower layers only. As for inexact match, transferring the layers up to the character LSTM layer achieved a F-measure very close to transferring all layers (67.47 to 67.51%), out-performing by ~0.02 the model without transfer learning (F-measure, 65.46%).

Discussion

In this paper, we proposed and evaluated a systematic pipeline to extract psychiatric stressors for suicide and suicidal ideations from Twitter. This pipeline had multiple steps: 1) Curation of a precise suicide related Twitter corpus by using keywords to collect and filter, and a deep learning based classifier to further select out suicide related tweets. This deep learning based classifier achieved a good F-measure at 83%, which is sufficient for practical application. 2) Leverage a state-of-art RNN based framework to extract stressors from suicide related tweets. This framework achieved the best F-measure by exact match at 53.25%. We also investigated the impact of transfer learning from clinical notes for the Twitter corpus. We found that transfer learning can achieve the same level of performance while reducing the annotation cost of tweets, in comparison with using only the Twitter data for training. For this RNN based framework, we found that transferring the parameters up to the character LSTM layer achieved the best F-measure by exact match (54.9%), 1.65% higher than the best model without transfer learning (F-measure: 53.25%).

To our best knowledge, this is the first effort to extract psychiatric stressors from Twitter data using deep learning based approaches. Compared with lexicon based text analysis, which often introduces much noise, this framework will facilitate more precise analysis. The deep learning based framework also saves great effort on feature engineering, compared to the conventional machine

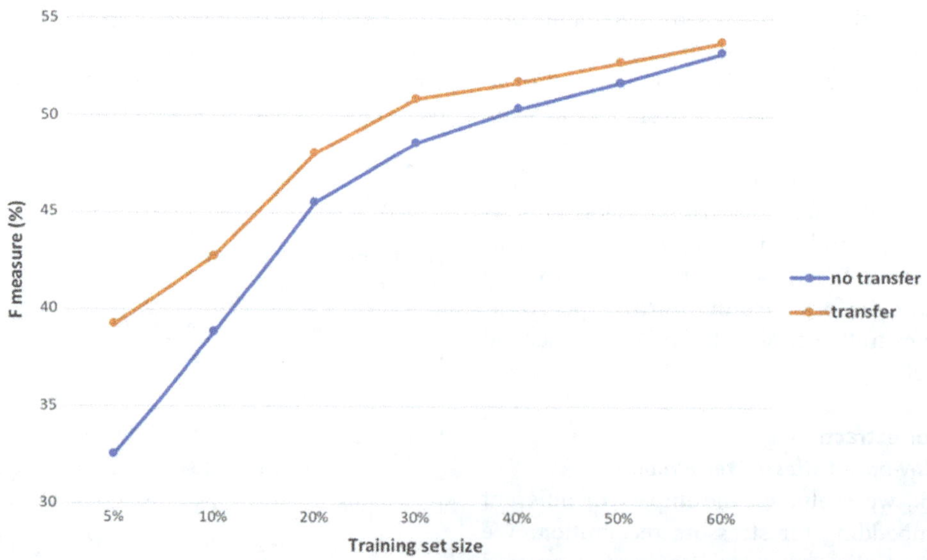

Fig. 4 Impact of transfer learning on the size of training data measured on F-1 measure by exact match

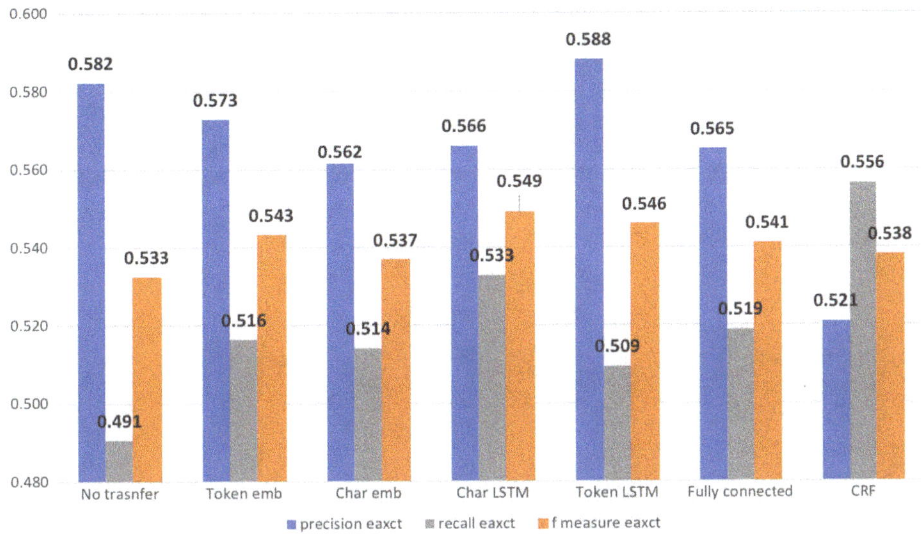

Fig. 5 Impact of transferring the parameters up to each layer of the RNN model for stressors recognition measured by exact match

learning based approaches that require many hand-crafted features. A common limitation of machine learning based Twitter data analysis is the highly imbalanced dataset [28, 36]. We mitigated the impact of imbalanced distributions of classes and entities by building a precise suicide related Twitter corpus using multiple steps. Using state-of-art deep learning based approaches and the transfer learning strategy, our pipeline o achieved a reasonable performance on both suicide related tweets prediction as well as psychiatric stressors extraction.

Certain limitations remain for our study. The major limitation of this study is the lack of ground truth data for the exact mental health status of the Twitter users. The annotations were based on the contents of the tweets. As tweet contents may not always reflect the true mental health status, our dataset may include some false positive suicide related tweets. In addition, due to the limitation of data collection, the current analysis is only based on a single tweet. The lack of context of tweets may introduce inexact interpretations of the contents. There also still exists room for performance improvement on stressor recognition task. The most common type of prediction error in stressor recognition is the boundary issue. As illustrated in Table 7, causes of prediction errors also include (1) missing annotations in the gold standard, (2) the lack of negation detection and (3) mistakenly predicting high-frequent mentions of stressors within a wrong context.

This study obtained a modest performance (exact match F-measure: 54.9%) on the stressors recognition

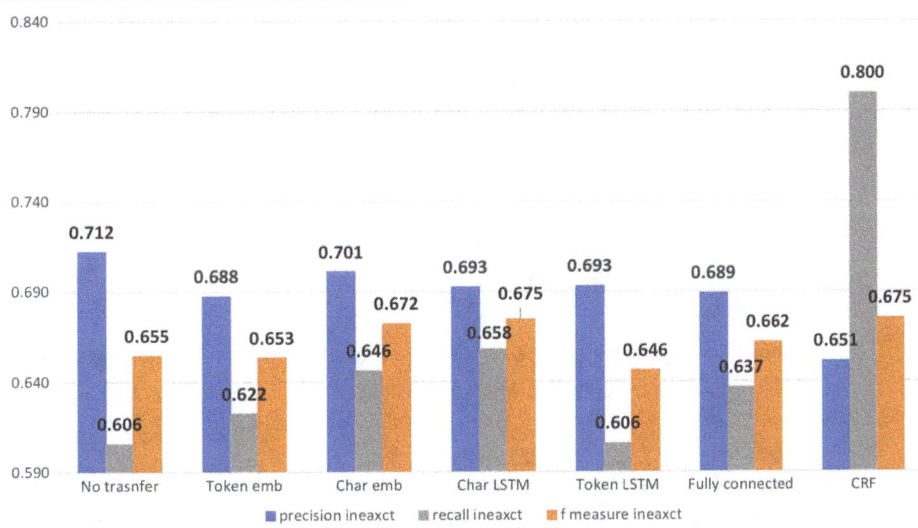

Fig. 6 Impact of transferring the parameters up to each layer of the RNN model for stressors recognition measured by inexact match

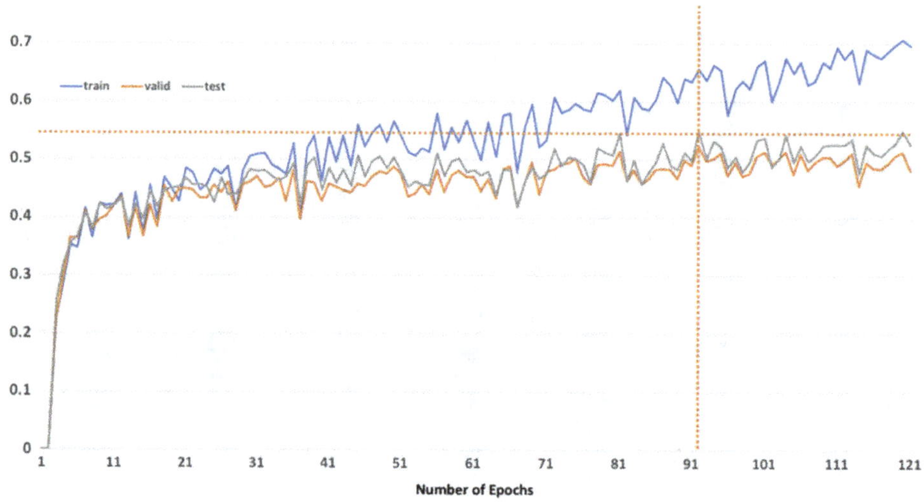

Fig. 7 Exact match F-1 measure by each epoch from the model transferring up to character LSTM layer

task using deep learning based methods. In fact, Twitter NER tasks appear to be more challenging than NER tasks in other domains. For example, in the recent two Twitter NER challenges [37, 38], most of the state-of-art systems achieved F-1 measure between 40 to 60% on various entity recognition tasks, including *person, location,* etc. Considering stressors recognition is an even more complicated problem (i.e. various lengths of boundary, sparseness of expression patterns), we posit that our result is comparable to the state-of-art performances achieved so far.

As for the future work, we're in the process of preparing a large-scale suicide related Twitter dataset. We will access the user level information by analyzing the historical tweets instead of the single tweet without any context. Ground truth data showing the mental health status of the users will be acquired by crowdsourcing or linkage to the users' electrical health record (EHR) data. To improve the performance of the stressors recognition, we will further refine the quality of the gold standard annotation. Moreover, the deep learning based NER systems will be augmented with domain knowledge based and context based rules for further performance improvement.

Conclusions

Few automated approaches have been proposed to extract psychiatric stressors from Twitter, mainly due to (a) the lack of annotated corpora that are time-consuming and costly to build, and (b) the inherent linguistic difficulties that stressors present beyond well-defined clinical concepts such as diseases. To our best knowledge, this is the first and comprehensive effort to extract psychiatric stressors from Twitter data using deep learning based approaches. We've build an annotated Twitter corpus on suicide related stressor recognition. We also performed extensive experiments to justify the use of the approaches presented. The comparison to traditional machine learning algorithms showed the superiority of deep learning based approaches. Our methods demonstrated good performance at identifying suicide-related tweets with a F-1 measure of 83%. In addition, stressor recognition obtained the best F-1 measure of 53.25% by exact match and 67.94% by inexact match. Moreover, transfer learning strategy was

Table 7 Common types of prediction errors. **Bold**: annotated entity; Underline: predicted entity

Boundary	• when the bottom of my **foot inches** i want death. • **allen high school** makes me want to kill myself for not allowing me to get out of a 2nd math class (that i don't need) knowing i work • **hormonal birth control** made me suicidal and acne-ridden! there's no winning against the beast within me
Annotation error: missing annotation	• harassment is not a thing you should have fun with. it almost killed me yesterday.
Negation	• im confident in my maths but **phys** makes me want to die i want
Entity in wrong context	• gonna kill myself after work today. Cant take the **bullying** no longer.
False negative	• when will my **best friend** stop telling me every little things she does with her boyfriend. i want death • i'd kill myself to make **everybody** pay

found to further improve the performance and show potential for saving annotation effort. The results indicate the potential to use deep learning based methods for automated stressor recognition in social media.

Abbreviations

Bi-LSTM: Bidirectional long short-term memory; CLAMP: Clinical language annotation, modeling, and processing toolkit; CNN: Convolutional neural networks; CRF: Conditional random fields; ET: Extra trees; LR: Logistics regression; LSTM: Long short-term memory; NER: Named entity recognition; NLP: Natural language processing; RBF: Radial basis function; RF: Random forest; RNN: Recurrent neural networks; SVM: Support vector machines

Acknowledgments

We thank the anonymous reviewers for their careful reading of our manuscript and their many insightful comments.

Funding

Research was partially supported by the National Library of Medicine of the National Institutes of Health under Award Number 2R01LM010681-05 and R01 LM011829, the National Institute of Allergy and Infectious Diseases of the National Institutes of Health under Award Number R01 AI130460, the National Cancer Institute of the National Institutes of Health under Award Number U01 CA180940, and the Cancer Prevention Research Institute of Texas (CPRIT) Training Grant #RP160015. The authors also acknowledge the support from the National Nature Science Foundation of China (Grant No.71501172), Zhejiang Provincial Nature Science Foundation of China (Grant No.LY18G020017), and the scholarship from the China Scholarship Council. Publication of this article was supported by National Institutes of Health under Award Number 2R01LM010681-05.

Disclaimer

The content is solely the responsibility of the authors and does not necessarily represent the official views of the National Library of Medicine and the Cancer Prevention and Research Institute of Texas.

Authors' contributions

JD and YZ designed the study, collected the data, performed the experiments and drafted the manuscript. JD, YZ, JL, YJ and QW designed the annotation guideline. JD, YZ, JL and YJ annotated the data. CT and HX supervised the study. Everyone read and revised the manuscript. All authors read and approved the final manuscript.

Competing interests

Dr. Hua Xu is a founder of Melax Technologies Inc., which licenses the CLAMP software.

Author details

[1]The University of Texas School of Biomedical Informatics, 7000 Fannin St Suite 600, Houston, TX 77030, USA. [2]Department of Management Science and Engineering, Zhejiang Sci-Tech University, Hangzhou 310018, China. [3]Department of Medical Informatics, School of Public Health, Jilin University, Changchun 130021, Jilin, China.

References

1. Wasserman D. Suicide: an unnecessary death. Oxford: Oxford University Press; 2016.
2. American Foundation for Suicide Prevetion. Suicide Statistics [Internet]. Available from: https://afsp.org/about-suicide/suicide-statistics/. Accessed Feb 2018.
3. Shepard DS, Gurewich D, Lwin AK, Reed GA, Silverman MM. Suicide and suicidal attempts in the United States: costs and policy implications. Suicide life-threatening Behav Wiley Online Library. 2016;46:352–62.
4. National Insitute of Mental Health. Suicide [Internet]. Available from: https://www.nimh.nih.gov/health/statistics/suicide/index.shtml. Accesses Feb 2018.
5. Jashinsky J, Burton SH, Hanson CL, West J, Giraud-Carrier C, Barnes MD, et al. Tracking suicide risk factors through twitter in the US. Crisis Hogrefe Publishing. 2014;35:51.
6. Homan CM, Johar R, Liu T, Lytle M, Silenzio V, Alm CO. Toward macro-insights for suicide prevention: analyzing fine-grained distress at scale. Acl. 2014;2014:107.
7. Mann JJ, Apter A, Bertolote J, Beautrais A, Currier D, Haas A, et al. Suicide prevention strategies: a systematic review. Jama. American Medical Association. 2005;294:2064–74.
8. Zhang OR, Zhang Y, Xu J, Roberts K, Zhang XY, Xu H. Interweaving Domain Knowledge and unsupervised learning for psychiatric stressor extraction from clinical notes. Int. Conf. Ind. Eng. Other Appl. Appl. Intell. Syst 2017. p. 396–406.
9. Feinberg T. Bullying prevention and intervention. Princ Leadersh Mag. 2003;4:10–4.
10. Zhang Y, Zhang O, Wu Y, Lee H-J, Xu J, Xu H, et al. Psychiatric symptom recognition without labeled data using distributional representations of phrases and on-line knowledge. J. Biomed. Inform. Elsevier. 2017;
11. Moorhead SA, Hazlett DE, Harrison L, Carroll JK, Irwin A, Hoving C. A new dimension of health care: systematic review of the uses, benefits, and limitations of social media for health communication, J Med Internet Res, vol. 15. Toronto, Canada: JMIR Publications Inc; 2013. p. 1–16.
12. Luxton DD, June JD, Fairall JM. Social media and suicide: a public health perspective. Am J Public Health American Public Health Association. 2012; 102:S195–200.
13. Wongkoblap A, Vadillo MA, Curcin V. Researching mental health disorders in the era of social media: systematic review. J Med Internet Res JMIR Publications Inc. 2017;19
14. Lv M, Li A, Liu T, Zhu T. Creating a Chinese suicide dictionary for identifying suicide risk on social media. PeerJ PeerJ Inc. 2015;e1455:3.
15. Coppersmith G. Wood a. Exploratory analysis of social media prior to a suicide attempt. In: Proc. 3rd work. Comput. Linguist. Clin. Psychol. From linguist. Signal to Clin. Real; 2016. p. 106–17.
16. Huang X, Zhang L, Chiu D, Liu T, Li X, Zhu T. Detecting suicidal ideation in Chinese microblogs with psychological lexicons. In: Proc - 2014 IEEE Int. Conf. Ubiquitous Intell. Comput. 2014 IEEE Int. Conf. Auton. Trust. Comput. 2014 IEEE Int. Conf. Scalable Comput. Commun. Assoc. Sy; 2014. p. 844–9.
17. Cheng Q, Li TMH, Kwok C-L, Zhu T, Yip PSF. Assessing suicide risk and emotional distress in Chinese social media: A text mining and machine learning study. J Med Internet Res JMIR Publications Inc. 2017;19:e243.
18. Zhang L, Huang X, Liu T, Chen Z, Zhu T, Li A, et al. Using linguistic features to estimate suicide probability of Chinese microblog users. Int Conf Hum Centered Comput 2014;1–11.
19. Smith RJ, Crutchley P, Schwartz HA, Ungar L, Shofer F, Padrez KA, et al. Variations in facebook posting patterns across validated patient health conditions:a prospective cohort study. J Med Internet Res. 2017;19:1–11.
20. O'Dea B, Wan S, Batterham PJ, Calear AL, Paris C, Christensen H. Detecting suicidality on twitter. Internet Interv Elsevier. 2015;2:183–8.
21. Abboute A, Boudjeriou Y, Entringer G, Azé J, Bringay S, Poncelet P. Mining twitter for suicide prevention. In: Int Conf Appl Nat Lang to Data Bases/ Information Syst; 2014. p. 250–3.
22. Burnap P, Colombo G, Amery R, Hodorog A, Scourfield J. Multi-class machine classification of suicide-related communication on twitter. Online Soc. Netw Media. Elsevier. 2017;2:32–44.
23. Du J, Zhang Y, Tao C, Xu H. A pilot study of mining association between psychiatric stressors and symptoms in tweets. IEEE Int Conf Bioinforma Biomed. 2017;2017:1254–7.
24. Soysal E, Wang J, Jiang M, Wu Y, Pakhomov S, Liu H, et al. CLAMP–a toolkit for efficiently building customized clinical natural language processing pipelines. J. Am. Med. In: Informatics Assoc; 2017.
25. LeCun Y, Kavukcuoglu K, Farabet C. Convolutional networks and applications in vision. Circuits Syst. In: (ISCAS), Proc. 2010 IEEE Int Symp, vol. 2010. p. 253–6.
26. Kim Y. Convolutional neural networks for sentence classification. arXiv Prepr. arXiv1408.5882. 2014;
27. Dos Santos CN, Gatti M. Deep convolutional neural networks for sentiment analysis of short texts. In: COLING; 2014. p. 69–78.
28. Nakov P, Ritter A, Rosenthal S, Sebastiani F, Stoyanov V. SemEval-2016 task 4: sentiment analysis in twitter. In: Proc SemEval; 2016. p. 1–18.

29. Conneau A, Schwenk H, Le Cun Y, Barrault L Very Deep Convolutional Networks for Text Classification arXiv Prepr arXiv160601781. 2016;
30. Paulus R. Script for preprocessing tweets [Internet]. Available from: http://nlp.stanford.edu/projects/glove/preprocess-twitter.rb. Accessed Feb 2018.
31. Dernoncourt F, Lee JY, Szolovits P NeuroNER: an easy-to-use program for named-entity recognition based on neural networks arXiv Prepr arXiv1705.05487. 2017;
32. Dernoncourt F, Lee JY, Uzuner O, Szolovits P. De-identification of patient notes with recurrent neural networks. J Am Med Informatics Assoc The Oxford University Press. 2016:ocw156.
33. Kermany DS, Goldbaum M, Cai W, Lewis MA, Valentim CCS, Liang H, et al. Identifying Medical Diagnoses and Treatable Diseases by Image-Based Deep Learning. Cell Elsevier. 2018;172:1122–1131.e9.
34. Lee JY, Szolovits P, Dernoncourt F, Szolovits P Transfer Learning for Named-Entity Recognition with Neural Networks arXiv Prepr arXiv1705.06273. 2017;
35. Stubbs A, Filannino M, Uzuner Ö. De-identification of psychiatric intake records: overview of 2016 CEGS N-GRID shared tasks track 1. J. Biomed. Inform. Elsevier. 2017;75:S4–S18.
36. Du J, Xu J, Song H, Liu X, Tao C. Optimization on machine learning based approaches for sentiment analysis on HPV vaccines related tweets. J Biomed Semantics. 2017;8:9.
37. Derczynski L, Nichols E, van Erp M, Limsopatham N. Results of the WNUT2017 shared task on novel and emerging entity recognition. In: Proc. 3rd work. Noisy user-generated Text; 2017. p. 140–7.
38. Lopez C, Partalas I, Balikas G, Derbas N, Martin A, Reutenauer C, et al. CAp 2017 challenge: Twitter Named Entity Recognition. arXiv Prepr. arXiv1707. 07568. 2017.

14

Automated extraction of Biomarker information from pathology reports

Jeongeun Lee[1], Hyun-Je Song[2], Eunsil Yoon[3], Seong-Bae Park[2], Sung-Hye Park[4], Jeong-Wook Seo[4], Peom Park[6] and Jinwook Choi[1,5*]

Abstract

Background: Pathology reports are written in free-text form, which precludes efficient data gathering. We aimed to overcome this limitation and design an automated system for extracting biomarker profiles from accumulated pathology reports.

Methods: We designed a new data model for representing biomarker knowledge. The automated system parses immunohistochemistry reports based on a "slide paragraph" unit defined as a set of immunohistochemistry findings obtained for the same tissue slide. Pathology reports are parsed using context-free grammar for immunohistochemistry, and using a tree-like structure for surgical pathology. The performance of the approach was validated on manually annotated pathology reports of 100 randomly selected patients managed at Seoul National University Hospital.

Results: High F-scores were obtained for parsing biomarker name and corresponding test results (0.999 and 0.998, respectively) from the immunohistochemistry reports, compared to relatively poor performance for parsing surgical pathology findings. However, applying the proposed approach to our single-center dataset revealed information on 221 unique biomarkers, which represents a richer result than biomarker profiles obtained based on the published literature. Owing to the data representation model, the proposed approach can associate biomarker profiles extracted from an immunohistochemistry report with corresponding pathology findings listed in one or more surgical pathology reports. Term variations are resolved by normalization to corresponding preferred terms determined by expanded dictionary look-up and text similarity-based search.

Conclusions: Our proposed approach for biomarker data extraction addresses key limitations regarding data representation and can handle reports prepared in the clinical setting, which often contain incomplete sentences, typographical errors, and inconsistent formatting.

Keywords: Biomarkers, Cancer disease knowledge representation model, Pathology reports, Natural language processing, Clinical decision-making

Background

Precision medicine is a newly emerging trend in medicine, whereby individualized medical treatments are designed based on the specific biologic information of each patient. Traditionally, tumors are classified based on their histological features. However, in the era of precision medicine, the biological behavior is interpreted in terms of not only histological morphology but also genomic features of the tumor.

For individualized diagnosis, pathologists currently rely substantially on immunohistochemistry (IHC) findings, which provide clues regarding genomic features in terms of relevant biomarkers [1]. Biomarkers reflect the biologic behavior of tumors, including pathogenicity and pharmacologic response [2, 3]. Thus, to ensure a reliable histologic diagnosis, it is important to have access to statistical data from pathology reports regarding similar patients, which can be achieved through the retrospective study of relevant reports describing biomarker

* Correspondence: jinchoi@snu.ac.kr
[1]Interdisciplinary Program for Bioengineering, Graduate School, Seoul National Universty, Seoul, Republic of Korea
[5]Department of Biomedical Engineering, College of Medicine, Seoul National University, Seoul, Republic of Korea
Full list of author information is available at the end of the article

findings, tumor staging, and morphologic features of the cancer [3–6].

Pathpedia (www.pathpedia.com) [7] is an online resource of pathology information providing statistical data including biomarker levels, anatomical pathology features, and clinical pathology features. The main advantages of Pathpedia include high-level, manual curation of data and the large number of information sources (up to 4000 references). However, there are disadvantages to using journal articles as the main source of reference data. Specifically, certain biomarkers are discussed in a limited number of journal articles, which precludes data verification. Moreover, there is limited coverage of various ethnic groups and uneven data distribution regarding race, life patterns, nutritional habits, geology, and climate, which precludes genomic-level comparisons based on data from Pathpedia.

The present study focused on the Korean population and involved careful review of 82,291 pathology reports, including IHC and surgical pathology (SP) reports, from Seoul National University Hospital (SNUH). In order to facilitate the detection of potential relationships between various immunologic biomarkers and pathologic diagnosis, we previously developed a web-based information system [8] designed to compute and display statistics of clinical data extracted from pathology reports (e.g., affected organ, diagnosis, cancer staging information, and IHC findings).

We further describe related work in the field of automated extraction of data from medical reports, and then introduce our information extraction approach specifically tailored to pathology reports. We then describe in detail the result of text processing via our proposed approach, as well as the relevance of the findings. Finally, we cover the limitations and implications of our proposed solution.

Most previous studies on automatic extraction of biomarker data focused on biomedical literature [9–11]. Yonesi et al. [9] suggested a system for improved recognition of biomarker names in published literature, which is implemented in ProMiner [10] and represents a rule-based system for gene name normalization. The BioNER [11] system uses a custom-made biomarker-specific disease dictionary to extract disease-related biomarkers from MEDLINE publications. However, the performance of these systems is insufficient for processing pathology documents because of intrinsic differences between such clinical documents and published scientific articles. Specifically, to enhance readability in the clinical setting, pathology reports generally do not follow formal grammar rules and are instead written in a keyword-oriented style and formatted using many line breaks, white spaces, and hyphens. This type of formatting makes it difficult to automatically detect the sentence boundary and apply normalization of term variation, which is particularly relevant because current solutions for biomarker data mining employ context to a substantial extent.

Although some studies have attempted to extract biomarker information, these typically focused on extracting cancer-related information (e.g., histologic type and stage) from pathology reports, and, in particular, from SP reports. Such studies [12–20] typically apply pattern-based natural language processing for extracting information on specific types of cancer (especially breast or lung cancer), which is not applicable to mining data on other types of cancer. On the other hand, Coden et al. [19] proposed a pan-cancer knowledge representation model for data from SP documents. Specifically, the Cancer Disease Knowledge Representation Model (CDKRM) defines what entities can be extracted and what relations these entities can have with each other. However, the CDKRM does not cover IHC findings and does not define how to combine biomarker information parsed from IHC reports with corresponding pathologic findings parsed from SP reports. For the same reason, the PEP [20] system, which follows the CDKRM for information extraction, cannot extract biomarker information by default and also requires modification to handle keyword-oriented SP reports typically encountered in clinical practice.

Unlike biomedical literature, clinical reports sometimes contain specific jargons and spelling errors [21], and therefore the identified medical terms require further normalization, i.e., ensuring that clinical terms with the same meaning are represented in the model using the same term. The cTAKES approach [22] is well known for its ability to recognize most medical terms (including anatomical sites and disease names) from clinical documents and to correctly normalize these terms to their Unified Medical Language System (UMLS) [23] identifiers. However, UMLS does not cover all variants of biomarker-related terminology used in IHC. Even though cTAKES can employ other dictionaries than UMLS for normalization, as it was designed to handle general clinical documents following formal English grammar, it is difficult to customize cTAKES for efficient normalization of keyword-based reports such as IHC.

Methods

Representation of biomarker knowledge

Our data model for representing biomarker knowledge is similar to the CDKRM [19], but it contains a new framework for handling IHC reports. Specifically, the CDKRM covers only microscopic pathologic findings from SP reports as model entities, whereas the model developed in the present study can represent biomarker test results extracted from IHC reports. Additionally, our model has the ability to define which biomarker test described in an IHC report represents evidence for which microscopic finding described in an SP report, which helps avoid incorrect assignment of IHC findings to pathology findings described in the SP report of another patient or of the same patient but for a different indication. For example, when the patient shows symptoms suggesting metastatic cancer, the physician may conduct the same IHC test for several tissue slides obtained from the same patient (Fig. 1a and b, Additional file 1: Figure S1a and S1b). The results of such an IHC test may be

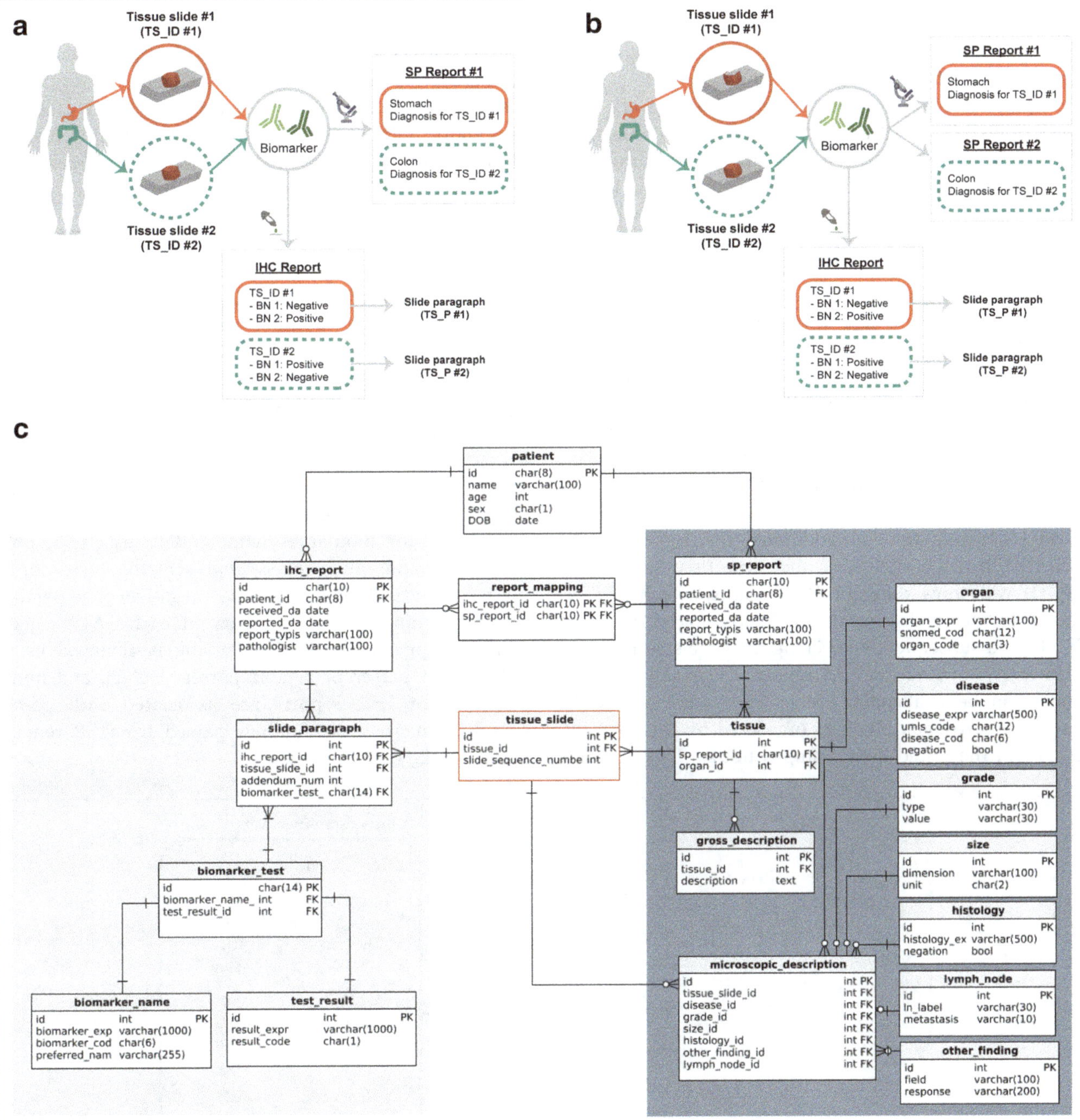

Fig. 1 Representation model for information extraction of biomarker. **a** Reporting system for multi biopsy samples from a patient. As same biomarker test can be conducted for tissue slide #1 and tissue slide #2 of the patient, a IHC report can contain multiple "slide paragraph (TS_P)". Also, multiple pathologic findings derived from multiple IHC tests can be reported in one SP report **b**) or in separate SP reports. **c** Representation model for information extraction of biomarker from pathology reports in Seoul National University Hospital. IHC:immunohistochemistry, SP:surgical pathologic, BN:biomarker name

reported either in an addendum to the original IHC and SP reports (Fig. 1a), or in an entirely new report (Fig. 1b, Additional file 1: Figure S1a and S1b) [24]. Thus, when designing the data representation model, it is important to take into account that the patient may have one or more SP reports with various microscopic findings for different tissue slides.

To facilitate appropriate association between the findings described in IHC reports and those described in SP reports, we assumed that a tissue slide represents the minimum unit for describing a pathologic finding. This assumption is based on the fact that almost every IHC report states the serial number of the target tissue slide at the top of the results of each analysis performed as the guidelines of College of American Pathologist (CAP) (Additional file 1: Figure S1c) [25, 26]. Furthermore, some descriptions of pathologic findings in the SP report explicitly state which tissue slide provides evidence for that particular finding. Thus, we associated IHC findings with microscopic findings based on tissue slide identifiers (TS_IDs), which represent the serial numbers of tissue slides; furthermore, we introduced the tissue slide paragraph (TS_P) to refer to a set of IHC findings corresponding to a single tissue slide.

Parsing IHC reports using TS_P provides another advantage for cases where the same IHC tests are repeated within a certain time interval because previous tests showed unstable results (Additional file 1: Figure S1a and S1b). In such situations, the same tissue slide (i.e., TS_ID) will show different IHC results, which can be traced easily by collecting all TS_Ps pointing to the same TS_ID, and subsequently checking the time stamps.

However, parsing the SP reports according to this model can be challenging. Most SP reports at SNUH describe microscopic findings organized by the anatomical site of the tested tissue sample, not by TS_ID which is consistent with guidelines of CAP (Additional file 2: Figure S2b and S2c) [24]. Therefore, when the SP report describes the microscopic findings in tissue samples from more than two different anatomical sites or in samples of the same tissue but with distinct pathological characteristics, it is not appropriate to simply map all tissue slides to the anatomical site first mentioned in the SP report. Instead, the system needs to determine the anatomical site of origin for each tissue slide. Fortunately, since one tissue sample is typically resected from each anatomical site, the algorithm steps for determining the anatomical site need to be triggered only when the SP report mentions more than two anatomical sites, thereby minimizing the computational burden of this procedure. A scheme describing our data representation model is given in Fig. 1c.

Information extraction from IHC reports

SNUH reports adopt a semi-structured style for describing IHC findings, further classified as list- or table-based style (Additional file 1: Figure S1a and S1b). We designed the information extraction system in consideration of this semi-structured style, to ensure simplicity and accuracy of parsing. After collecting a set of patterns for each style (i.e., list- or table-based) from training set, we defined a context-free grammar to identify which tokens stand for biomarker names (BNs; e.g., p53, p63, Cyclin-D1) and which tokens represent the corresponding test results (TRs; e.g., positive, negative). The parsing also takes note of the boundary of each TS_P tagged with the appropriate TS_ID. Parsing is achieved using either a list parser or a table parser (Fig. 2), and items parsed from IHC reports are associated with corresponding microscopic findings parsed from SP reports based on TS_ID.

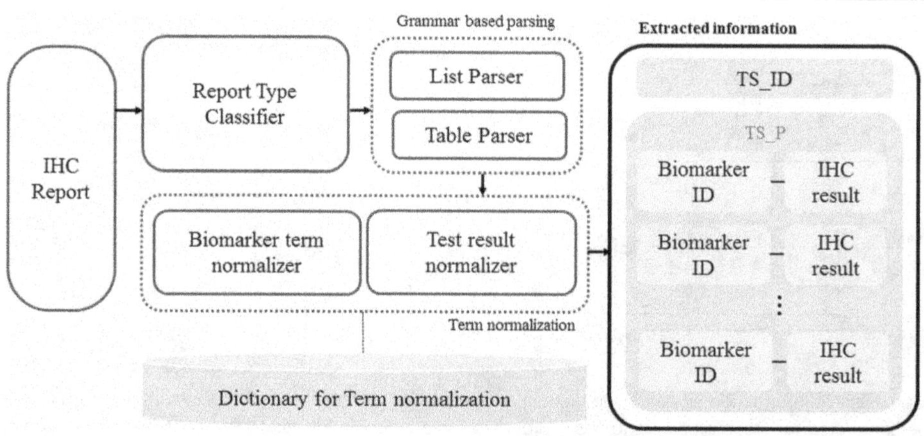

Fig. 2 Flow chart of information extraction from IHC report with an example. Step #1) Classify type of IHC report and choose appropriate parser for the input. Step #2) Normalize biomarker names recognized from step #1 using BN dictionary. Step #3) Normalize test results recognized from step #1 using TR dictionary. BN: biomarker name, TR: test result

Biomarker term normalization handles terminology variation in BNs and ensures that, for example, 'Wilms' tumor 1 protein', 'WT-1', 'Wilms tumor 1-protein', and 'WT1 (4)' are converted into the single representative form 'Genes, Wilms Tumor'. To facilitate term normalization, we created a BN dictionary for dictionary look-up and text similarity-based search. The dictionary is based on a list of official product names of biomarkers used at SNUH, comprising 184 original BNs, which we annotated with Preferred Terms (P_BN) of Medical Subject Headings (MeSH) codes. If there was no MeSH entry for a given BN, the P_BN assigned by the pathologists was used as the general term. The list of BNs was then automatically expanded with a set of hand-crafted rules to cover simple variations in notation, such as addition of hyphens or white spaces. This type of dictionary expansion was designed to make text similarity-based searching fast and efficient.

The rules applied to expand the BN dictionary (Table 1) are similar to those described by Bravo et al. [11] for term normalization of gene/biomarker protein names in the biomedical literature, except we remove laboratory-related terms included in parenthesis, so that 'WT-1 (4)' and 'WT-1 (Repeat)' are normalized to 'WT-1'. Consequently, the number of entries in the expanded BN dictionary was 3370. This BN dictionary was cross-checked by three pathologists at SNUH.

Term variations in TRs were also considered. For example, 'positive in mesothelial cells' and 'positive in tumor cells' are normalized to 'Positive', whereas and 'focal weak positive' and 'a few positive cells' are normalized to 'Focal positive'. Unfortunately, as TR normalization requires background knowledge about the tested biomarkers, it was not feasible to create a TR dictionary by applying the same rule-based approach as that used for creating the BN dictionary. Therefore, three pathologists manually created a TR dictionary based on all TRs from training set to assign the normalized TR terms: "Positive", "Focal Positive", "Negative", or "Error" (i.e., failed IHC test or spelling error that precludes normalization of the detected TRs). This TR dictionary was then used for normalization of TR terms by dictionary look-up.

Table 1 Term expansion rules for biomarker names

Rule	Example
1) Replace Roman numbers with the corresponding Arabic numbers	Factor VIII → Factor 8
2) Replace Greek symbol with the corresponding letters	CD79 α → CD79 alpha
3) Remove laboratory related terms	CD10(repeat) → CD10
4) Generate new variants	GAL3 = GAL-3 = GAL 3
5) Convert to lowercase	DESMIN→ desmin

Information extraction from SP reports

SP reports are parsed and processed in a similar manner as that employed for handling IHC reports. However, unlike IHC reports, SP reports are rather unstructured in terms of reporting style, and thus, the grammar-based parsing approach used for parsing IHC reports was not adequate for parsing SP reports, as it could not account for all patterns of reporting styles employed in SP reports. Fortunately, in most SP reports archived at SNUH, the first few lines typically mention what organ the tissue sample originated from, whereas the subsequent lines describe the pathologic findings for that tissue [24]. Additionally, when pathologic findings are reported for a specific disease, these findings are grouped under the disease name with an indentation which is consistent with recommendation of CAP for visual separation (Additional file 2: Figure S2b and S2c) [24]. We took this behavioral tendency into account when designing the parser, aiming to reduce the search space for each item and improve parsing accuracy. Specifically, we implemented a tree-based parsing approach of the SP reports, whereby the tree root node is designated in terms of the organ name. In the example illustrated in Fig. 3, the organ name "Breast" appears on the first line of the SP report, so the system creates a tree with the root node containing the first line. Because the next line is numbered and starts with the disease name "1. INFILTRATING DUCT CARCINOMA, multiple, residual (see note)", this line is assigned as the first sub-node of the root node, at the same level as other numbered lines, such as "2. Fibrocystic change with microcalcification". Because the lines below the first sub-node have indentations, the system assigns them as sub-nodes of the first sub-node. In this way, the system can generate candidate boundaries for organs, diseases, and specific pathologic findings.

In other words, to create a tree with the root node represented by the organ, the parser must recognize the organ name correctly. To implement such a parser, we first created a dictionary based on terms corresponding to organ names from the Systematized Nomenclature of Medicine-Clinical Terms (SNOMED-CT). The system performs a dictionary look-up operation and calculates a look-up score as the linear sum of the Edit distance, string kernel, Jaro-Winkler distance, and soft term frequency-inverse document frequency statistic. If the look-up score is above a certain threshold, the system registers the term into the organ terminology database, which consists of a normalized set of terms describing organs. We used a training set of SP reports to build the organ terminology database according to this method, which was then verified and curated by two clinicians at SNUH. When parsing the SP reports, the system applies a similar approach to recognize and normalize disease names with UMLS disorder names. If a node corresponding to a disease name is

a

DIAGNOSIS:

Breast, right, breast conserving surgery:

1. INFILTRATING DUCT CARCINOMA, multiple, residual (see note)
 - Post-neoadjuvant chemotherapy status
   (C12-1567, 1568: Infiltrating duct carcinoma)
 - Invasive tumor size: up to 2.4 x 2.0 x 1.0cm
 - Tumor extent including DCIS: 4.6 x 2.0 x 2.5cm
 - Nuclear grade: 3/3
 - Histologic grade: II/III
 - DCIS component: present,
   around the tumor, non-comedo type, high grade
 - Tumor border: infiltrative
 - No involvement of nipple
 - Microcalcification: present
 - Lymphatic emboli: present
 - Vascular emboli: absent
 - Surgical margins
   superior margin: clear (Fro#2)
   inferior margin: clear (Fro#3)
   medial margin: clear (Fro#1)
   lateral margin: clear (Fro#4)
   superficial margin: clear
   deep margin: clear (safety margin: 2mm)
 - Lymph node: metastasis in one out of five lymph nodes
   ("level 1", 1/5)
2. Fibrocystic change with microcalcification

b

<ORGAN> Breast, right, breast conserving surgery: **SNOMED-CT: 76752008**
- **<DIAGNOSIS>** INFILTRATING DUCT CARCINOMA, multiple, residual **UMLS: C1134719**
  - **<OTHER_FINDING>** Post-neoadjuvant chemotherapy status (C12-1567, 1568: Infiltrating duct carcinoma)
  - **<SIZE>** Invasive tumor size: up to 2.4 x 2.0 x 1.0cm
  - **<OTHER_FINDING>** Tumor extent including DCIS: 4.6 x 2.0 x 2.5cm
  - **<GRADE>** Nuclear grade: 3/3
  - **<GRADE>** Histologic grade: II/III
  - **<OTHER_FINDING>** DCIS component: present, around the tumor, non-comedo type, high grade
  - **<OTHER_FINDING>** Tumor border: infiltrative
  - **<OTHER_FINDING>** No involvement of nipple
  - **<OTHER_FINDING>** Microcalcification: present
  - **<OTHER_FINDING>** Lymphatic emboli: present
  - **<OTHER_FINDING>** Vascular emboli: absent
  - **<OTHER_FINDING>** Surgical margins
    superior margin: clear (Fro#2)
    inferior margin: clear (Fro#3)
    medial margin: clear (Fro#1)
    lateral margin: clear (Fro#4)
    superficial margin: clear
    deep margin: clear (safety margin: 2mm)
  - **<LYMPH_NODE>** Lymph node: metastasis in one out of five lymph nodes ("level 1", 1/5)
- **<DIAGNOSIS>** Fibrocystic change with microcalcification **UMLS: C0016034**

Fig. 3 **a** Excerpt of a SP report, **b** corresponding parsing tree of SP report in 3a

found to have a sub-tree, all its sub-nodes are considered to represent detailed microscopic findings regarding that disease. Finally, for recognition of negation and metastasis terms, we used a set of patterns manually created based on the same training set of SP reports.

Merging IHC and SP information

Biomarker information extracted from IHC reports and corresponding microscopic findings extracted from SP reports are matched according to TS_P and TS_ID.

Datasets and performance evaluation

We obtained 41,772 IHC reports and 40,519 SP reports archived at SNUH between 2007 and 2012 (Table 2). Subsequently, reports created between 2007 and 2011 were used as the training data set, whereas later reports were used as a validation data set. Additionally, in order to create a gold standard for the evaluation, we randomly selected 400 patients for whom we manually annotated the reports (508 IHC reports and the corresponding 831 SP reports) using the BRAT tool [27]. There were three trained annotators. Each document of patient was annotated by two annotators for normalization of BNs and TRs along with recognition of boundaries of entity mentions. Inter-annotator agreement was measured by F-measure [28]. (Additional file 3: Table S1).

Table 2 Statistics of SNUH dataset

Type of report	2007	2008	2009	2010	2011	2012	Total
IHC	0	6370	7611	8067	10,889	8830	41,772
SP	160	6338	7507	7893	10,341	8280	40,519

IHC Immunohistochemistry reports, *SP* Surgical pathology reports

For validation, we selected only those IHC reports for which the corresponding SP reports described information regarding only one organ and one diagnosis, so as to assess solely the issue of data extraction itself. The issue of discriminating findings that refer to multiple organs or diagnoses listed in the SP report will be covered in future work, as this aspect also involves the processing of SP report data without corresponding IHC findings (e.g., findings of the gross examination).

The training data was mainly used to generate patterns while making hand-crafted rules for parsing. Also, we used the training set to manually curate the dictionaries for normalization of BNs and TRs. Validation of information extraction was performed on the gold standard set we manually made.

Results

The IHC report parser extracts TS_ID, BN, and corresponding TRs. The ability of the parser to recognize the boundaries of these entities was evaluated by exact matching, which indicated that the parser recognized the entity boundaries well, with F-1 scores of 1, 0.998, and 0.9978 for TS_ID, BN and TR, respectively (Table 3). After parsing each entity, the system normalized term variants to a single representative term, which was also achieved with high performance, namely with F-1 scores of 0.972 and 0.969 for BN and TR, respectively.

On the other hand, the SP report parser was evaluated only in terms of term boundary recognition for organ and diagnosis, as the data set used for training only contained such information. The exact matching test indicated good performance for organ name recognition but poor performance for diagnosis recognition (Table 3). Because the boundaries of the disease term showed some differences between annotators, we also applied overlap matching to evaluate the performance of the parser regarding term boundary recognition. Although the exact matching test results indicated low performance (F-1 score 0.556), the overlap matching test results indicated higher performance (F1 score 0.773).

When applying the developed system to all pathology reports (i.e., including the reports used as a validation data set), 45,999 TS_Ps were found within 41,765 IHC reports. The remaining 7 IHC reports could not be parsed because they did not include TS_ID. Furthermore, 4135 of 45,999 TS_Ps identified were ignored because their corresponding SP reports were not included in our target dataset. Within the 41,864 TS_Ps analyzed, the system recognized 206,534 BNs and successfully normalized 205,759 BNs into 215 P_BNs. Each extracted BN was associated with a corresponding TR. All but 105 TRs were correctly normalized. Finally, we obtained 205,627 BN-TR pairs.

When applying the system to parse 37,211 SP reports corresponding to 41,864 TS_Ps extracted from IHC reports (Fig. 4), a total of 5012 SP reports were found to describe no microscopic diagnosis. Furthermore, only SP reports mentioning a single organ and a single diagnosis were retained (21,090 SP reports), within which 21,090 candidates for organ names were recognized. With the exception of 277 organ name candidates, all other candidates were successfully normalized into 46 representative organ names. Subsequent parsing of disease names resulted in 20,758 candidate disease names, of which 68.11% were successfully normalized. The reason for this relatively lower success rate of the normalization is likely related to including inappropriate candidates of disease names, as well as to the high term variation for disease names. The process of parsing SP reports is illustrated in Fig. 4, with the main graph showing statistics for total BNs, and the corner graph showing statistics for total SP reports.

Finally, we compared the statistics provided by our proposed approach for information extraction with the statistics provided by Pathpedia (Fig. 5) regarding the positive rate of biomarker assays. The first important difference between the SNUH- and Pathpedia-based findings is the composition of the set of biomarkers employed for such analyses. For example, the mean number of assay attempts for ErbB-2, thymidylate synthase, EGFR, p53, FOXP3, PDPN, MLH-1, ERCC1, CDH17, CD44, CK 7, and CK 20 is 469 based on SNUH data, compared to only 132 based on Pathpedia data. Moreover, although the number of ErbB-2 assays was similar (720 and 650 assays for SNUH and Pathpedia, respectively), the rate of positives (including focal positive) was substantially different, with 290/720 for SNUH and 26/650 for Pathpedia.

Table 3 Extraction performance for IHC and SP

A	Recognition			Normalization		
	Recall	Precision	F1	Recall	Precision	F1
TS_ID	1	1	1	–	–	–
BN	0.999	1	0.999	1.000	0.946	0.972
TR	0.998	0.998	0.998	1.000	0.939	0.969
B	Exact Matching					
	Recall	Precision	F1			
Organ	0.896	0.953	0.924			
Diagnosis	0.794	0.427	0.556			
C	Overlap matching					
	Recall	Precision	F1			
Organ	0.901	0.961	0.930			
Diagnosis	0.794	0.754	0.773			

TS_ID Tissue slide ID, *BN* Biomarker name, *TR* Test result

Discussion

The proposed approach for automated extraction of biomarker data showed high performance for parsing IHC reports (very high F1-scores), which is due to the very stable reporting format used at SNUH. Specifically, since 2008, SNUH pathologists have written IHC reports using one of only two reporting formats (i.e., list- or table-based). Although there were spelling errors in writing, detecting certain formatting determinants such as semi-colon (";"), colon (":"), or vertical bar ("|") was extremely helpful in accounting for report format variations while still using relatively simple grammar; in fact, we were able to update the internal database of IHC report templates with a new version.

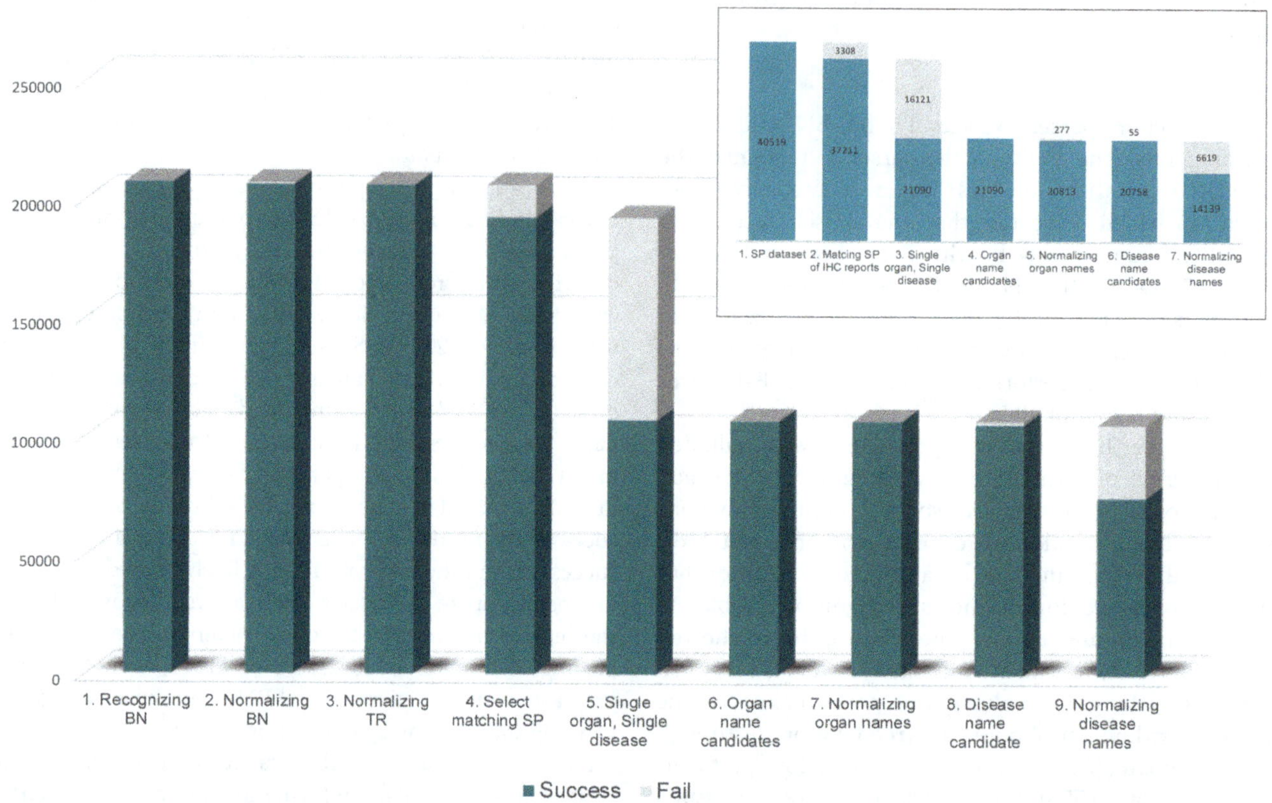

Fig. 4 The process of parsing SP reports; the main graph showing statistics for total BNs, and the corner graph showing statistics for total SP reports

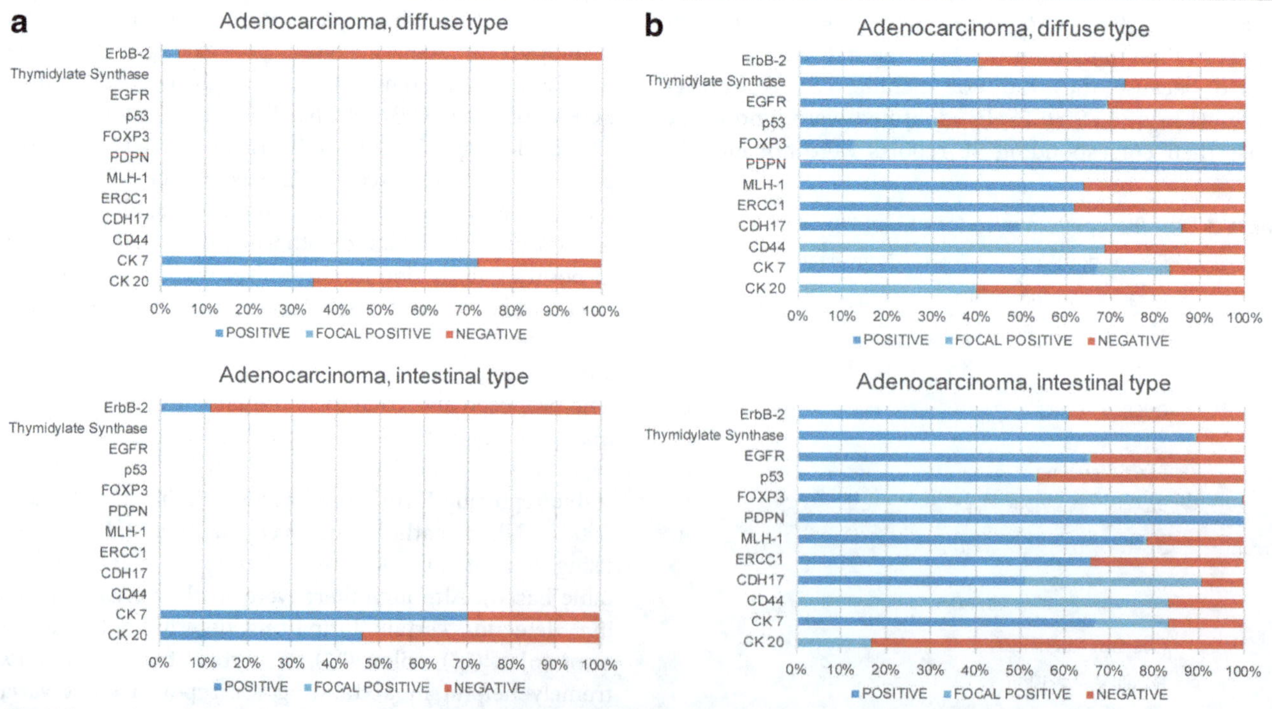

Fig. 5 Comparison of the statistics provided by our proposed approach for information extraction with the statistics provided by Pathpedia regarding the positive rate of biomarker assays. **a** statistics provided by Pathpedia, **b** the statistics provided by our proposed approach for adenocarcinoma, diffuse type and intestinal type in stomach

Our approach involves using dictionaries for recognizing and normalizing BNs and TRs, which we created based on initial processing of the training data set. As depicted in Fig. 6, a similar number of new IHC tests (described as BN-TR pairs) were performed each year at SNUH, and the number of BN terms increased steadily every year. This finding is related to the fact that, every year, SNUH purchased a new type of biomarker. Moreover, SNUH received and archived IHC reports prepared by pathologists at other hospitals regarding patients referred to SNUH for consultation. Fortunately, most variations were covered by the expanded BN dictionary, but terms related to the new biomarkers had to undergo normalization according to UMLS terminology. Notably, there was substantially higher variation in TR terminology, and the parser required almost ten times longer to recognize and normalize TRs than to do so for BNs. Moreover, as some BNs have numeric TRs whose ranges may differ with cell type, classifying the TRs into four categories (positive, focal positive, negative, and error) resulted in some controversy between consulting pathologists.

Unlike IHC reports, SP reports at SNUH showed high variability in reporting style and format, and creating the SP report parsing tree with a single organ root node was sometimes difficult because some SP reports contained a description of findings of the macroscopic or frozen section evaluations, which are commonly performed during surgery. When pathologists deem that further tests are necessary or they lack sufficient evidence for a definite diagnosis, they report several candidate disease names. As the goal of extracting IHC and SP data in this manner is to facilitate detection of potential relationships between IHC profiles and pathologic diagnosis, further study is warranted to develop an automated framework for discriminating between final and intermediate diagnosis. Here, we chose to include in the validation data set only SP reports describing a single sample with a single, explicitly stated diagnosis.

Parsing the SP reports produced the name of the organ of origin of the tissue sample, and the diagnosis based on microscopic findings. Under the assumption that the pathologic findings are described after the organ is mentioned, we could discriminate the lines describing the organ of origin from the lines describing the disease, as well as from the lines describing the actual findings, and organized this information into a tree-like structure. We then used dictionaries based on SNOMED-CT and UMLS to further normalize the recognized organ names and disease names, but these dictionaries did not cover all parts of the disease or organ names. For example, because UMLS had an entry only for "gastric carcinoma", whereas the SP report was found to refer to "multiple gastric carcinoma" or "early gastric carcinoma", we normalized both disease terms to the same identifier. By recording the entire line containing the disease name (part of which likely corresponds to at least one UMLS term), we aimed to preserve as much information as possible.

Because we have parsed IHC and SP reports based on assumptions that may apply only to reports from SNUH,

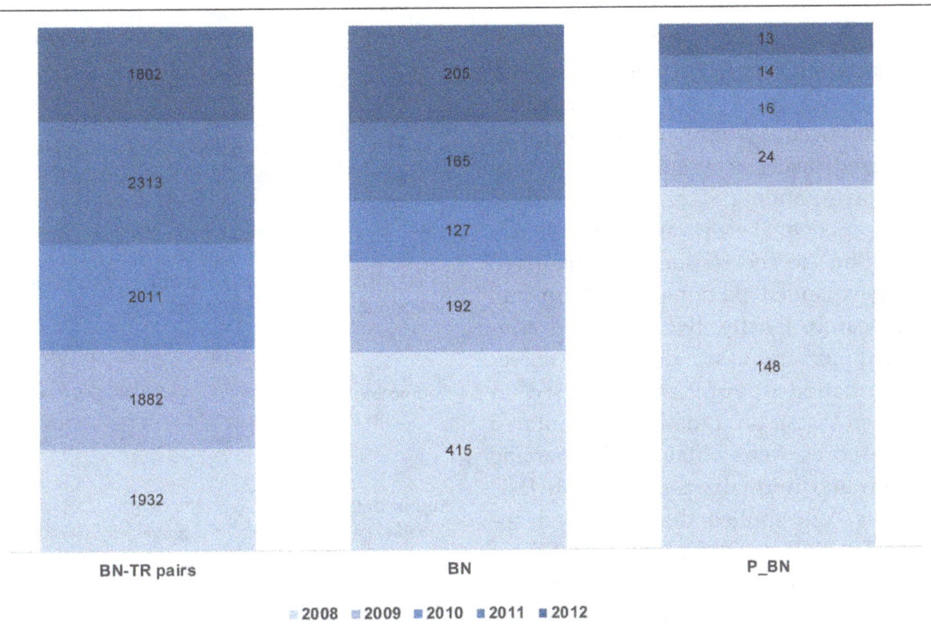

Fig. 6 The creation rate of new BN term variants per year. Although a similar number of new IHC tests (described as BN-TR pairs) were performed each year at SNUH, the number of new biomarker name (BN) variants increased steadily every year. This increase is partially related to the increase of a new type of biomarkers (described as P_BN) which SNUH analyzes

our approach may not be as easily applied to other hospital data. As we checked two branch hospitals of SNUH which operate independent hospital information system, both of which adopt the closely matched reporting format with SNUH. It is likely that this result comes from a policy that adheres to guidelines of CAP that recommend to display multiple diagnostic findings with visual separation such as an indentation for indicating a subordinate relationship or (checklist item: response) style [24]. Thus, if a hospital is referring to guidelines of CAP, the representation model we propose would be reasonable choice when localization efforts for rule-based parsing such as adjusting formatting determinants for visual separation could be made.

In this study, we proposed a representation model and developed the system from scratch to apply the model for information extraction of SNUH pathology reports. Although our parsing approach is not remarkably innovative, we could get data that reveals the differences between the Korean population and the other ethnic group of literature, as we defined the entity-relationship model for reliable associations between IHC results and microscopic findings and developed a systematic strategy. Also, in addition to that the web-based information system which calculates multi-conditional statistics of the extracted data from this study showed stable performance, 25 pathologists confirmed that the statistics is reliable in the previous study [8]. Accordingly, we could say that our representation model is reasonable for presenting the entities for pathology reports.

Conclusion

We proposed a systematic approach to mine and corroborate biomarker information from IHC reports and SP reports. According to our new data representation model for biomarker knowledge from pathology records, IHC reports are parsed using a grammar-based approach, whereas the corresponding SP reports are parsed using a tree-based approach. Term variations are resolved by normalization to corresponding preferred terms determined by expanded dictionary look-up and text similarity-based search. Finally, IHC data and relevant pathological findings are associated with corresponding clinical information from SP reports based on TS_ID and TS_P. When tested on a manually annotated dataset, acceptable F-scores were obtained for parsing (with term recognition and normalization) of both IHC reports and SP reports. We applied the developed approach to process 41,772 IHC reports and 40,519 SP reports archived between 2007 and 2012 at SNUH, and obtained information on 221 unique biomarkers, which is consistent with biomarker profiles obtained from the literature but provides more comprehensive statistics regarding biomarker use.

Additional files

Additional file 1: Figure S1. a) list-style of IHC report of a patient, b) table-style of IHC report of the same patient reported later in a separate document, c) excerpt of synoptic report template from College of American Pathologists (CAP) which shows that tissue block number should be described on the IHC report. (TIF 898 kb)

Additional file 2: Figure S2. Comparison of SP report styles between SNUH and report templates from CAP. a) SP report at SNUH which shows the combination of synoptic report style and non-synoptic report style. b) synoptic report template for ductal carcinoma in situ of the breast which presents organ information on the first line and describes microscopic findings in the following lines. The synoptic report template shows the grouping of pathologic findings using indentation for better visual separation. c) non-synoptic report template provided by CAP. The first line contains organ information and the second line contains the diagnosis information with indentation for visual separation. (TIF 985 kb)

Additional file 3: Table S1. Inter-Annotator Agreement (IAA) for gold standard set. (XLSX 8 kb)

Abbreviations

BN: Biomarker Names; BRAT: Brat Rapid Annotation Tool (developed by Stenetorp et al.); CAP: College of American Pathology; CDKRM: Cancer Disease Knowledge Representation Model (a knowledge model proposed by Coden et al.); cTAKES: Clinical Text Analysis Knowledge Extraction System (an apache based open source natural language system for information extraction from EMR); IHC: Immunohistochemistry; P_BN: Preferred term of the Biomarker Name in MeSH; PEP: Pathology Extraction Pipeline (developed by Ashish et al.); SNOMED: Systematized Nomenclature of Medicine Clinical Terms; SNUH: Seoul National University Hospital; SP: Surgical Pathology; TR: Test Result; TS_ID: Tissue Slide Identifier; TS_P: Tissue Slide Paragraph; UMLS: Unified Medical Language System; WT-1: Wilms' Tumor 1 protein

Funding

This study was financially supported by a grant of the Korean Health Technology R&D project, Ministry of Health & Welfare, Republic of Korea (A112005) and by the National Research Foundation of Korea (NRF) grant funded by the Korea government (MSIP) (2010-0028631).

Authors' contributions

JL and EY contributed in collecting and cleansing data, also in generating code sets for anatomical region. JL, HJS and SBP developed a pipeline for text processing. SHP and JWS contributed in reviewing the clinical contents and making gold standard for the evaluation. PP participated in its design and coordination. JL was a major contributor in writing the manuscript. JC participated in coordination and helped to draft the manuscript. All authors read and approved the final manuscript.

Competing interests

The authors declare that they have no competing interests.

Author details

[1]Interdisciplinary Program for Bioengineering, Graduate School, Seoul National Universty, Seoul, Republic of Korea. [2]School of Computer Science and Engineering, Kyungpook National University, Daegu, Republic of Korea. [3]PAS1 team, TmaxSoft, Gyeonggi-do, Republic of Korea. [4]Department of Pathology, College of Medicine, Seoul National University, Seoul, Republic of Korea. [5]Department of Biomedical Engineering, College of Medicine, Seoul National University, Seoul, Republic of Korea. [6]Department of Industrial Engineering, Ajou University, Suwon, Republic of Korea.

References

1. Abeloff MD, Armitage JO, Niederhuber J, Kastan M, McKenna W. Abeloff's clinical oncology. Philadelphia: Churchill Livingstone/Elsevier; 2008.
2. Biomarkers Definitions Working G. Biomarkers and surrogate endpoints: preferred definitions and conceptual framework. Clin Pharmacol Ther. 2001; 69(3):89–95.
3. Ray P, Le Manach Y, Riou B, Houle TT. Statistical evaluation of a biomarker. Anesthesiology. 2010;112(4):1023–40.
4. Evans DG, Lalloo F, Cramer A, Jones EA, Knox F, Amir E, Howell A. Addition of pathology and biomarker information significantly improves the performance of the Manchester scoring system for BRCA1 and BRCA2 testing. J Med Genet. 2009;46(12):811–7.
5. Siegal T. Clinical impact of molecular biomarkers in gliomas. J Clin Neurosci. 2015;22(3):437–44.
6. Yotsukura S, Mamitsuka H. Evaluation of serum-based cancer biomarkers: a brief review from a clinical and computational viewpoint. Crit Rev Oncol Hematol. 2015;93(2):103–15.
7. PathPedia http://www.pathpedia.com/. Accessed 11 July 2017.
8. Yun JM, Hwang SJ, Anh SY, Lee SM, Kang P, Lee JE, Yoon ES, Choi JW, Park SH, Seo JW, et al. Development of biomarker positivity analysis system for cancer diagnosis based on clinical data. Biomed Mater Eng. 2015;26(Suppl 1):S2101–11.
9. Younesi E, Toldo L, Muller B, Friedrich CM, Novac N, Scheer A, Hofmann-Apitius M, Fluck J. Mining biomarker information in biomedical literature. BMC Med Inform Decision Making. 2012;12:148.
10. Hanisch D, Fundel K, Mevissen HT, Zimmer R, Fluck J. ProMiner: rule-based protein and gene entity recognition. BMC Bioinformatics. 2005;6(Suppl 1):S14.
11. Bravo A, Cases M, Queralt-Rosinach N, Sanz F, Furlong LI. A knowledge-driven approach to extract disease-related biomarkers from the literature. Biomed Res Int. 2014;2014:253128.
12. Xu H, Anderson K, Grann VR, Friedman C. Facilitating cancer research using natural language processing of pathology reports. Stud Health Technol Inform. 2004;107(Pt 1):565–72.
13. Nguyen AN, Lawley MJ, Hansen DP, Bowman RV, Clarke BE, Duhig EE, Colquist S. Symbolic rule-based classification of lung cancer stages from free-text pathology reports. J Am Med Inform Assoc. 2010;17(4):440–5.
14. Napolitano G, Fox C, Middleton R, Connolly D. Pattern-based information extraction from pathology reports for cancer registration. Cancer Causes Control. 2010;21(11):1887–94.
15. Martinez D, Li Y. Information extraction from pathology reports in a hospital setting. In: International conference on information and knowledge management, proceedings, vol. 2011; 2011. p. 1877–82.
16. Buckley JM, Coopey SB, Sharko J, Polubriaginof F, Drohan B, Belli AK, Kim EM, Garber JE, Smith BL, Gadd MA, et al. The feasibility of using natural language processing to extract clinical information from breast pathology reports. J Pathol Inform. 2012;3(1):23.
17. Strauss JA, Chao CR, Kwan ML, Ahmed SA, Schottinger JE, Quinn VP. Identifying primary and recurrent cancers using a SAS-based natural language processing algorithm. J Am Med Inform Assoc. 2013;20(2):349–55.
18. Spasic I, Livsey J, Keane JA, Nenadic G. Text mining of cancer-related information: review of current status and future directions. Int J Med Inform. 2014;83(9):605–23.
19. Coden A, Savova G, Sominsky I, Tanenblatt M, Masanz J, Schuler K, Cooper J, Guan W, de Groen PC. Automatically extracting cancer disease characteristics from pathology reports into a disease knowledge representation model. J Biomed Inform. 2009;42(5):937–49.
20. Ashish N, Dahm L, Boicey C. Pathology extraction pipeline: the pathology extraction pipeline for information extraction from pathology reports. Health Inform J. 2014;20(4):288–305.
21. Moon S, McInnes B, Melton GB. Challenges and practical approaches with word sense disambiguation of acronyms and abbreviations in the clinical domain. Healthc Inform Res. 2015;21(1):35–42.
22. Savova GK, Masanz JJ, Ogren PV, Zheng J, Sohn S, Kipper-Schuler KC, Chute CG. Mayo clinical text analysis and knowledge extraction system (cTAKES): architecture, component evaluation and applications. J Am Med Inform Assoc. 2010;17(5):507–13.
23. Bodenreider O. The unified medical language system (UMLS): integrating biomedical terminology. Nucleic Acids Res. 2004;32(Database issue):D267–70.
24. Definition of Synoptic Reporting http://www.cap.org/ShowProperty?nodePath=/UCMCon/Contribution%20Folders/WebContent/pdf/cp-synoptic-report-definition-and-examples.pdf. Accessed 28 Jan 2018.
25. Template for Reporting Results of Biomarker Testing of Specimens From Patients With Carcinoma of the Breast http://www.cap.org/ShowProperty?nodePath=/UCMCon/Contribution%20Folders/WebContent/pdf/cp-breast-biomarker-template-14.pdf. Accessed 28 Jan 2018.
26. Hammond MEH, Hayes DF, Dowsett M, Allred DC, Hagerty KL, Badve S, Fitzgibbons PL, Francis G, Goldstein NS, Hayes M, et al. American Society of Clinical Oncology/College of American Pathologists Guideline Recommendations for Immunohistochemical testing of estrogen and progesterone receptors in breast Cancer. J Clin Oncol. 2010;28(16):2784–95.
27. Stenetorp P, Pyysalo S, Topić G, Ohta T, Ananiadou S, Tsujii J. brat: a Web-based Tool for NLP-Assisted Text Annotation. Proceedings of the Demonstrations at the 13th Conference of the European Chapter of the Association for Computational Linguistics, April 2012; Avignon: Association for Computational Linguistics. 2012;102-107.
28. Deleger L, Li Q, Lingren T, Kaiser M, Molnar K, Stoutenborough L, Kouril M, Marsolo K, Solti I. Building gold standard corpora for medical natural language processing tasks. In: AMIA annual symposium proceedings. Chicago: American Medical Informatics Association; 2012;144-53.

15

What do emergency medicine and burns specialists from resource constrained settings expect from mHealth-based diagnostic support?

Iona Crumley*, Lisa Blom, Lucie Laflamme and Helle Mölsted Alvesson

Abstract

Background: Traumatic injury is a serious global health burden, particularly in low- and middle-income countries where medical care often lacks resources and expertise. In these contexts, diagnostic telemedicine could prove a cost effective tool, yet it remains largely underused here, and knowledge on its potential impact is limited. Particularly scarce is the view of the expert user physicians, and how they themselves relate to this technology.

Methods: This qualitative study investigated tele-experts' ($n = 15$) views on the potential for image based teleconsultation to be integrated in trauma and emergency care services. A semi-structured interview guide was used to gather data concerning an mHealth app for burns diagnostics in the acute care setting, in the Western Cape, South Africa. Questions examined challenges and opportunities in user acceptance and outcomes, in specific case management and in the wider healthcare system. Resulting data were subject to qualitative content analysis.

Results: Experts perceived remote diagnostic support through mHealth as linking directly to several key ideas in medicine, including barriers to care, medical culture and hierarchy, and medical ethics within a society. Ideas running through the data pertained to the widening and narrowing of inherent gaps in the healthcare system, and the formalisation of processes, practices and relationships, effected by the introduction of an app. Wide consensus was stated on positive outcomes such as increased education opportunities, improved professional relationships and a better ability to advise and diagnose, all further facilitated through greater ease of access. The belief was that these could achieve a narrowing of systemic divides within healthcare, although it was acknowledged that the possibility to induce the opposite effect also arose. Differing opinions were voiced relating to the involvement of allied health professionals and feedback.

Conclusion: Experts see several aspects to an mHealth app for remote diagnostic support which could enhance provision of trauma and emergency care in a resource poor setting, relating to reduced delays, streamlined care and improved outcomes. Attention is also drawn, however, to specifics of the environment which would demand further and careful consideration for success – time pressure, intensity and the wide range of subspecialties to be considered.

Keywords: Emergency medicine, Remote consultation, South Africa, Burns, mHealth, Qualitative research

* Correspondence: Iona.crumley@amsterdam.msf.org
Department of Public Health Sciences, Karolinska Institutet, Tomtebodavägen 18A, SE-171 77 Stockholm, Sweden

Background

Traumatic injury is responsible for more than five million deaths each year, and accounts for around 11% of Disability-Adjusted Life Years (DALYs) globally [1]. Low- and middle-income countries (LMICs) currently bear an unequal brunt of this burden; estimates suggest that up to 90% of deaths due to injury occurs in LMICs, and cases may continue to rise as socio-economic transitions continue apace [2]. Trauma and emergency medicine in these contexts is subject to many challenges typical of health care systems in LMICs, overburdened, and constrained by limited financial, human and physical resources.

Specific characteristics which complicate trauma and emergency cases can also be exacerbated in such settings, such as the following three which are critical for both research and intervention. *Remote Presentation*; Often the initial presentation of these cases is outside of the emergency department, to poorly resourced or remote facilities, a situation compounded by a lack of pre-hospital emergency services [3], and inadequate road and transportation systems [4]. Where specialists exist they are often clustered in major cities, thus expert knowledge is not widely dispersed. *A Vast Array of Cases;* Emergency Medicine (EM), a well-developed specialty itself, entails interaction with all medical specialties [5], as cases are diverse in cause and consequence. *The Time Critical Factor;* in trauma and emergency medicine, every second is critical, and immediacy of care has repeatedly been shown to be paramount [5]. Increased response time, or hesitance in diagnosis and initiating treatment, may lead to diminished outcomes for the patient.

Telemedicine, 'the delivery of health care services, where distance is a critical factor, using information and communication technologies...' [6] has the potential to help address these challenges. Studies from high income countries (HICs) show a positive correlation between use of diagnostic telemedicine and reduced patient time in the emergency room, reduced time to transfer to specialist services, reduced costs incurred by the patient or health service and fewer medical errors [7–9]. Diagnostic tools much relied upon in the emergency environment such as Computed Tomography, Plain Film Radiography and Echocardiography are well suited to electronic transfer for remote assessment [10], and studies into burns show that diagnosis can be effectively made through transmitted images reducing both patient transfers and costs associated with treatment [11–13]. Research suggests that interpersonal connections facilitated by telemedicine can diminish professional isolation [14, 15], improve communication, and build professional relationships. Further, an educational benefit is perceived in the exchange of advice and information between very experienced doctors and more junior colleagues [16–21].

mHealth, a sub-segment of telemedicine involving 'medical and public health practices supported by mobile devices such as mobile phones...', has seen substantial growth in recent years [22]. As developments in mHealth further explore the potential of smartphone technology, such devices become more affordable, available and applicable in the resource limited context [13, 23]. With these factors in conjunction, diagnostic mHealth could reap similar benefits in outcomes for patients and physicians in low resource settings, as those previously demonstrated by telemedicine in HICs.

As with the introduction of any intervention or technology into a medical setting however, proving its efficacy is only one part of the challenge for adoption into practice. For mHealth, issues to consider for implementation include telecommunications policy, confidentiality of patient data, and financing [1, 24], as well as complex behavioural barriers regarding the motivation to accept a new way of work [24, 25]. Research abounds into both telemedicine, and more specifically mHealth, both quantitative, and, to a lesser extent, qualitative. However, to the best of our knowledge there is little research which explores diagnostic mHealth for acute care in a resource limited setting [26–28]. A knowledge gap was thus identified relating to diversity of situations where mHealth may be applicable, acceptance and outcomes for users, strategies for successful introduction and implementation and the wider challenges and benefits to patients and the health care system.

Further to this, an additional knowledge gap was identified related to expert users' perspectives in remote advice technology. Diagnostic telemedicine usually implies a three way interaction involving patient, point-of-care (POC) user physician, and remote tele-expert, of whom the latter appear less represented in existing research. As users, these specialists' experiences of such systems are key, further, they are a great resource regarding the detailed medical specifics which must be addressed by these technologies, because of their vast knowledge and experience.

The study aim was thus to understand expert users' perceptions of impacts, challenges and opportunities of an mHealth clinical diagnosis system prior to implementation for acute burns in a resource constrained setting, and the specific implications for diagnostic trauma and emergency telemedicine within this context.

Methods

As a large middle-income country, South Africa faces many challenges in health care at the present time, and is reported to be suffering a quadruple burden of disease - violence, AIDS/HIV, infectious diseases and non-communicable diseases [29]. While excellent health care exists, the public system, which covers up to 84% of the population, suffers from chronic underfunding and shortages, and often struggles to cope with demand [30]. Access to health care is thus limited in a population of 56 million inhabitants, many subject to high levels of poverty, unemployment and limited education, and where much of the population inhabits rural areas poorly served by existing health care facilities [29].

The burden of traumatic injury in South Africa is extensive, with approximately a third of admissions to the emergency department due to injuries, a figure far higher than in many other countries [29]. Of these cases, a substantial proportion is burn injuries; estimates suggest that 3.2% of South Africa's population suffer burns annually, with burns injuries the third highest cause of injury fatality in the under 18 s. In adults, assault is responsible for the highest percentage (37%) of injuries, followed by accidents, shack fires, and stoves; in children, burns relate more to accidents in the home [31]. In both age groups, consequences of high levels of poverty such as overcrowded housing, unsafe cooking facilities, fuel and power supply are without doubt exaccerbatory factors. [31]

'mHealth for Burn Diagnostics and Care in South Africa' is one telemedicine project, specifically developed to help improve outcomes for acute burns patients, through its deployment in the trauma and emergency setting [32]. Using smart phone technology, the project involved the development of an app which allows doctors in rural, resource poor areas, or secondary level emergency departments, to send images and textual descriptions of burns cases to an on call tele-expert, who then replies via the app with management and referral advice. The mHealth app had been tested and was about to be implemented in a pilot phase across eight hospitals within the Western Cape Province. By conducting interviews prior to implementation, we hoped to take the opportunity to explore perceptions of a telemedicine system in a hypothetical context, allowing for examination unclouded by the particular issues of a system currently in use.

The data collected for this study originally related to the care of acute burns injury patients, but for this paper, was analysed through the lens of an emergency care perspective. As upmost medical emergencies with specific treatment requirements, burns injuries embody many of the challenges within EM, and thus this data was considered highly suited to such an investigation.

Data collection

An extensive literature review was undertaken pertaining to research into existing telemedicine projects and pilots, evaluation and implementation, outcomes and user acceptability [12, 33–35], with themes arising from these works organised into broad categories of physician impact, patient impact and health system impact. Inspiration was originally drawn from the Information Ecologies Framework, whose holistic approach describes *'a system of people, practices, values, and technologies in a particular local environment',* all aspects of which should be considered for successful implementation of new technology [36]. The interview guide (Additional file 1) was developed from the matrix presented in this framework, using broad questions to facilitate open discussion and capture the issues most relevant to the experts. The interview began with descriptions of current working situation and practices, then moved to investigate formal and informal experiences with apps, and finally explored expectations of the current mHealth app. Two pilot tests were undertaken to ensure comprehensibility and content validity.

Purposive sampling was used to identify the sample, thus physicians working in the Western Cape Province who were qualified to act as tele-experts according to the criteria of the mHealth project were invited to participate. This sample comprised consultant physicians at all stages of their career, and included both emergency medicine and burns medicine experts, allowing representation of the concerns of both specialties. A 'next generation' view was sought by also including registrars completing specialist training to become a consultant in either burns or emergency medicine, currently in year 3 or 4 of their training. One further expert participant was included from a different province and unaffiliated to the project in order to gain an outsider perspective, identified by consensus recommendation of several primary interviewees. Of 18 physicians approached to participate in the study, 15 agreed to do so, and written informed consent from each participant was obtained prior to the interview. Participants' years of experience ranged from 3 to 35 and a range of professional qualification levels was represented. Interviews took place over a period of approximately 2 months. Further details related to the interviews conducted are listed in Table 1; years of experience and professional level have been removed to protect participants' identities.

All participants were interviewed individually using the same interview guide by a team of two interviewers, a UK masters student with a clinical background, and a Swedish PhD student with a public health background. One researcher had been involved in the early phases of the project with project planning, and data collection and presentation to some of the potential expert users. This researcher was therefore known to some participants, but was not one of the project leaders and was not involved in decisions related to development of the app. The second researcher was previously unknown to

Table 1 Participant characteristics

ID	Gender	Specialty	Length of interview (in minutes)	Previous knowledge of the app to be implemented
1	M	Emergency Medicine	44	Yes
2	M	Emergency Medicine	79	Yes
3	F	Emergency Medicine	53	Yes
4	M	Burn Surgery	53	Yes
5	F	Emergency Medicine	50	Yes
6	M	Emergency Medicine	90	Yes
7	M	Emergency Medicine	92	No
8	M	Emergency Medicine	95	No
9	F	Burns Surgery	78	Yes
10	M	Burns Surgery	76	Yes
11	F	Emergency Medicine	76	Yes
12	F	Burns Surgery	80	No
13	M	Burns Surgery	56	No
14	F	Burns Surgery	76	Yes
15	F	Burns Surgery	71	No

all participants and had no involvement to the project prior to the study. It was hoped that this team would allow a balance between an 'insider' and an 'outsider' perspective, and allow the study to benefit from the positives to be gained from these two positions [37]. Ethical approval for this study was granted by Stellenbosch University Health Research Ethics Committee (N15/01/008).

Interviews, lasting between 44 and 95 min were conducted at a time and place chosen by the participant. Recordings were transcribed verbatim or intelligent verbatim, and verified for content by the interviewers. Subsequent to transcription of the material, a summary of topics of each interview was made. Any interviews containing themes which required further clarification or elaboration were identified, and corresponding participants were requested to take part in a brief member check [38].

Every effort was made to enhance trustworthiness of the data [39]. It was hoped that the team of 2 interviewers with differing professional disciplines, experiences, and knowledge of the project allowed two very different approaches to understanding the data. Researchers took care to invest in a process of reflexivity to try to identify any areas in which their previous experiences would cloud the process and adapt for this. Constant discussion between the interview team and wider research team in developing the guide, coding and analysing the data was conducted. Member checks allowed for clarification and uniformity in process for all participants [38], and observational notes allowed us to compare processes as described and as witnessed, such as regarding referral processes.

Data analysis

The transcriptions, member-check and observational notes were subjected to a qualitative content analysis, driven by the processes described by Graneheim and Lundman [40]. Each interview was listened to and read extensively to allow immersion in the data. Throughout the data set, meaning units were identified, abbreviated to condensed meaning units and allocated a code. After initial coding of the first interview was completed, this was discussed at length among the two interviewers for consensus and amended accordingly. Coding of the full data set was then completed, with continued input and discussion from the wider research team. Codes were studied and collated in sub-categories, and then wider categories. Following this process of organizing and compartmentalizing the manifest ideas, the sense or meanings behind the categories and their associations was explored. From here, two latent themes interconnecting the categories were elucidated. In addition, the material was explored as related to the two distinct specialist groups questioned, and their views on topics were compared for evidence of consensus or disparity.

Results

In reflecting upon their work, the experts raised the idea of inherent, systemic gaps or divides which hindered their ability, beyond scarce resources, to provide the level of care they idealised. These 'gaps' or 'divides' were developed as categories in the analysis, and infiltrated many characteristic concerns of trauma and emergency - the immediacy, the inability to refuse a patient, and the emotional and psychological challenges for clinician and patients. The two themes found running through the data were (i) the inherent potential for mHealth to bridge these gaps, or conversely, widen them, and (ii) the formalisation of processes and practices that confer these changes. A summary of the final analysis in table format demonstrating the sub-categories, categories and themes is presented below in Fig. 1, followed by elucidation of the categories identified.

In addition, the different perspectives afforded from the two specialties were investigated, and while there was much coherence in opinion found, the focus of the specialties differed on some key areas.

Gold standard practice and achievable practice

The first category on "power and personality" included three sub-categories of 'Emotional dilemmas', 'Sensitivity and ethics' and 'Tools for the future', capturing areas in which a discrepancy was highlighted between a 'gold standard' practice, and that which was achievable within the realities of the setting (Fig. 1).

Emotional dilemmas

In a resource poor setting, and in treating patients with traumatic injuries, there can be a gap between the care health professional's wish to provide for their patient, and what they are able to do in practice, for reasons more diverse than the scarcity of resources. These dilemmas and their emotional and psychological impact came up frequently, both for the experts themselves, and as they envisaged from the perspective of the POC doctors.

> *"I think most of these guys, especially at the primary care facilities, urban and non-urban, are really functioning quite a long way beyond where any human being should be functioning to be, sustainably productive" –ID.2*

Pressure to maintain a high turn-over and 'task fragmentation' required to address the needs of many patients at once was mentioned as a prominent challenge of the emergency setting. The implications for telemedicine according to the participants were clear; speed, reliability and user friendly design are non-negotiable for success [14, 41]. Such is the relentless intensity of the trauma and emergency field, a system for this arena must be, *"analogous to battlefield apps".-(ID.2)*, and unreliable service or delayed response could lead to the system being rejected. As one expert described: *"... in an environment like that, you can't have long delays, you can't sort of let the patient lie there while you see if the expert replies. So I think rapid, expert feedback is key, because if people use it once and get back a delayed response, they won't use it a second time." –ID.4*

Trauma and emergency can involve treating terrible injuries, whilst dealing with patients in pain, fearful and vulnerable. In addition, the socioeconomic context of some cases can also be emotionally challenging for the medics, where they occur as a consequence of poverty or violence. In the study setting, as described above, domestic abuse and burns resulting from poor housing conditions were commonly reported mechanisms of injury. Speaking of assessing acute burns patients, one expert commented: *"It's always just that emotional aspect, it's getting sort of past that, and, sort of the horror of it all, actually having, it's, I think it's probably one of the most, em, emotive things that you can see." –ID.3*

For doctors with limited trauma and emergency experience, often 'out of their comfort zones' in terms of subspecialty, the demands of treating these injuries can be overwhelming. In the case of burns, some have only one day's training before taking up post, often alone.

Some experts expressed a belief that the presence of a senior colleague via an mHealth app, albeit remote, constituted a 'moral support component' that could be of comfort to inexperienced doctors. All believed that in taking difficult decisions such as to palliate rather than to resuscitate, expert concurrence was valuable both emotionally as well as medically. Decisive instruction, decision support and trustworthy advice facilitated by interaction with experts was seen as key to limiting

Themes	Bridging or widening gaps and divides Formalisation within healthcare							
Categories	Gold standard practice vs. achievable practice			Power and personalities		Physical divides within the trauma journey		
Sub categories	Emotional dilemmas	Sensitivity and ethics	Tools for the future	Hierarchy	Experts as gatekeepers	Disparity of setting	Assessment at a distance	Moving pts over distance

Fig. 1 Themes, categories and sub-categories in the content analysis of expert perspectives on the app

inherent pressures within trauma and emergency, whilst not being able to eliminate them.

Sensitivity and ethics

All but one expert described how informal 'telemedicine' practices were already used extensively, in that images are shared via mobile phone messaging apps in order to consult with colleagues. While confirming the value of image sharing as a concept, some expressed worry around ethical and legal implications in the current system, and saw benefit to a more formalised arrangement. The ability to regulate users for greater security of patient data was one specific advantage listed of such systems, another, the data storage capacity and a legal documentation of having sought help. It was also suggested that using such image records to demonstrate visual improvement to patients, can have a psychological role to play in trauma recovery.

Even in a regulated system however, ethics around photographing injuries, particularly in trauma and emergency where consent may be an issue, are complex. It was suggested that innovations such as apps can exacerbate these issues, making medical practice seem too familiar and removed from the clinical setting.

> *"..and so it was easier when you had to dig out your big camera, because it kind of forced you into that cognitive space of being aware that you're taking pictures of people" –ID.1*

Effective communication with patients and carers is seen as crucial to remedy such problems. One expert suggested 'pop-up prompts' within systems, reminding users to explain various stages of the process before use.

Tools for the future

Many experts saw education as a vital component of their role, and most viewed telemedicine as an opportunity to enhance their capacity as educators. Teleconsultation's potential for education is well documented, [21, 42] and has been rated in other studies by POC users as one of the most important aspects to influence their satisfaction in its use [3, 16].

The importance of providing feedback on patient treatment and outcome proved a more divisive issue. Many questioned its necessity to job satisfaction at the expert level, and commented that due to the transient nature of the patient journey through EM, feedback is often inevitably lower priority in this specialty. While some did welcome it, many expressed sentiments such as:

> *"for the experts, as heartless as it sounds, no, because I've got my own patient load, I've got my own patients that I'm dealing with that are complex and that's enough for me to handle..." –ID.15*

Discrepancies did not lie between specialties, and seemed idiosyncratic or related to personal preference. Other studies have found that expert physicians find patient follow up notifications to be beneficial [25, 43], although these studied experts in HICs providing advice to resource poor settings, potentially acting in a voluntary capacity and through interest or desire for reciprocal learning.

Despite questions raised over the additional workload burden that feedback provision could incur for tele-experts, agreement was complete on its value for POC staff, for their development and encouragement as well as learning opportunities.

Overall, in terms of being able to lift practice from that which was currently achievable to that which was envisaged as gold standard, the potential for telemedicine was believed to relate strongly to educational opportunities, and greater access to support and information, whilst formalising many aspects of technology use already in place through interaction with Whatsapp and other similar services.

Power and personality

The second category on "power and personality" included two sub-categories both capturing hierarchical dimensions of the health care system (Fig. 1).

Hierarchy

Many experts spoke of the hierarchical system that exists within medicine. There was acknowledgment that ingrained systemic fear of seniors could lead to hesitation to seek advice, with subsequent critical delays in patient care, and the effect was imagined to be amplified for nursing and allied health staff. One expert described his first years in medicine:

> *"That's part of medical training, you're made to feel stupid and there's always someone smarter than you, so it doesn't create a culture of openness and asking for help... It was very much the sense I don't want to disturb anyone, what if my question is stupid, what if they ask me something I don't know."- ID.11*

Telemedicine's possible contributions in spanning these professional divides included its potential anonymity, reducing anxiety in calling, and an allocated expert per shift reducing the sense of 'bothering someone.' One expert clarifies:

> *"I think it will probably just help in building more positive relationships, because it's another way of*

saying we are reachable, you can approach us and I think that helps a lot for doctors who are on the periphery dealing with major problems."-ID.10

From the expert level, it was proposed that an app could incorporate an allocated 'shift system' – with specific time slots during which an assigned expert was responsible for queries directed to them thought the app. This was viewed as potentially more psychologically manageable than the 'endless on call' of an informal system, making experts more amenable to queries, and improving communication as a result.

Both EM and burns experts were split in their opinion on whether nursing staff should also be able to seek advice through such a system. Some thought their inclusion to be crucial; in the primary health care facilities nurses tended to be permanent and experienced, in contrast to the short term junior doctors. Many others, however, doubted their ability to engage with such a system, although their reservations related to nurses' perceived lack of familiarity with smart phone technology rather than ability to use telemedicine per se. A previous study analysing telemedicine referrals from nurses, physiotherapists and other health care workers, found little difference between their responses and those of physicians [29, 44], however, the position of allied staff, their professional standing and potential for role extension varies widely between different countries.

Another related issue that was raised pertained to the idea of hierarchy extending not only to individuals but to institutions and specialties. Some participants queried the relative merits of systems which solely included tele-experts attached to the tertiary burn unit, as opposed to those employing experts from a variety of secondary and tertiary level facilities. Others raised the question of specialty, and on what grounds somebody would be deemed and remain an 'expert' within such systems, in terms of credentials or experience.

"I think that it might be, it's something that, that would need to be quite carefully, trod around, in terms of who's going to be the experts... I just think it needs to be strategically done. And I was thinking maybe, I mean, maybe there could be like an, exam, or something, some sort of qualification before you actually are allowed to be an expert."-ID.3

In a system which combines the talents of two specialties, as in many trauma and emergency situations, this is a question which may require consideration at implementation. Simultaneously however, potential was seen to reduce a professional gap at this expert level; greater collaboration between specialties and institutions could enhance partnerships, and foster deeper mutual respect. In general it was perceived that telemedicine could be used to counteract negative effects of a hierarchical system, but would neither dispel nor entrench the hierarchical structure itself.

Experts as gatekeepers

A connected discussion involved issues of communication and trust, in a system where the expert can be viewed as the 'gatekeeper' to scarce resources. Related to this was the proposed benefit of images adding 'proof' or 'evidence' to a query. Many of the experts suspected an exaggeration or underplaying of the severity of cases during telephone consultation by POC staff, in order that the patient would fit the criteria for referral.

"when a burn patient comes in, is this patient going to get that golden bed....like what is it about this patient that I can package them in a way, and sell them in a way to get them into that bed"-ID.11

Many experts expressed empathy towards the motivation behind such misrepresentations of a patient's condition. Simultaneously, however, many viewed this 'tactic' as furthering the crisis in referral and resources, leading to patients directed to inappropriate levels of care. It was thought that the validity and that an app could bring was essential for appropriate disposition, but also for long term relationship building between colleagues and institutions as this 'evidence' component eroded previous suspicion and distrust. The possibility was raised however, that such systems could be underused at POC for this exact same reason.

Here, the key elements for interaction with such a technology to effectively elevate practice related to improved relationships, greater transparency of communication a more formalised access to colleagues and definition of their roles.

Physical divides within the trauma journey

One of the greatest divides related to tangible gaps; the physical distance between where trauma cases first present to medical services and where they can best be treated, between the resources and facilities of the primary health care facilities and the specialist tertiary units, and potentially between the experience and skills of their respective staff.

Here, huge potential for diagnostic telemedicine systems to bridge these gaps was anticipated. Suggested benefits pertained to a greater understanding and appreciation of the difficulties and roles between the primary health care facilities and tertiary units, better information exchange leading to enhanced ability to advise, and greater confidence in doing so. Consequential to these crucial enhancements was better initial treatment so vital in trauma and emergency, greater adherence to referral criteria ensuring the right patients selected for transfer, and an overall uplifting of the service. Challenges still remained however related to how new pathways for referral would fit into existing systems, and how inexperienced doctors would respond to greater information. However, the key anticipated areas of potential improvement relating to formalisation of information exchange, and a corresponding increase in the experts' confidence in their ability to advise were strongly echoed by many of the participants.

Much of the specific information gleaned within this category is beyond the scope of this paper, and has been discussed in greater detail in another work relating to specialists' expectations of image based teleconsultation [45].

Discussion

Directly addressing the tele-experts and taking a broad approach to the subject matter provided both corroboration of previous findings and extension of existing knowledge. While limited studies from HICs have found positive potential for Trauma and Emergency telemedicine [7–9], others have suggested prerequisite conditions of strong infrastructure for success, or where this does not exist, introduction through 'simple' functions such as video conferencing [46]. The view of the South African experts would seem to strongly disagree with this. While acknowledging the additional demands resource constrained settings put on such systems, the expert view appeared overall optimistic.

Many of the findings touched on interdependencies of different users and how evolution will occur organically in response to new technology. Improved information exchange allows experts to advise better, this allows POC to treat better, patients arrive to tertiary care more optimised allowing experts better treatment options, affording them, too, the capacity to improve the standard of care they provide.

Telemedicine's inherent ability to span borders and contexts means much knowledge is transferable even between vastly differing contexts; the main areas of impact presented here indicate that many of the tele-experts' concerns and expectations correlate with those of POC users, and those found in HIC systems. Areas where consensus was found on opportunities, such as education and relationship building, have been previously cited as strong benefits of telemedicine [10]. It is important to note, however, that the experts - would be educators and participants in these relationships - agree that these findings apply to the acute resource restrained context, and are keen to engage with these functions. Areas of lower consensus in the study, notably the role of feedback and the inclusion of allied health professionals, perhaps pinpoint areas needing greater attention on a case by case basis for implementation.

Formalisation and the effect on 'gaps' in the system

It is hoped that the interviews, exploring both daily working practice, and relationships with technology such as apps, revealed how this technology could be best utilised to reduce some of the challenges of working in such settings.

Running across all themes was an idea of 'gaps' in the system creating barriers. Within the 'gold standard practice vs achievable practice' theme, we elucidate gaps such as those in staff experience from POC to referral center, and resources available, gaps between the desire to care and the ability to do so, and from the Power and Personality category the effects of distance on relationship, as well as status and seniority.

A formalisation of processes and practices emerged as an important aspect in the latent potential for telemedicine to bridge gaps of inequality in the trauma and emergency system, with aspects relating to the themes which were uncovered. Some are more apparent, the formalisation of queries through a technology interface means data is provided efficiently and systematically, facilitating the exchange of information and advice. The formalisation of data storage is effective for managing cases in continuous care, research, and legal documentation. Further, formalised systems may standardise care, so inherent inequalities are reduced.

Less obvious perhaps are the benefits of formalisation of relationships and interpersonal exchanges, relating to some of the ideas explored under the 'power and personality' theme. Such formalisation can reduce intimidation founded in hierarchy and open communication channels, increasing options for new professionals who lack the contacts to approach colleagues informally. Awareness of the option to seek help is enhanced, and the resilience and self-reliance required to manage the professional and personal challenges described in such a setting could be diminished. More, a formalisation of the role of the experts and access to them enhances their capacity to provide essential education and support.

One possible key benefit then of such apps, may be to harness the potential of technology to formalise processes, reducing gaps and inequalities within systems. Our data suggested the potential for this process through technology in this setting related to 4 key areas of impact– increased access, the ability to advise, education and relationships. Such information could allow focus on these aspects, which if considered forefront in development and introduction of new technologies, could increase their positive impact on practice, and thus their acceptability and uptake.

The importance attached to formalisation is perhaps unsurprising within medical culture and the trauma and emergency environment where accuracy and attention to detail can be critical. Respecting pre-defined 'rules' within medicine could prove key in technology implementation, and as previously noted, telemedicine needs to work within the system for maximum effect, rather than aiming to change it.

It is also acknowledged however, that informal processes developed organically as solutions to problems, and in some cases formalisation could have the opposite of the desired effect on the issues it seeks to address. As with any change, formalisation can be opposed initially, hit teething problems and inevitably involve 'trade off' in some areas rather than straight out gains, but these were concessions which most experts seemed willing to entertain.

Figure 2 illustrates the proposed main opportunities of our results, interplay between effects and outcomes, and how key themes and categories relate.

Implications for implementation of telemedicine systems in trauma and emergency

The tensions highlighted in the study are presented in the hope that, in implementation of design of such systems, benefit can be gained from prior consideration of these factors. In many examples, there is no given solution as the context of the locality will widely impact positive resolutions to the challenges highlighted. For example, issues around ethics and sensitivities will obviously vary widely according to cultural context. In some settings, the very idea of photography will be a barrier to overcome, in others, gender issues may require consideration. In cultures with a high use of internet technology, suspicion around the use and secure storage of data may prove a growing concern.

In some areas however, recommendations can be made addressing certain recurring concerns. Looking at the ideas within the theme of 'power and personality' a number of opportunities exist to address challenges and enhance interpersonal relations; training should underline the experts' acknowledgement of the challenges at

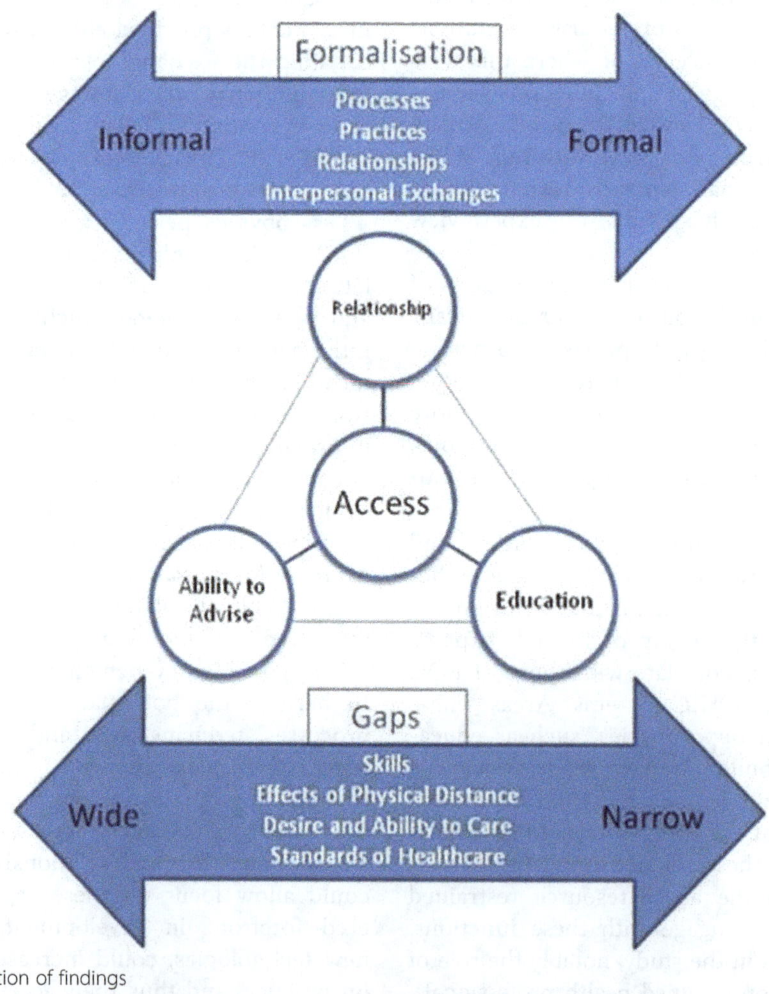

Fig. 2 Graphical representation of findings

POC and demonstrate the experts' willingness to participate and reduce stress around communications for their junior colleagues. It is also interesting that experts questioned how 'the experts' of such systems would be defined, and remain current. Practical examples could include a test for inclusion as a system expert, with great transparency, giving reassurance to both experts and POC users of the advice provided. This will also be particularly pertinent in assessing the role of allied health profession and nursing staff.

Other practical solutions can be proposed relating the challenges outlined in the 'gold start practice vs achievable practice' theme. In a system where remote consultation already occurs via informal solutions, these technologies, must not only impress, but compete with informal alternatives. To address the inevitable competition from apps such as WhatsApp, it is suggested that unique aspects are developed and highlighted at implementation, such as the ability to store and organise case data, the inclusion of additional diagnostic tools, and the legal benefits of patient confidentiality. In terms of addressing the issues around sensitivity and care, and the dehumanisation associated with the greater use of technology, the technology itself can be used to counteract such effects. For example, the suggested use of 'pop-up prompts' within tele-medicine systems, or the idea of using a thumb print onto the screen to demonstrate patient consent.

The differences in focus between burns and emergency specialists are interesting to consider. The differently weighted emphases perhaps points to potential gains at the conceptual design and implementation stages of such tools through addressing both specialties, and further to consider which specialist input is best sought when addressing particular features. For example; heeding emergency physicians' warnings on system issues relating to speed, reliability and user friendly design may include incorporating ringtone rather than text alerts, delivery reports, and installation on personal devices or static units within the department which could not be lost or misplaced. Simultaneously, seeking subspecialty expert advice on technical details of how best to capture the most pertinent specific injury details, such as in the case of burns, a circumferential component or airway involvement.

As stated at the outset, a complex area of this study was the many subspecialties that are called on within the field of trauma and emergency, burns being just one. This raises a major challenge; each subspecialty is very diverse and specifics such as those above can be unique to each, but from the physician point of view, maintaining countless apps each pertaining to a different subspecialty would be challenging. Rather than being a limiting factor, perhaps key is to identify such specifics and envisage systems in trauma and emergency which, whilst functioning as one streamlined application, contain areas of input tailored to each specialty and are thus adaptable to the emergency at hand. Further work in applicable subspecialties would be required to identify common areas and those requiring particular input, and then to collate this information. The positive results found in acute burns, however, suggest that other subspecialties may stand to benefit similarly, and thus work in this area could be extremely productive.

Strengths and limitations

The capture of only one subspecialty within trauma and emergency, and only the expert user view are limiting factors to the study; comparisons with the view of a 'referrer user' and with experts of another trauma and emergency subspecialty would add interest and validity. It is hoped however that the method allows for transferability of results to similar contexts which can relate to the challenges of limited expert knowledge on site, and great distances between point of care and referral facilities. Methodologically, the possibility of project bias must be highlighted, as the interviewees, as experts within the project, may have a vested interest in its success and positive portrayal. As noted above, some had previous knowledge of the app, had contributed in some way to various elements of the conceptual design or participated in user training. At this early stage in the process prior to the emergence of concrete issues, an element of 'over positive' or 'wishful' thinking may emerge and positively skew results in favour of the possible impacts of the app. Conversely, experts may also have the incentive to over emphasis possible issues, with the objective of resolving any such problems prior to implementation. However, the wide exploration of the challenges and positives points to a willingness for free thinking on the subject, and critical analysis of the possible problems to be encountered.

Given the small sample size, participants may have feared identification through their opinions, despite every effort being made to protect anonymity. Further, the possibility of social desirability bias, and of elite participants speaking for an institution or ideal rather than indulging a personal view cannot be excluded [40].

Conclusions

Experts perceive many potential implications of the introduction of mHealth support for diagnosis and advice, including enhanced opportunity to fulfil their role as experts, and ensuing positive impact for other users and patients. It was believed that aspects of such apps could improve provision of trauma and emergency care in a resource constrained setting, in terms of reduced delays, quality, and outcomes. Such settings can bring exacerbated and extended challenges to acute trauma care telemedicine however, and in the view of expert users, there are specifics of the environment which would demand further and careful consideration for successful implementation – time pressure, intensity, and the wide range of subspecialties to be considered.

The overriding view of the tele-experts was that there is a place for clinical diagnosis telemedicine systems within trauma and emergency. Although special considerations are required, diagnostic telemedicine has the potential to bridge gaps in healthcare provision, which translate to inequalities in care in the current system.

Abbreviations

App: Mobile application software; DALYs: Disability-Adjusted Life Years; EM: Emergency Medicine; HICs: High-income countries; LICs: Low-income countries; LMICs: Low- and middle-income countries; POC: Point-of-care; SA: South Africa

Acknowledgements

We would like to thank all the participants for their time and invaluable input, which made the study possible.

The paper is based on a master's thesis in Global Health at Karolinska Institutet, entitled 'Remote Expert Diagnosis in Trauma and Emergency Medicine: Understanding Perspectives from the Tele-Experts in a Resource Constrained Setting, with Regards to Acute Burn Care.

Funding

The study was conducted based on a grant from the Marianne and Marcus Wallenberg Foundation.

Authors' contributions

The research question and design were largely determined by LL and HMA, the data collection grid was developed by all authors. LB and IC took responsibility for the data collection. IC, HMA and LB participated in the data treatment. All authors took part in the interpretation of the results and made significant contribution to the manuscript, including the drafting and the revising of the manuscript for critical intellectual content. All authors read and approved the final manuscript.

Competing interests

The authors declare that they have no competing interests.

References

1. Institute for Health Metrics and Evaluation. Global Burden of Disease Data. http://www.healthdata.org/gbd/data Accessesed 09.11.14.
2. Hofman K, Primack A, Keusch G, Hrynkow S. Addressing the growing burden of trauma and injury in low- and middle-income countries. Am J Public Health. 2005; https://doi.org/10.2105/AJPH.2004.039354.
3. Al-Kadi A, Dyer D, Ball CG, McBeth PB, Hall R, Lan S, et al. User's perceptions of remote trauma telesonography. J Telemed Telecare. 2009; https://doi.org/10.1258/jtt.2009.081007.
4. Hanewinckel R, Jongman HP, Wallis L, Mulligan TM. Emergency medicine in Paarl, South Africa: a cross-sectional descriptive study. Int J Emerg Med. 2010; https://doi.org/10.1007/s12245-010-0185-9.
5. Bebarta V, Cairns C. Emergency care research - A primer. Dallas: American College of Emergency Physicians; 2012.
6. World Health Organisation. Telemedicine. In: Opportunities and Developments in Member States. Report on the second survey on Ehealth. Geneva: WHO; 2009.
7. Duchesne JC, Kyle A, Simmons J, Islam S, Schmieg RE, Olivier J, et al. Impact of telemedicine upon rural trauma care. J Trauma. 2008; https://doi.org/10.1097/TA.0b013e31815dd4c4.
8. Keane MG. A review of the role of telemedicine in the accident and emergency department. J Telemed Telecare. 2009; https://doi.org/10.1258/jtt.2009.003008.
9. Dharmar M, Kuppermann N, Romano PS, Yang NH, Nesbitt TS, Phan J, et al. Telemedicine consultations and medication errors in rural emergency departments. Pediatrics. 2013; https://doi.org/10.1542/peds.2013-1374.
10. Kim YS. Telemedicine in the U.S.a. with focus on clinical applications and issues. Yonsei Med J. 2004;45(5):761–75. https://doi.org/10.3349/ymj.2004.45.5.761.
11. Boissin C, Laflamme L, Wallis L, Fleming J, Hasselberg M. Photograph-based diagnosis of burns in patients with dark skin types: the importance of case and assessor characteristics. Burns. 2015; https://doi.org/10.1016/j.burns.2014.12.014.
12. Saffle JR, Edelman L, Theurer L, Morris SE, Cochran A. Telemedicine evaluation of acute burns is accurate and cost-effective. J Trauma. 2009; https://doi.org/10.1097/TA.0b013e3181ae9b02.
13. den Hollander D, Mars M. Smart phones make smart referrals. Burns. 2016; https://doi.org/10.1016/j.burns.2016.07.015.
14. Gagnon M-P, Fortin J-P, Landry R. Telehealth to support practice in remote regions: a survey among medical residents. Telemed J E Health. 2005; https://doi.org/10.1089/tmj.2005.11.442.
15. Martínez A, Villarroel V, Seoane J, del Pozo F. A study of a rural telemedicine system in the Amazon region of Peru. J Telemed Telecare. 2004; https://doi.org/10.1258/1357633041424412.
16. Van der Heijden JP, de Keizer NF, Voorbraak FP, Witkamp L, Bos JD, Spuls PI. A pilot study on tertiary teledermatology: feasibility and acceptance of telecommunication among dermatologists. J Telemed Telecare. 2010; https://doi.org/10.1258/jtt.2010.091205.
17. Scott RE, Jennett P, Yeo M. Access and authorisation in a glocal e-health policy context. Int J Med Inform. 2004; https://doi.org/10.1016/j.ijmedinf.2003.11.020.
18. Sidhoum N, Sandy D, Abeer A, Herlin C, Raphael S. WhatsApp: improvement tool for surgical team communication. Br J Plast Surg. 2016; https://doi.org/10.1016/j.bjps.2016.06.005.
19. Johnston MJ, King D, Arora S, Behar N, Athanasiou T, Sevdalis N, et al. Smartphones let surgeons know WhatsApp : an analysis of communication in emergency surgical teams. Am J Surg. 2015; https://doi.org/10.1016/j.amjsurg.2014.08.030.
20. Gulacti U, Lok U, Hatipoglu S, Polat H. An analysis of WhatsApp usage for communication between consulting and emergency physicians. J Med Syst. 2016; https://doi.org/10.1007/s10916-016-0483-8.
21. Lund S, Boas IM, Bedesa T, Fekede W, Nielsen HS, Sørensen BL. Association between the safe delivery app and quality of care and perinatal survival in Ethiopia: a randomized clinical trial. JAMA Pediatr. 2016; https://doi.org/10.1001/jamapediatrics.2016.0687.
22. World Health Organisation. mHealth. New horizons for health through mobile technologies. Based on the findings of the second Global Health series. In: Global observatory for eHealrh series – Volume 3. Geneva: WHO; 2011.
23. Mars M, Scott RE. WhatsApp in clinical Practice : a literature review. In: Promise New Technol an Age New Heal Challenges; 2016. https://doi.org/10.3233/978-1-61499-712-2-82.
24. Opoku D, Stephani V, Quentin W. A realist review of mobile phone-based health interventions for non-communicable disease management in sub-Saharan Africa. BMC Med. 2017; https://doi.org/10.1186/s12916-017-0782-z.
25. Gagnon M-P, Godin G, Gagné C, Fortin J-P, Lamothe L, Reinharz D, et al. An adaptation of the theory of interpersonal behaviour to the study of telemedicine adoption by physicians. Int J Med Inform. 2003; https://doi.org/10.1016/S1386-5056(03)00094-7.
26. Ali EE, Chew L, Ya KY-L. Evolution and current status of mhealth research: a systematic review. BMJ Innovation. 2016; https://doi.org/10.1136/bmjinnov-2015-000096.
27. Howitt P, Darzi A, Yang GZ, Ashrafian H, Atun R, Barlow J, Blakemore A, Bull AM, Car J, Conteh L, Cooke GS, Ford N, Gregson SA, Kerr K, King D, Kulendran M, Malkin RA, Majeed A, Matlin S, Merrifield R, Penfold HA, Reid

SD, Smith PC, Stevens MM, Templeton MR, Vincent C, Wilson E. Technologies for global health. Lancet. 2012; https://doi.org/10.1016/S0140-6736(12)61127-1.
28. Opoku D, Stephani V, Quentin W. A realist review of mobile phone-based health interventions for non-communicable disease management in sub-Saharan Africa. BMC Med. 2017; https://doi.org/10.1186/s12916-017-0782-z.
29. Wallis L, Garach SR, Kropman A. State of emergency medicine in South Africa. Int J Emerg Med. 2008; https://doi.org/10.1007/s12245-008-0033-3.
30. Naidoo S. The south African national health insurance: a revolution in health-care delivery. J Public Health. 2012; https://doi.org/10.1093/pubmed/fds008.
31. Rode H, Berg AM, Rogers A. Burn care in South Africa. Ann Burn Fire Diasters. 2011;24(1):7–8.
32. Wallis LA, Fleming J, Hasselberg M, Laflamme L, Lundin J. A Smartphone App and Cloud-Based Consultation System for Burn Injury Emergency Care; 2016. https://doi.org/10.1371/journal.pone.0147253.
33. Demiris G, Speedie SM, Hicks LL. Assessment of Patients' acceptance of and satisfaction with Teledermatology. J Med Syst 2004; doi.org/https://doi.org/10.1023/B:JOMS.0000044959.71456.df .
34. Foy ME, Marbrey LE, Grambow SC, Ph D, Dudley TK, Stat M, et al. Patient and clinician satisfaction with a store-and- forward Teledermatology consult system, Telemed J E-Health; 2004. https://doi.org/10.1089/tmj.2004.10.422.
35. Wootton R, Vladzymyrskyy A, Zolfo M, Bonnardot L. Experience with low-cost telemedicine in three different settings. Recommendations based on a proposed framework for network performance evaluation. Glob Health Action. 2011; https://doi.org/10.3402/gha.v4i0.7214.
36. Nardi B, O'Day V. Information ecologies: using technology with heart. Cambridge: MIT Press; 1999.
37. Dwyer SC, Buckle J. The space between: on being an insider-outsider in qualitative research. Int J Qual Methods. 2009;8(1):54–63.
38. Green J, Thorogood N. Qualitative methods for Health Research. 2nd ed. Los Angeles: Sage; 2009.
39. Malterud K, Dirk Siersma V, Dorrit Guassora A. Sample size in qualitative interview studies: guided by information power. Qual Health Res. 2015; https://doi.org/10.1177/1049732315617444.
40. Graneheim UH, Lundman B. Qualitative content analysis in nursing research: concepts, procedures and measures to achieve trustworthiness. Nurse Educ Today. 2004; https://doi.org/10.1016/j.nedt.2003.10.001.
41. Bergrath S, Rörtgen D, Rossaint R, Beckers SK, Fischermann H, Brokmann JC, et al. Technical and organisational feasibility of a multifunctional telemedicine system in an emergency medical service - an observational study. J Telemed Telecare. 2011; https://doi.org/10.1258/jtt.2011.110203.
42. Khanna V, Sambandam SN, Gul A, Mounasamy V. "WhatsApp"ening in orthopaedic care: a concise report from a 300-bedded tertiary care teaching center. Eur J Orthop Surg Traumatol. 2015; https://doi.org/10.1007/s00590-015-1600-y.
43. Halton J, Kosack C, Spijker S, Joekes E, Andronikou S, Chetcuti K, et al. Teleradiology usage and user satisfaction with the telemedicine system operated by Médecins Sans Frontières. Front Public Heal. 2014; https://doi.org/10.3389/fpubh.2014.00202.
44. Patterson V, Wooton R. A web based system for telemedicine system for low resource settings 13 years on. Glob Health Action. 2013; https://doi.org/10.3402/gha.v6i0.21465.
45. Blom L, Laflamme L, Mölsted Alvesson H. Expectations of medical specialists about image-based teleconsultation – a qualitative study on acute burns in South Africa. PLoS One. 2018; https://doi.org/10.1371/journal.pone.0194278.
46. Moehr JR, Schaafsma J, Anglin C, Pantazi SV, Grimm N, Anglin S. Success factors for telehealth-a case study. Int J Med Inform. 2005; https://doi.org/10.1016/j.ijmedinf.2005.11.001.

16

A machine learning model to predict the risk of 30-day readmissions in patients with heart failure: a retrospective analysis of electronic medical records data

Sara Bersche Golas[1*†], Takuma Shibahara[4†], Stephen Agboola[1,2,3†], Hiroko Otaki[4], Jumpei Sato[4], Tatsuya Nakae[4], Toru Hisamitsu[4], Go Kojima[4], Jennifer Felsted[1], Sujay Kakarmath[1,2,3], Joseph Kvedar[1,2,3] and Kamal Jethwani[1,2,3]

Abstract

Background: Heart failure is one of the leading causes of hospitalization in the United States. Advances in big data solutions allow for storage, management, and mining of large volumes of structured and semi-structured data, such as complex healthcare data. Applying these advances to complex healthcare data has led to the development of risk prediction models to help identify patients who would benefit most from disease management programs in an effort to reduce readmissions and healthcare cost, but the results of these efforts have been varied. The primary aim of this study was to develop a 30-day readmission risk prediction model for heart failure patients discharged from a hospital admission.

Methods: We used longitudinal electronic medical record data of heart failure patients admitted within a large healthcare system. Feature vectors included structured demographic, utilization, and clinical data, as well as selected extracts of un-structured data from clinician-authored notes. The risk prediction model was developed using deep unified networks (DUNs), a new mesh-like network structure of deep learning designed to avoid over-fitting. The model was validated with 10-fold cross-validation and results compared to models based on logistic regression, gradient boosting, and maxout networks. Overall model performance was assessed using concordance statistic. We also selected a discrimination threshold based on maximum projected cost saving to the Partners Healthcare system.

Results: Data from 11,510 patients with 27,334 admissions and 6369 30-day readmissions were used to train the model. After data processing, the final model included 3512 variables. The DUNs model had the best performance after 10-fold cross-validation. AUCs for prediction models were 0.664 ± 0.015, 0.650 ± 0.011, 0.695 ± 0.016 and 0.705 ± 0.015 for logistic regression, gradient boosting, maxout networks, and DUNs respectively. The DUNs model had an accuracy of 76.4% at the classification threshold that corresponded with maximum cost saving to the hospital.

Conclusions: Deep learning techniques performed better than other traditional techniques in developing this EMR-based prediction model for 30-day readmissions in heart failure patients. Such models can be used to identify heart failure patients with impending hospitalization, enabling care teams to target interventions at their most high-risk patients and improving overall clinical outcomes.

Keywords: Heart failure, Machine learning, Deep learning, Deep unified networks, Readmission reduction, Value-based care

* Correspondence: sgolas@partners.org
†Sara Bersche Golas, Takuma Shibahara and Stephen Agboola contributed equally to this work.
[1]Partners Connected Health Innovation, Partners HealthCare, 25 New Chardon St., Suite 300, Boston, MA 02114, USA
Full list of author information is available at the end of the article

Background

As of 2013, heart failure affects (HF) 5.7 million Americans with annual costs of $30.7 billion [1]. It is one of the leading causes of hospitalization in the United States (US), particularly in patients aged 65 years and above [2]. 1 in 4 heart failure patients are readmitted within 30 days of discharge, and risk-adjusted all-cause readmission rates declined only slightly from 2009 (20%) to 2012 (19%) in Medicare beneficiaries [3].

In recognition of this troubling trend, the Center for Medicare & Medicaid Services (CMS), the largest payer for medical services in the US, instituted penalties for hospitals with excess readmissions for heart failure. This policy change resulted in a shift from the traditional model of fee-for-service to value-based care [4]. In response, major hospitals and healthcare systems have been implementing strategies to decrease risk of readmission following hospital discharge. The outcomes thus far are encouraging: a pre-post analysis of changes in readmission rates before and after Medicare's Hospital Readmissions Reduction Program (HRRP) showed that HF-specific risk-standardized readmissions decreased after HRRP by 84.7 per 10,000 discharges per year (compared with an increase of 5.1 per 10,000 discharges per year before HRRP) [5]. However, as of 2013, the rate of all-cause readmission for heart failure index admissions was still 23.5%, the highest rate of readmission following an index stay for a high-volume condition (higher than that for chronic obstructive pulmonary disease (20.0%), pneumonia (15.5%), and acute myocardial infarction (14.7%) [6].

To control rising hospitalization cost and improve outcomes in HF management, an area of promise is predictive analytics. Within healthcare, prediction models may be used to develop disease- or event-related risk assessment tools. While advances in big data solutions now allow for storage, management, and mining of large volumes of structured and semi-structured data such as healthcare data, leveraging these advances to build prediction models in healthcare poses challenges. Healthcare data is notoriously noisy and heterogeneous [7], existing in multiple databases across even a single healthcare delivery system. However, big data analytics tend to be tolerant of poor data quality, though applications are naturally more valid and clinically useful when applied to higher quality data [8]. Additionally, methods such as data mining and machine learning can make use of all variables available in a data set without presumed associations between variables or predictive power of any particular variables. These methods allow for identification of potentially highly predictive variables that otherwise may have gone unexplored using more traditional methods such as logistic regression.

Despite challenges, and in light of the great need to improve quality of care and patient outcomes, effort continues in developing prediction models to assess patient risk for complications or adverse events [9]. Overall, the literature reports modest performances of predictive models for readmissions in heart failure patients, with few models demonstrating an area under the curve (AUC) of ≥0.70 [9, 10]. Citing the mixed results of readmission prediction models for HF patients which use traditional methods, recent studies [7, 11–14] are testing whether machine learning methods, which can take into account higher-order and nonlinear interactions between predictors, might demonstrate higher performance. Results show modest improvements over traditional statistical methods when compared directly, though AUCs demonstrate a comparable range of performance (0.54 [12] to 0.78 [13]). The mixed results of big data models highlight the need for further research to add clarity to the existing body of literature, as well as more approaches to demonstrate the ability to implement these models (if appropriate) into clinical practice, and provide more evidence that the application of these models can translate into improved healthcare quality, outcomes, and lower healthcare costs.

A great majority of efforts to develop predictive models frequently rely on structured data. Given the volume and richness of data available in unstructured clinical notes or reports, machine learning models may benefit from leveraging text mining tools to enhance the model. In this paper, we describe the development of a risk prediction model using structured and unstructured electronic medical record (EMR) data to predict the risk of 30-day readmission in HF patients, capitalizing on admission data available at discharge.

Methods

Aims

The primary aim of this study was to develop a machine learning model to predict the risk of all-cause 30-day readmission for HF patients.

Our secondary aim was to estimate the potential healthcare utilization cost savings that could be achieved if a telemonitoring intervention is selectively offered to patients at high risk of 30-day readmission.

Design

This retrospective study used de-identified structured and unstructured patient data from the EMR of a large healthcare delivery network, applying a deep learning method to develop a model to predict the risk of 30-day readmission for HF patients discharged from a hospital admission. Records included in the derivation dataset were from HF patients who were discharged alive from an inpatient hospital admission between 2014 and 2015.

Settings

All study data were generated from inpatient and outpatient encounters which took place within the Partners Healthcare System (PHS), a not-for-profit network of seven major hospitals, including two large academic centers in the Boston Metro area, and several community health centers across eastern Massachusetts. To be included, all patients had to have had at least one HF hospital encounter and have been discharged alive from an inpatient encounter (i.e. admission) at least once from any PHS facility.

Data sources

There are 2 sources of data for this study: i) Enterprise Data Warehouse (EDW): The EDW aggregates structured data from multiple PHS source systems – clinical, operational, financial, and claims – to create a consistent view of data collected across these systems; ii) Research Patient Data Repository (RPDR): The RPDR is a centralized clinical data warehouse that gathers structured and unstructured data from multiple hospital EMR systems and stores it in one place. Data content includes demographic and clinical data only; it does not include operational, financial, or claims data.

Data selection

To be considered a 'HF patient' in this study, we considered patients who were aged 18 years or older and diagnosed with heart failure as designated by any hospital encounter with a principal diagnosis of HF (International Classification of Diseases (ICD)-9 Codes: 402.01, 402.11, 402.91, 404.01, 404.03, 404.11, 404.13, 404.91, 428.xx) anytime between fiscal years 2011-2015 (Oct 2010 – Sept 2015). Medical records were extracted for those patients who were discharged alive from an inpatient admission at least once anytime during the study period: fiscal years 2014-2015 (Oct 2013 – Sept 2015).

Qualifying patients were identified using the above criteria with no methods applied to balance the readmission ratio of the patient populations. We then extracted the following structured data elements: demographics, hospital utilization information, diagnoses, procedures, labs, and medications; and the following unstructured data elements: physician notes and discharge summaries.

Outcomes

The outcome of interest was all-cause 30-day readmission. Every hospitalization was designated an index admission with potential for a readmission. An index admission may be flagged as having a 30-day readmission if the number of days between discharge of the index admission and its subsequent readmission is ≤30 days. Not all index admissions have readmissions. Readmissions may themselves be index admissions if the readmission is followed by a subsequent readmission within ≤30 days of discharge. Within-hospital transfer, patient leaving against medical advice, and planned admissions (e.g. chemotherapy, radiation, dialysis, birth/delivery) were all excluded from the readmission counts.

Statistical plan

Data from the EDW and RPDR were extracted and managed using structured query language (SQL) within Microsoft SQL Server Management Studio 2016 (SSMS). All data was de-identified using the "Safe harbor" method: removal of 18 identifiers recommended by the Health Insurance Portability and Accountability Act (HIPAA), including names, dates, contact information, ages > 89, ID numbers, etc. of patients or relatives, employers, or household members of patients, as well as device identifiers, serial numbers, and policy numbers. Text-mining techniques were used to de-identify unstructured data using a combination of SQL Server Management Studio and SweetScape Text Editor 010. Statistical analysis of baseline patient social and clinical demographics was completed using R version 3.2.2 in RStudio. Vector data generation was completed using Apache Spark 2.1.0. Text processing was completed using Python v2.7.13 and Stanford core NLP library v.3.5.2. Python v.2.7.13 was used to build three prediction models: logistic regression (Scikit-learn v0.18.1), gradient boosting (XGBoost v0.6), deep learning (Keras v1.2.1 and Theano v0.9.0 backend). Hyperopt v0.1 library was used to optimize hyper parameters of the prediction methods [15].

Feature vector generation and model building

Feature vectors for the prediction model were calculated by medication information code mapping, HF-relevant well-known factors (WKF) mapping, text data selection, and variable coding. To build a high accuracy readmission prediction model, we developed a new architecture of deep learning: deep unified networks (DUNs). The details of each process are explained in the subsections below.

Medication information code mapping

All names of prescribed drugs were mapped to anatomical therapeutic chemical (ATC) classification codes to have the active ingredient as an independent variable of the feature vector. ATC classification codes have five levels based on efficacy, action site, and scientific features. The variables of the feature vector were composed of the fifth level of the ATC classification code that expresses the active ingredient. First, RxNorm codes (a naming system developed by the National Library of Medicine which normalizes US generic and brand drug names) were mapped by matching drug names from the medication master data set to RxNorm drug names. The RxNorm codes were then converted to fifth level ATC classification codes by using information about the relationship between RxNorm codes and ATC classification codes. Using this strategy, we allocated ATC classification codes to 88.9% of the drug names present in the medication master data set.

Heart failure relevant well-known factors mapping

Our prediction model used WKFs relevant to HF according to the American College of Cardiology Foundation (ACCF) and American Heart Association (AHA) guidelines, and a previous study by Sun J et al. [16, 17]. Codes to create the WKFs were extracted from three types of data elements: diagnoses, clinical laboratory tests (labs), and medications.

For diagnoses, diseases associated with HF (e.g. pneumonia, hypertension, diabetes mellitus) were identified from the ACCF/AHA guideline and mapped by their ICD-9 diagnosis codes. For clinical laboratory tests, brain natriuretic peptide (BNP) and N-terminal pro b-type natriuretic peptide (NT-proBNP) codes were used as well-known biomarkers of HF, in addition to codes from tests frequently used during hospital stays: hematological codes such as hemoglobin, white blood cell count, and alanine aminotransferase (ALT), and urinalysis codes. All test names were mapped to logical observation identifiers names and codes (LOINC). For medications, drugs associated with HF, such as aldosterone antagonists and thiazides, were identified according to the ACCF/AHA guideline and Sun J et al., followed by mapping based on the ATC classification.

Text data selection and pre-processing

The data set contained two types of unstructured patient notes – physician notes and discharge summaries – which contain information about the cause of admission, the patients' hospital course, and discharge conclusions and instructions. Text data were divided into sections by content header. The contents of each document vary with each section. We selected sections which were present in 50% or more of notes posted during inpatient admissions. Physicians' notes contained sections pertaining to patients' social history (e.g. smoking/drinking history, description of family network). Discharge summaries contained sections pertaining to hospital course and treatment; allergic reactions, intolerances and sensitivities; history of present illness and reason for hospitalization, and significant findings.

Text data were converted numerically before the application of machine learning. The bag-of-words (BOW) model was employed to express the text as feature vectors of numerals. The feature vectors regard the frequency of appearance of each word in each document and the presence/absence of its appearance (binary). Words were transformed to standard word form using lemmatization techniques. A part-of-speech (POS) filtering technique extracted specific words including nouns, adjectives, and prepositions. Because words with low frequencies of appearance in the entire document could have less contribution to the prediction model, we deleted words that appeared less than or equal to 5 times.

Feature variable coding

Each variable was stored in a unique element of a feature vector. Target periods, data sources, and value expressions for each data type were set as shown in Table 1.

Demographic data included patient characteristic and socioeconomic variables such as age, race, marital status, level of education, employment status, and median

Table 1 Target periods and value expressions of each data type

Data Type	Data Source	Target periods	Value expression
Demographics	EDW	*Patient-level, no applicable target period*	Binary (0 or 1); Continuous/discrete value
Admissions	EDW	Admission date to discharge date	Continuous/discrete value
Diagnoses	EDW	2 years pre-discharge date to discharge date	Binary of occurrence in the target period
Labs	EDW	Admission date to 1 week after admission date; 1 week before discharge date to discharge date	Number of occurrences in the target period [a]
Medications	EDW/ RPDR	Admission date to discharge date	Number of occurrences in the target period
Procedures	EDW	Admission date to discharge date	Number of occurrences in the target period
Notes	RPDR	Admission date to discharge date [b]	Binary of occurrence in the target period [c]

[a] abnormal occurrences, [b] except Social History = penultimate to admission date, [c] except Allergies = number of occurrences in the target period

income. Admissions data included variables such as the dates of admission and discharge, length of stay, re-admission status, principal diagnosis, admission source, and discharge disposition. Diagnosis data included the date of the encounter (inpatient admission or outpatient visit), number of diagnoses, and ICD-9 codes for up to 20 diagnosis positions where applicable. Labs data included the name of the lab test, LOINC, date of the order, text or numeric result of the test, and out-of-range status of the result. Medications data consisted of prescription (not claims) information detailing name of the medication, date of the prescription update, and dose and strength of the drug. Procedures data included the date of the encounter (inpatient admission or outpatient visit), number of procedures, and ICD-9 codes for up to 20 procedure positions where applicable. Notes data included the type of note (discharge summary or physician note), date the note was initiated, subject of the note, and the text extract corresponding to the section of interest (e.g. reason for hospitalization, hospital course, social history, allergies, etc.).

1-of K expression converted the quantitative variables to elements of the feature vector [18]. To deal with missing data, interpolation techniques such as zero, median, and mean filtering were tested and found to be comparable, thus missing values in each variable were treated as zero. Additionally, to improve the numerical stability of the prediction modeling, each variable was rescaled in the range from 0.0 to 1.0 by using min-max normalization.

We reduced the number of variables to avoid overfitting and to decrease computational memory requirements. The number of admissions (i.e. samples) and variables were $n = 27{,}334$ and $p = 34{,}621$, respectively. As such, the number of variables p was much larger than the number of samples n. Such a situation where p> > n may lead to overfitting [18]. Additionally, a substantially high amount of GPU memory is required to train a deep-learning based predictive model with a large number of variables. To reduce the number of variables (p), we used the total Kullback-Leibler (KL) divergence method to evaluate the differences between the 30-day readmission group and the non-30-day readmission group [19]. Total KL divergence measures the difference between two distributions of a variable. If the two distributions are similar, the value of total KL divergence is small, and the redundant variable can be removed. Variables with a total KL divergence equal to or higher than the mean + 1/2 × standard deviation of all variables were retained for use in the prediction models, resulting in a final total of 3512 variables.

Deep unified networks (DUNs)

We used artificial neural networks (NN), also known as deep learning, to build the prediction models. Ravì et al. introduced six different deep learning architectures: deep neural network (DNN), deep autoencoder, deep belief network, deep Boltzmann machine, recurrent neural network, and convolutional neural network (CNN) [20]. Generally, DNN is used for the task of early readmission prediction [21, 22]. In the case of the DNN architecture, it is difficult to train the lower inner layers [20]. Yan et al. showed that the HF readmission prediction performances of logistic regression and DNNs were almost equivalent (logistic regression: AUC 0.657 and DNN 0.662) [22]. So far, it has not been possible to use the DNN architecture successfully in the areas of computer vision and natural language processing, where CNNs have shown impressive results. Addressing this problem, *deep unified networks* (DUNs) are a newly developed architecture of deep learning characterized by the binding of each network layer's neurons in a mesh-like form as shown in Fig. 1. The architecture of DUNs is different from the six conventional architectures of deep learning described above. Using vertical and horizontal

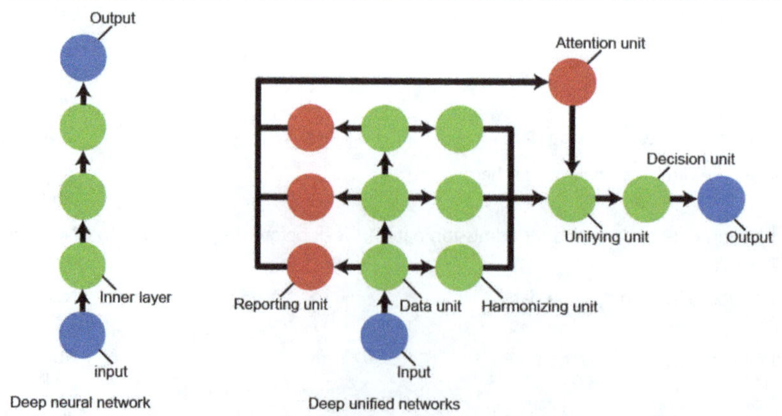

Fig. 1 Network architectures of deep neural network and deep unified networks. Demonstrates the network architecture of deep unified networks (right side) compared to deep neural networks (left side)

connections of neurons, all inner layers of DUNs can learn the prediction task from the training data to avoid over-fitting. The DUNs architecture has horizontally shallow and vertically deep layers to prevent gradient vanishing and explosion. No matter how many layers deep the architecture is vertically, there are only two horizontal layers from the data unit nodes to the output node as shown in Fig. 1. Only the harmonizing and decision units have learning parameters. If a linear relationship can explain feature variables and 30-day readmissions, a deep learning architecture that has many layers is not suitable to avoid overfitting. On the other hand, if there is a nonlinear relationship between them, linear models such as logistic regression cannot predict the patient's risk of readmission with high accuracy. The DUNs' attention unit selects the appropriate inner layers (i.e., data units) depending on the complexity of the data available. For a more detailed explanation of how DUNs were applied in this present work, please see Additional file 1: Appendix A.

Evaluation methodology

Prediction accuracy validation

The readmission prediction models were built using logistic regression, gradient boosting and maxout networks (existing deep learning), and DUNs (the proposed method described above). [18]. *Gradient boosting* is an ensemble learning composed of weak prediction models (decision trees in many cases) [18]. A software library of XGBoost for gradient boosting has a suitable balance between calculation speed and predictive performance [23]. *Maxout networks* are network architectures having neurons grouped into each inner layer. The architecture of maxout networks covers a standard DNN with dropout. When the number of maxout is one, the maxout networks are equivalent to DNN that was used by the previous studies of early readmission prediction tasks [21, 22]. Maxout networks empirically have higher predictive performance as the number of maxout increases [24].

We used area under curve (AUC) to evaluate the effectiveness of each prediction model. AUC was determined by setting thresholds according to the probability for prediction of readmission within 30 days calculated from the test data, then calculating true positive (TP) and false positive (FP) ratios sequentially while shifting the threshold level serially. Where the threshold level at which $\sqrt{FP^2 + (1-TP)^2}$ was minimal, the presence/absence of readmission within 30 days was labeled, followed by calculation of accuracy, precision, recall, and fl-measure (fl).

Machine learning techniques have tuning parameters (such as a number of neurons in deep learning) that are also called the hyper-parameters [18]. Note that the hyper-parameters do not contain the learning parameters. Using all data samples to tune hyper-parameters may cause overfitting. Nonlinear machine learning, including gradient boosting and deep learning, are at especially high risk of overfitting. In this study, hyper-parameter tuning and prediction model evaluation were carried out by sampling 10% of data at random from the entire dataset, followed by 100 iterations of optimization of each technique's hyper-parameters with the use of the tree-structured parzen estimator of the hyperopt library [15]. In each iteration of hyper-parameter optimization, the mean AUC was calculated by 10-fold cross validation (10-fold CV) as an indicator of prediction accuracy. The predictive accuracy of each technique also was evaluated with 10-fold CV. The optimized results of hyper-parameters in each method are described in the "Hyper-parameter optimization results" section below.

Cost saving evaluation

PHS offers heart failure telemonitoring (Connected Cardiac Care Program (CCCP)) to heart failure patients with recurrent hospitalizations [25]. We evaluated the economic benefits that could be generated by using the prediction models for selecting CCCP enrollees based on readmission risk. Net savings from readmission reduction were calculated for each classification threshold based on the receiver operating characteristic (ROC) curve of each round of 10-fold CV using the following equation.

$$\begin{aligned}&\textit{Net savings from readmission reduction}\\&= \textit{Total saved readmission cost} - \textit{Total CCCP cost}\\&= \textit{Readmission cost per patient} \times \textit{Number of true positives}\\&\times \textit{CCCP response rate} - \textit{CCCP cost per patient}\\&\times \textit{Number of predicted positives}\end{aligned}$$

where *readmission cost per patient* and *CCCP cost per patient are* \$9655 and \$1500 respectively [25]. *CCCP response rate* is the possibility of successfully preventing a readmission by applying CCCP to a patient who would be readmitted within 30 days without CCCP, which is set to 50% [26]. *Number of predicted positives* is the number of index admissions that were classified as positive (i.e., 30-days readmission occurs) by the prediction model.

We derived the maximum *net savings from readmission reduction* and the accuracy at the corresponding classification threshold for each round of the 10-fold CV. Then the mean and the standard deviation of the maximum net savings and the accuracy were derived.

Results

Patient population

Figure 2 below summarizes the patient selection process. Of 28,031 patients identified as having a hospital encounter with HF as the principal diagnosis between 2011

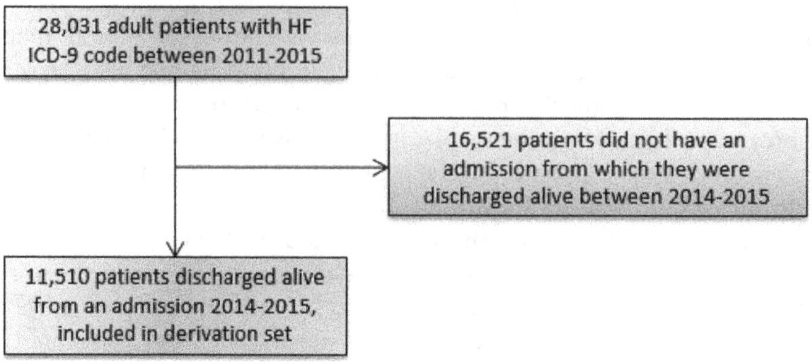

Fig. 2 Patient selection flowchart. Summarizes the patient selection process

and 2015, 11,510 (41%) were discharged alive from a hospital admission during the study period (between 2014 and 2015).

Table 2 below summarizes the patient demographics. The age distribution was skewed, with 75% of patients being 65 years of age or older. There were slightly more men (53%) than women (47%), and the cohort was primarily white (84.5%). A higher proportion of patients were married or partnered (45.6%), and roughly half the cohort (51.4%) had no higher than a high school education. The majority of patients (57.3%) were retired. Patients were also likely to be managing more than one health condition: 77.2% of patients presented to a hospital with one or more comorbidities during the study period, including hypertension (37.3%), other cardiovascular disease (32.5%), and chronic kidney disease (26.1%).

In comparing patients who did (30.4%) versus did not (69.6%) have readmissions, we see the two groups did not differ significantly in age ($p = 0.75$), gender ($p = 0.74$), race ($p = 0.16$), or marital status ($p = 0.07$). However, they did differ significantly in level of education, employment status, and number of comorbidities (all $p = < 0.01$). Specifically, patients with readmissions were less likely to have had education above high school ($p = < 0.01$), less likely to be employed ($p = < 0.01$) and more likely to be on disability ($p = < 0.01$), and more likely to have ≥3 comorbid conditions.

Inpatient hospital utilization by disease group

For the following analysis, we grouped the principal ICD-9 codes by disease category according to designations by the Health Cost and Utilization Project (HCUP) Clinical Classifications Software (CCS), which characterizes diagnoses into clinically meaningful categories making it easier to see diagnosis data patterns [34]. The top 10 diagnosis categories for the 27,334 inpatient admissions in descending order were as follows: HF (non-hypertensive; 22.3%), dysrhythmia (5.3%), septicemia (3.9%), device complications (3.7%), pneumonia (4.6%), hypertension (with complications; 3.3%), COPD (2.8%), acute renal failure (2.5%), urinary tract infection (2.2%), and acute myocardial infarction (2.1%). Of the device complications, 43% were related to cardiac devices.

Readmission rates

To account for the likelihood of a readmission for HF regardless of index admission cause, we allowed for all-cause index admissions in our dataset. Of 27,334 inpatient admissions, 6374 (23.3%) were associated with 30-day readmissions. Of these 6374 admissions with a readmission, 1448 (22.7%) of the index admissions were flagged as HF-related, and 1461 (22.9%) of the readmissions were flagged as HF-related, with an overlap of 552 (8.7%) where both the index and its readmission were HF-related. Therefore, of the 1461 HF-specific readmissions, only 38% had index admissions which were HF-related.

Common medications, labs, and procedures

The top 5 most commonly prescribed medications for this population during the study period, determined by percentage of patients with a prescription record for the drug anytime between 2014 and 2015, were Furosemide (60% of patients), Metoprolol (43%), Aspirin (43%), Omeprazole (39%), and Lisinopril (37%).

The top 5 most commonly ordered lab tests for this population during the study period, determined by a lab order date occurring during the target window described in Table 1, were electrolyte/renal/glucose panels (e.g. estimated glomerular filtration rate, glucose, potassium; 25% of labs), complete blood counts (e.g. hematocrit, white blood cell, red blood cell; 23%), blood differential absolute/percentage (e.g. nucleated red blood cell, lymph, eosinophil; 18%), general chemistries (e.g. calcium, magnesium, phosphorous; 8%), and routine coagulation (e.g. prothrombin time, international normalized ratio, partial thromboplastin time; 4%).

The top 5 most commonly performed principal procedures for this population during the study period,

Table 2 Patient Cohort Demographics

Patient Characteristics	Whole Cohort N = 11,510	Patients with readmissions n = 3502	Patients without readmissions n = 8008	p-value
Age Distribution				0.75
Median (1, 3 quartile)	75.7 (64.3, 84.7)	76.0 (64.4, 84.6)	75.5 (64.2, 84.7)	
Gender, n (%)				0.74
Male	6073 (52.8)	1839 (52.5)	4234 (52.9)	
Race, n (%)				0.16
White	9490 (84.5)	2872 (83.8)	6618 (84.9)	
Black or African American	889 (7.9)	297 (8.7)	592 (7.6)	
Hispanic or Latino (all races)	423 (3.8)	141 (4.1)	282 (3.6)	
Asian	221 (2.0)	61 (1.8)	160 (2.1)	
Other, or more than one race	202 (1.8)	58 (1.7)	144 (1.8)	
Unknown (excluded in calculations)	*n = 285*	*n = 73*	*n = 212*	
Marital status, n (%)				0.07
Married / Partnered	5125 (45.6)	1516 (44.3)	3609 (46.2)	
Widow	2360 (21.0)	718 (21)	1642 (21)	
Single	2274 (20.2)	715 (20.9)	1559 (19.9)	
Divorced / Separated	1069 (9.5)	323 (9.4)	746 (9.5)	
Other	412 (3.7)	148 (4.3)	264 (3.4)	
Unknown (excluded in calculations)	*n = 270*	*n = 82*	*n = 188*	
Highest educational attainment, n (%)				< 0.01*
Some High School or Less	1117 (12.7)	392 (14.2)	725 (12)	
High School Graduate/GED	3418 (38.7)	1127 (40.7)	2291 (37.8)	
Some College/Vocational/Technical Program	492 (5.6)	134 (4.8)	358 (5.9)	
Graduate of College or Postgraduate School	2911 (33.0)	864 (31.2)	2047 (33.8)	
Other	887 (10.1)	253 (9.1)	634 (10.5)	
Unknown (excluded in calculations)	*n = 2685*	*n = 732*	*n = 1953*	
Employment status, n (%)				< 0.01*
Retired	4338 (57.3)	1329 (57.7)	3009 (57.1)	
Employed [a]	2067 (27.3)	556 (24.1)	1511 (28.7)	
Disability	656 (8.7)	259 (11.2)	397 (7.5)	
Unemployed	467 (6.2)	149 (6.5)	318 (6)	
Other	49 (0.6)	12 (0.5)	37 (0.7)	
Unknown (excluded in calculations)	*n = 3933*	*n = 1197*	*n = 2736*	
Number of comorbidities, n (%) [b]				< 0.01*
0	2619 (22.8)	578 (16.5)	2041 (25.5)	
1	3032 (26.3)	840 (24)	2192 (27.4)	
2	2684 (23.3)	841 (24)	1843 (23)	
≥ 3	3175 (27.6)	1243 (35.5)	1932 (24.1)	

[a]Includes part-time and self-employment

[b]The following list of comorbidities was selected based on a literature review of comorbidities frequently found in patients with heart failure [27–33], in addition to clinical opinion of study staff physicians. Please see Additional file 3: Appendix B for a complete list of ICD-9 codes used to identify each condition. Each condition evaluated is listed here with the percentage of the study population who presented to a PHS facility with the condition as the principal diagnosis for either an inpatient or outpatient encounter at least once between 2014 and 2015. Hypertension (37.3%), cardiovascular disease (32.5%), chronic kidney disease / renal insufficiency (26.1%), non-secondary diabetes mellitus (22.8%), anemia (19.2%), chronic obstructive pulmonary disease (9.8%), osteoarthritis (9.1%), mental health conditions (7.2%), back pain (3.3%), osteoporosis (3.2%), obesity (2.3%)

determined by a procedure date occurring between admission and discharge date, were procedures of the cardiovascular system (e.g. hemodialysis, cardiac catheter, coronary artherectormy; 36% of procedures), miscellaneous diagnostic and therapeutic procedures (e.g. non-invasive mechanical ventilation, packed cell transfusion, heart ultrasound; 29%), procedures of the digestive system (e.g. small bowel endoscopy, abdominal paracentesis, esophagogastroduodenoscopy; 13%), procedures of the musculoskeletal system (e.g. knee replacement, hip replacement, arthrocentesis; 9%), and procedures of the respiratory system (e.g. thoracentesis, endoscopic bronchial biopsy, insertion of intercostal catheter, 5%).

Feature category variables

After reducing features via total KL divergence (method described above under Feature Variable Coding), the final algorithm included 3512 variables represented over 25 feature categories derived from demographic, admissions, diagnosis, procedure, medication, lab, and unstructured text data. Table 3 shows the number of feature categories and variables per category for each data type.

Prediction model evaluation

Hyper-parameter optimization results

The hyper-parameters for the logistic regression were the coefficient λ of the L1 or L2 norm of the weights, used to avoid multicollinearity. The logistic regression models with L1 and L2 norm regularization are equivalent to lasso and ridge regression models, respectively [18]. For hyper-parameter tuning, λ was varied in the range [− 15, 0] over the log-uniform distribution (= exp.(lower, upper)). The best results were obtained using the L2-norm for $\lambda = 6.931 \times 10^{-6}$ with AUC 0.628. In the case of gradient boosting, Table 4 shows each hyper-parameter of the XGBoost library and its range of adjustment. For the parameters not shown in Table 4, gradient boosting used the standard values given in the library. The best AUC of gradient boost was 0.639.

Table 4 also shows the hyper-parameters of maxout networks and DUNs. Stochastic Gradient Descent (SGD) used a learning rate of 0.01 with momentum 0.9, and a batch size 100. Maxout networks selected three inner layers with 914 neurons. The inner layers and neurons of DUNs corresponded to those of the data unit, respectively. DUNs selected five layers with 759 neurons. Number of maxout is the number of inner layer groups. The best number of the groups was three. Activation function is the type of activation function for the inner layer of maxout networks, as well as the data units and harmonizing units of DUNs. Maxout networks and DUNs selected the sigmoid function. Dropout rate is a parameter of the dropout ratio for the input and the inner layers. Maxout networks and DUNs selected about 40% defect rate for the input and inner layers. The best AUC for maxout networks and DUNs were 0.624 and 0.636 respectively.

10-fold cross validation results

Table 5 shows the mean ± standard deviation (std.) for 10-fold CV yielded from evaluation with each technique. The mean AUCs in Table 5 were calculated from the area under the receiver operating characteristic (AUROC) curves shown in Fig. 3, which displays the curve for each fold of the cross validation for each method. Only DUNs exceeded AUC 0.70 and marked the best value in each evaluation. The second-best result was obtained with maxout networks (AUC 0.695). There was no large turbulence in the ROC curve of DUNs, and the true positive rate rose slowly as the false positive rate rose with each technique. The AUC in the final 10-fold CV evaluation was improved from that in hyper-parameter tuning for all techniques. In the results of hyper-parameter optimization, gradient boosting marked the best performance (AUC 0.639), however, it was the worst performance (AUC 0.650) in the final 10-fold CV evaluation. On the other hand,

Table 3 Description of contributing variables and results of variable reduction post-processing, by data type

Data Type	Major Variables	Number of feature categories	Variable reduction from → to
Demographics	Marital status, education, gender, language	2	39 → 15
Admissions	Total cost of index admission, age at admission, cumulative number of 30-day readmissions, length of stay	2	217 → 53
Diagnoses	ICD-9 codes, WKF	4	8101 → 1297
Labs	WKF at admission, WKF at discharge	2	94 → 58
Medications	RXCUI, Medication name, WKF	7	16,779 → 1107
Procedures	ICD-9 codes	1	1833 → 95
Notes	Words from: social history, hospital course, hospital reason, allergies	7	7558 → 887
Total		*25*	*34,621 → 3512*

Table 4 Hyper-parameters of Gradient Boosting (XGBoost), Maxout networks, and DUNs

		GRADIENT BOOSTING (XGBOOST)		
Parameter name		Distribution and search range	Best parameter	
learning_rate		Log-uniform [−5.0, −0.5]	0.007	
max_depth		Discrete uniform [3, 25]	5	
min_child_weight		Discrete uniform [1, 10]	1	
n_estimators		Discrete uniform [100, 1000]	398	
gamma		Log-uniform [−10, 0]	0.042	
alpha		Log-uniform [−10, 0]	0.0003	
lambda		Log-uniform [−10, 0]	0. 116	
subsample		Discrete uniform (units of 0.05) [0.5, 1.0]	0.70	
colsample_bytree		Discrete uniform (units of 0.05) [0.5, 1.0]	0.80	
		MAXOUT NETWORKS and DUNs		
Parameter name		Distribution and search range	Best parameter	
			Maxout networks	*DUNs*
Number of epochs		Discrete uniform [20, 100]	22	100
Number of inner layers		Discrete uniform [2, 5]	3	5
Number of inner neurons		Discrete uniform [100, 1000]	914	759
Number of maxout		Discrete uniform [2, 5]	5	–
Activation function		Random choice from: sigmoid, tanh, softplus, softsign	Sigmoid	Sigmoid
Dropout rate of:	- input layer	Uniform [0.001, 0.5]	0.446	0.397
	- inner layers	Uniform [0.001, 0.5]	0.394	0.433

with deep learning, the difference in AUC of 10-fold CV from that during hyper-parameter optimization was 0.071 higher for maxout networks and 0.069 higher for DUNs.

Figure 4 is a boxplot of the attention unit output for DUNs. As shown in Fig. 1, the attention unit generates weights to mix the output values obtained by the inner units for each input feature vector. The weights indicate the measure of difficulty of the 30-days readmission prediction task for each patient. DUNs calculate nonlinear features as a multiple feature combination by increasing the inner layer (i.e., data units). Thus, the upper layers' features have a more complex nonlinearity than that of the lower layers. To improve prediction accuracy, DUNs' attention unit selects the best features for each patient's readmission case. For example, if a patient's readmission prediction task does not have a nonlinear relationship between the input variables and the target variable, the attention unit generates strong weights for the lower inner layers. The mathematical mechanism of the attention unit is further described in Additional file 1: Appendix A.

Figure 4 plots the attention unit (0.0-1.0; Y axis) against the layer number (X axis). Layers yielding the strongest output were layer 3 (mean 0.226 ± std. 0.006) and layer 6 (mean 0.218 ± std. 0.005). The layer yielding the lowest output was layer 5 (mean 0.170 ± std. 0.011). The attention unit output from each layer ranged between 0.0 and 1.0, with the sum total of output from all layers being 1.0.

Calculating importance of feature variables

Logistic regression and gradient boosting enable the calculation of the importance of feature variables, as determined by the frequency with which the variable was used for decision making during XGBoost. Because the AUC of logistic regression was higher than that of gradient boosting, we selected logistic regression to obtain the importance of feature variables. Logistic regression

Table 5 10-fold CV Results

	AUC mean ± sd	Accuracy mean ± sd	Precision mean ± sd	Recall mean ± sd	f1 mean ± sd
Logistic regression	0.664 ± 0.015	0.626 ± 0.020	0.336 ± 0.014	0.616 ± 0.029	0.435 ± 0.012
Gradient boosting	0.650 ± 0.011	0.612 ± 0.013	0.325 ± 0.008	0.615 ± 0.032	0.425 ± 0.010
Maxout networks	0.695 ± 0.016	0.645 ± 0.016	0.354 ± 0.016	0.631 ± 0.016	0.454 ± 0.016
DUNs (proposed)	0.705 ± 0.015	0.646 ± 0.018	0.360 ± 0.015	0.652 ± 0.036	0.464 ± 0.013

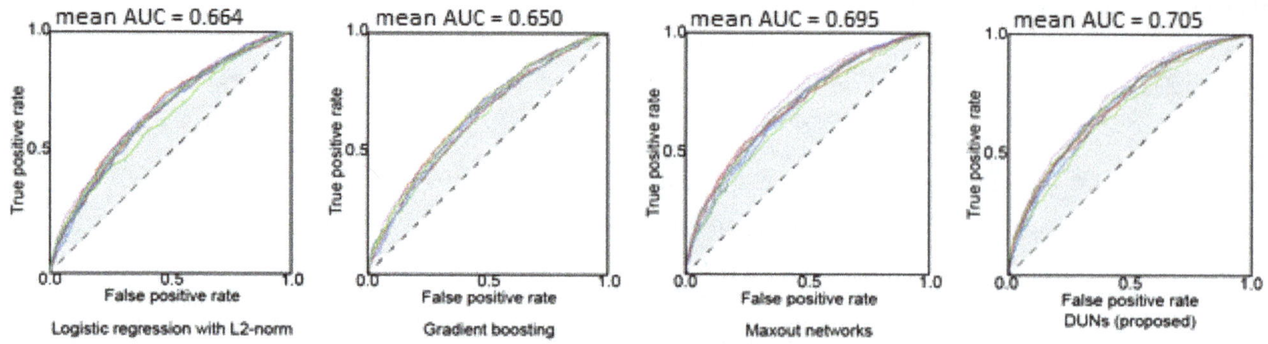

Fig. 3 ROC curves of 10-fold CV. Demonstrates the ROC curve for each predictive modeling technique

calculated the absolute values (magnitude) of the learning parameters (weight coefficients) as the feature importance. Table 6 shows the top 15 most important features in the logistic regression. More information about all feature variables (names, data types, importance) will be made available on our website as of July 2018 (HitachiPartnersAIproject.com).

Cost evaluation results

Figure 5 shows the net savings from readmission reduction, calculated by changing the number of CCCP enrollees along with the classification threshold, assuming the CCCP enrollees were selected for 2 years from 2014 to 2015, using the ROC curves of 10-fold CV of DUNs, maxout networks, logistic regression, and gradient boost models as shown in Fig. 3. The series of R0 to R9 represent the round number of the 10-fold CV. The 10 circles in the chart correspond to the point where the net savings reached the maximum in each round.

Table 7 shows the mean ± standard deviation of the maximum net savings and accuracy at the classification threshold corresponding to the maximum net savings which were derived from the 10-fold CV for each technique. DUNs demonstrated the maximum net savings at

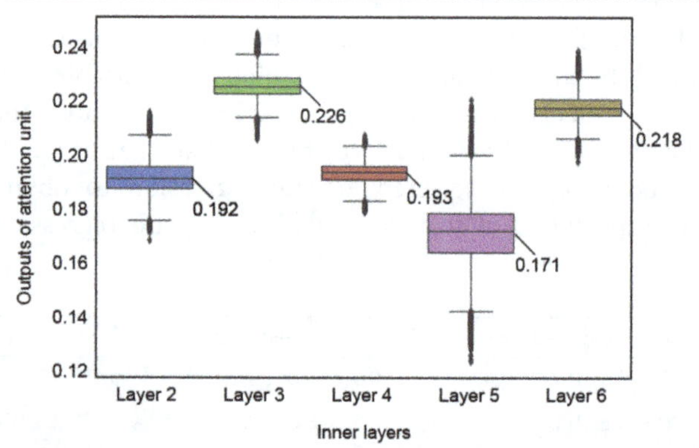

Fig. 4 Layer importance of DUNs. Shows the boxplot distributions of the attention unit output (Y axis) against each layer number (X axis)

3.403 ± 0.536 million. The mean ± standard deviation of the accuracy at the classification threshold that corresponds with the maximum cost savings was 76.4 ± 1.4%.

Discussion

This was a retrospective study which applied deep learning to structured and unstructured patient data from the EMR of a large healthcare delivery network to create a risk prediction model to predict 30-day readmissions in patients with HF. With an AUC of 0.705, the developed model performs moderately well, with results within the upper range compared with previously published models.

The DUNs AUC marked the best result of 10-fold CV compared to logistic regression, gradient boosting, and maxout networks. The mean AUCs in the final 10-fold CV for deep learning-based techniques were about 0.07 points higher compared to hyper-parameter optimization results. Hyper-parameter overfitting occurred in gradient boosting, as demonstrated by its having the highest AUC in the hyper-parameter optimization results but the lowest AUC in the final 10-fold CV results. This suggests that prediction models that have many hyper-parameters need a particular validation scheme to measure actual prediction accuracy.

For the prediction task of early readmission after hospitalization for HF, Futoma, et al. and Yang, et al. independently compared logistic regression with DNN using three inner layers [21, 22]. For the 10-fold CV results evaluated by Futoma, et al., the AUC of the DNN (0.676) was 0.022 points higher than that of the logistic regression (0.654) [21]. For the 10-times random split validation results evaluated by Yang, et al., the AUC of the DNN (0.662) was 0.005 points higher than that of the logistic regression (0.657) [22]. The 10-fold CV results in Table 5 show that the AUC of maxout networks and DUNs were, respectively, 0.031 and 0.041 points higher than that of logistic regression. This suggests that if deep learning-based techniques are applied to cases where a large training data set is available, the

Table 6 Feature importance ranking of logistic regression

Rank	Feature description
1	Cumulative number of *30-day readmissions*
2	Presence of *acute respiratory failure* ICD-9 code
3	Number of *abnormal sodium level* laboratory tests
4	Presence of *pneumonia (organism unspecified)* ICD-9 code
5	Number of *abnormal chloride level* laboratory tests
6	Presence of *acute kidney failure (unspecified)* ICD-9 code
7	Presence of *diabetes (with other specified manifestations)* ICD-9 code
8	Presence of *acute kidney failure (any)* ICD-9 code
9	Presence of *respiratory failure*, WKF
10	Presence of *disorders of fluid electrolyte and acid-base balance (any)* ICD-9 code
11	Presence of *disorders of fluid/electrolyte/acid-base*, WKF
12	Number of *abnormal albumin level* laboratory tests
13	Presence of *asphyxia and hypoxemia* ICD-9 code
14	Presence of *anemia of chronic illness* ICD-9 code
15	Presence of *hypokalemia* ICD-9 code

automated generation of feature variables – a capability unique to deep learning – works sufficiently, yielding higher accuracy when compared to the other techniques.

Because of the DUNs' attention unit's ability to maximize prediction accuracy by selecting an inner layer depending on the level of nonlinearity between the input variables and the target variable for each readmission case, the architecture of DUNs was more suitable compared to conventional DNNs and other traditional classifiers for this readmission prediction task, due to the dataset containing both linear and nonlinear relationships. The AUC of 0.665 achieved with logistic regression solved simpler cases i.e. cases where a linear relationship could explain feature variables and 30-day readmissions. The higher AUC of 0.695 achieved with maxout networks suggests the more complex cases had a nonlinear relationship. Maxout networks selected three inner layers (the optimization range is two from five), suggesting that high-dimensional feature variables with four or more layers are not necessary for all readmission cases. As shown in Fig. 4, the DUN attention unit weights were higher for layers three and six, indicating that the 30-day readmission events consisted of a mixture of cases which could be explained by the feature variables of the dimension similar to maxout networks, and cases which could be explained by the high-dimensional six-layer feature variables.

The calculated importance of feature variables (Table 6) highlighted a number of characteristics representative of symptoms related to HF and its frequent comorbidities. Four features pertained to pulmonary disease and distress (#2 and 9: respiratory failure ICD-9 code and WKF, #4: pneumonia ICD-9 code, and #14: asphyxia and hypoxemia ICD-9 code), all potentially symptomatic of COPD, which was present more frequently as a comorbidity in the patient segment with readmissions compared to those without (13% vs. 8.5%, $p < 0.001$). Eight pertained to renal disease and monitoring (#6 and 8: acute kidney failure ICD-9 codes, #3, 5, and 12: abnormal sodium, chloride, and albumin labs, #10 and 11: disorders of fluid/electrolyte/acid-base ICD-9 code and WKF, and #15: hypokalemia), the labs in particular all being part of a basic renal panel. Chronic kidney disease was also more represented in the patient segment with readmissions compared to those without (36.5% vs. 21.6%, $p < 0.001$). Similarly, features #7 and 14 – diabetes and anemia – were more represented in patients with readmissions compared to those without (respectively: 26.1 vs. 21.4%, $p < 0.001$; and 24.8 vs. 16.7%, $p < 0.001$).

Following external validation to assure efficacy, the developed model has promising clinical uses. Healthcare organizations and providers might consider using such a model to monitor their patients with HF, to assess their likelihood of readmission following discharge from an inpatient admission. Using predictive analytics to select high readmission risk patients to receive telemonitoring intervention may help to save on intervention costs to the hospital. Upon identification of readmission risk, the patient's care team may consider an enhanced review of the patient's current comorbidities and care plan at discharge, to determine if there are any care gaps which can be filled to potentially avoid readmission. Additionally, knowledge of one's risk for readmission may also provide patients with important decision-making

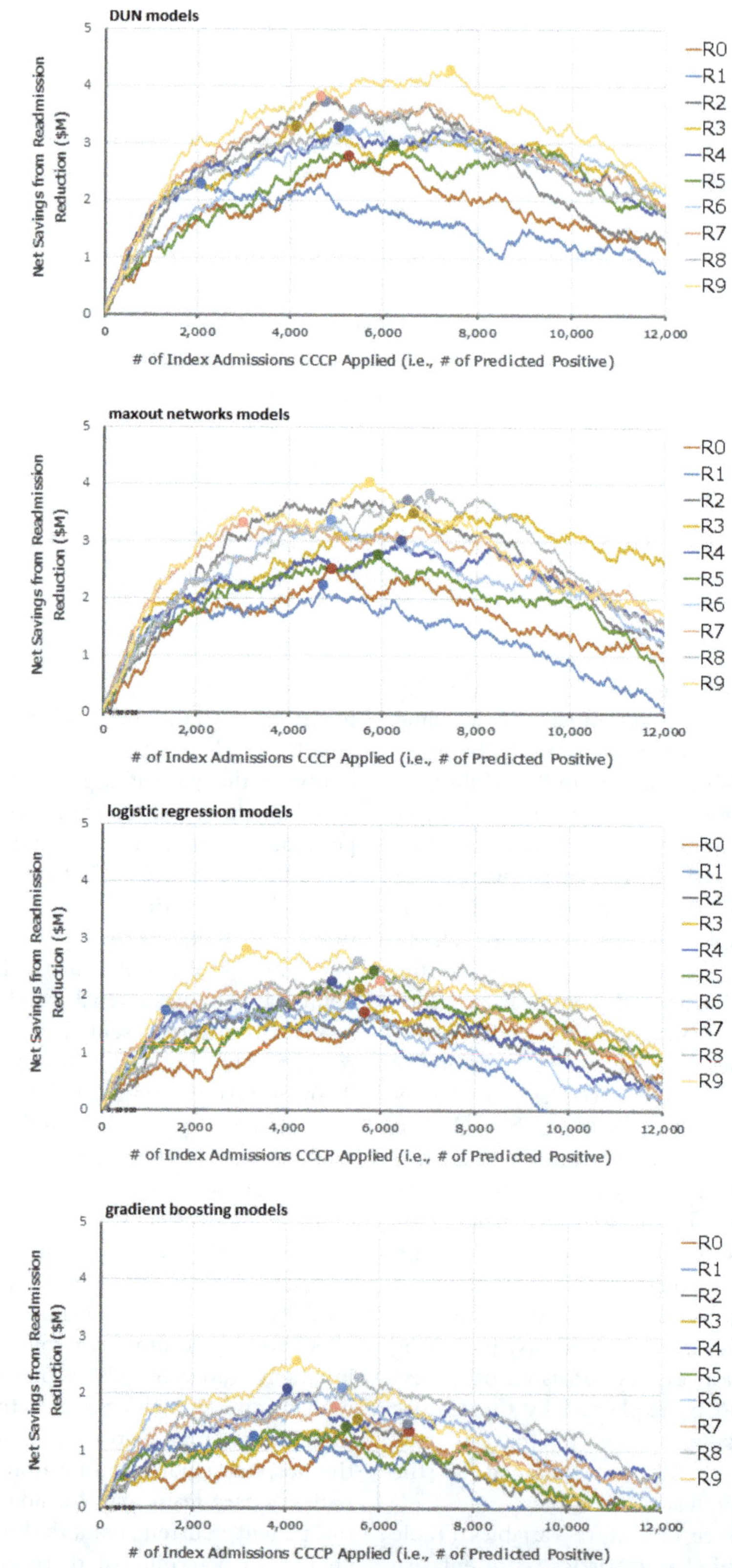

Fig. 5 Projected net savings from readmission reduction by using prediction models to select CCCP enrollees. Shows the net savings from readmission reduction, calculated by changing the number of CCCP enrollees along with the classification threshold, using the ROC curves of 10-fold CV of 1) DUNs, 2) maxout networks, 3) logistic regression, and 4) gradient boosting as shown in Fig. 3

Table 7 Maximum net savings and corresponding accuracies

	Max net savings ($M)	Accuracy
DUNs (proposed)	3.403 ± 0.536	0.764 ± 0.014
Maxout networks	3.241 ± 0.561	0.754 ± 0.014
Logistic regression	2.173 ± 0.357	0.750 ± 0.018
Gradient boosting	1.787 ± 0.428	0.739 ± 0.016

information about their own health, such as adopting health changes (e.g. diet, medication adherence) or increased communication with their care team.

Strengths, limitations, and challenges

The model was developed on a HF patient population and included HF-specific WKFs as features, however, the index event itself need not be HF-specific. By including all-cause index as well as all-cause readmissions, a strength of this study may be increased generalizability of the model to any encounter the HF patient experiences. The readmission rates in this study suggest that in the event of a readmission, patients are as likely to be readmitted for HF regardless of index admission as they are to have an index HF admission. This finding corresponds to insights from previous studies. In an analysis of re-hospitalization patterns using Medicare claims data, Jencks et al. found that HF was the most frequent cause of readmission regardless of index admission diagnosis [35]. Similarly, Dharmarajan et al. found a high occurrence of HF readmissions regardless of index diagnosis in their analysis of Medicare claims data, and further emphasize that any admission places a patient in a position of heightened vulnerability to a variety of conditions throughout the post-discharge period [36]. In this study, the finding that *cumulative number of 30-day readmissions* is ranked first among logistic regression feature importance (Table 6) further suggests that any admission is itself a contributor to readmission risk. Thus, for patients with heart failure, focusing only on HF index admissions may result in missed opportunities to intervene to prevent any readmission, including that for HF itself. The remaining top-ranked 14 features, as discussed above, likewise highlight the importance of monitoring HF patients for their common comorbidities which also put them at risk for readmission.

Another strength of this study is the inclusion of both structured and unstructured clinical data. To our knowledge, this is the first model to apply deep learning to a readmission prediction algorithm for heart failure patients featuring both structured and unstructured data. By including both structured and unstructured data as features, the algorithm utilizes more robust data available on a given patient at the time of discharge, including important patient information not generally available in a structured format, such as patient's current living situation (available as social history), and details about the patient's course through the hospital during admission (available through hospital course and history of present illness).

The vertically deep and horizontally shallow architecture of DUNs prevented overfitting of both the hyper- and learning parameters, and constructed a high accuracy prediction model (AUC 0.705). However, DUNs do not mathematically calculate the importance of feature variables. Logistic regression provided the feature importance as shown in Table 6, although it could not achieve an AUC higher than 0.700. Thus, a limitation of deep learning, including DUNs, is the lack of 'explainability' of the prediction models [37, 38]. The DUNs' prediction model might contain unknown and nonstandard knowledge which could possibly improve the treatment of HF patients. Future work will focus on developing explainable deep learning to provide tailored feedback to physicians.

There are limitations to the study. With regards to algorithm development, KL-divergence filtering - a supervised feature selection process - was the first step in our experiments, meaning the feature selection procedure had access to the entire dataset to pre-select a subset of features that were predictive of the outcomes, which could potentially lead to overfitting (i.e., an exaggerated performance). Some feature selection methods use supervised classifiers such as logistic regression and random forests. The classifier-based methods have much higher feature selection ability than the total KL-divergence filtering. There might be a trade-off between the feature selection ability and the risk of overfitting (i.e. accuracy decreasing in a test dataset). We used the total KL-divergence filtering as the conservative approach. Additionally, we used an external dataset to measure the overfitting effect of variable preprocessing and prediction model construction (described in Additional file 2: Appendix C). In this experiment, using the total KL-divergence method for feature selection did not lead to overfitting. The AUC of the 10-fold CV described above and of this external evaluation was 0.705 (as shown in Table 5) and 0.720, respectively. This suggests the DUNs demonstrate consistent prediction ability in this retrospective study. We will plan a prospective study to evaluate the use of the DUNs' prediction model in our future research.

Missing data is a well-known limitation of utilizing EMR data for research [8]. Specifically within the PHS network, until 2014, various facilities used separate EMR systems, which collect data in different ways. Since 2014, facilities have updated their EMR to a single system, and each facility adopted this new EMR on their own schedule. This means that data was collected for patients in multiple ways across multiple systems over several years. The treatment of missing values is described above under Feature Variable Coding. An important next step for this work is to validate the algorithm on current data now that all PHS network facilities are on the same EMR system. The increased consistency of data collected within a single EMR system may have an effect on the performance of the model.

An additional limitation is that the data contains only episodes of care which occurred within the PHS network, meaning any admissions to out-of-network facilities are not captured in the data. Relatedly, results may not be generalizable to other healthcare systems, due to specifics of the patient population demographics (see Table 2) and the nature of being a large integrated healthcare delivery network.

Future work will consider the use of scaled exponential linear unit (SELU), a recently developed activation technique [39], to examine its effect on the performance of neural networks. Additionally, to improve the prediction accuracy of DUNs, future work may consider other techniques of deep learning such as activation functions (e.g. SELUs with alpha-dropout [39]), normalization techniques (ext. batch, weight, and layer normalization [40]), and faster SGDs (e.g. YellowFin [41], entropy-SGD [42]).

Conclusions

The value of this model is its ability to identify heart failure patients with an impending hospitalization regardless of cause of index admission. This enables care teams to target interventions at their most high-risk HF patients and improve overall clinical outcomes by treating the whole picture of the patient, not just a single diagnosis, which is important in a population with high rates of comorbidity and readmission. In the next stage of this project, we aim to validate this model on a new set of patient data. Like the present study, this new data set will utilize data generated by PHS patients, but will exclude patient data generated by patients whose data was included as part of algorithm development or the experiment described in the limitations above and in Additional file 2: Appendix C. Data will also be more recent, being generated from mid-2017 to present, to assure all data was collected within a single EMR system, as discussed in the limitations section above.

Additionally, we will conduct a multi-stage feasibility and usability study which will examine in detail what inputs, sources, computational requirements, and cost are necessary to functionally implement a predictive tool such as the one described herein into care provider workflow. The evaluation will include interviews with key stakeholders to determine perceived clinical value and relevance, desired output and user interface, and how the tool will be integrated into clinical workflow. Finally, we will conduct a comprehensive impact assessment to better understand the potential cost savings and value addition of the tool to an integrated healthcare network.

Successful implementation of a readmission risk prediction model could give care teams valuable insights to their patient pool, identifying high-risk patients and permitting the opportunity to target early clinical interventions to these patients with the aim of reducing the likelihood of readmission.

Abbreviations

ACCF: American College of Cardiology Foundation; AHA: American Heart Association; ALT: Alanine Aminotransferase; ATC: Anatomical Therapeutic Chemical; AUC: Area Under the [Receiver Operating Characteristic] Curve; AUROC: Area Under the Receiver Operating Characteristic; BNP: Brain Natriuretic Peptide; BOW: Bag of Words; CCCP: Connected Cardiac Care Program; CCS: Clinical Classifications Software; CMS: Center for Medicare & Medicaid Services; CNN: Convolutional Neural Network; COPD: Chronic Obstructive Pulmonary Disease; CV: Cross Validation; DNN: Deep Neural Network; DUN: Deep Unified Network; EDW: Enterprise Data Warehouse; EMR: Electronic Medical Record; HCUP: Health Cost and Utilization Project; HF: Heart Failure; HIPAA: Health Insurance Portability and Accountability Act of 1996; HRRP: Hospital Readmissions Reduction Program; ICD: International Classification of Diseases; IRB: Institutional Review Board; KL: Kullback-Leibler; LOINC: Logical Observation Identifiers Names and Codes; NLP: Natural language processing; NN: Neural Network; NT-proBNP: N-terminal pro b-type natriuretic peptide; PHS: Partners HealthCare System; POS: Parts of Speech; ROC: Receiver Operating Characteristic Curve; RPDR: Research Patient Data Repository; SELU: Scaled Exponential Linear Unit; SGD: Stochastic Gradient Descent; SQL: Sequential Query Language; SSL: Secure Sockets Layer; SSMS: Microsoft SQL Server management Studio; WKF: Well-Known Factors

Acknowledgements

Mahesh Agarwal PhD provided invaluable advice and edits to the manuscript. Siyu Tian MS, Mursal Atif BA, and Nils Fisher MPH contributed to the deidentification of study data prior to analysis. Hideo Aoki and Mika Takata provided their valuable advice on improving the management system of the feature variables. Finally, we would like to thank Ken Naono PhD for valuable scientific advice for our study.

Funding

Hitachi, Ltd. provided funding and did not play a role in the design of the study or collection of study data. Hitachi, Ltd. participated in the analysis and interpretation of data, as well as writing portions of the manuscript.

Authors' contributions

SBG and TS contributed equally to this work. SA and KJ designed the research. SBG extracted the data and performed the statistical analyses for patient cohort demographics and hospital utilization; HO processed the medication information code and text information. JS constructed the HF-relevant WKFs. GK processed the feature variable coding and extraction. TS designed the architecture of DUNs and statistically evaluated the prediction models. TN evaluated the cost saving benefit of the prediction model. TH conducted the conception and design; SA, KJ, JK, JF, SK provided feedback on analyses and interpretation of results; SBG, SA, TS, HO, JS, TN, TH, GK, JF, SK, JK, and KJ wrote the paper; SBG and SA had primary responsibility for the final content. All authors read and approved the final manuscript.

Competing interests

Hitachi Ltd. funded the study. Takuma Shibahara, Hiroko Otaki, Tatsuya Nakae, and Toru Hisamitsu work for Hitachi Ltd. Jumpei Sato and Go Kojima are currently with the University of Tokyo and Teradata Corporation in Japan, respectively. This study was done while they were with Hitachi, Ltd.

Author details

[1]Partners Connected Health Innovation, Partners HealthCare, 25 New Chardon St., Suite 300, Boston, MA 02114, USA. [2]Massachusetts General Hospital, Boston, MA, USA. [3]Harvard Medical School, Boston, MA, USA. [4]Research and Development Group, Hitachi, Ltd, Tokyo, Japan.

References

1. Adams KF, et al. Characteristics and outcomes of patients hospitalized for heart failure in the United States: rationale, design, and preliminary observations from the first 100,000 cases in the acute decompensated heart failure National Registry (ADHERE). Am Heart J. 2005;149(2):209–16. https://doi.org/10.1016/j.ahj.2004.08.005.
2. Mozzaffarian D, Benjamin EJ, Go AS, on behalf of the American Heart Association Statistics Committee and Stroke Statistics Subcommittee, et al. Heart disease and stroke statistics—2016 update: a report from the American Heart Association. Circulation. 2016;133:e38–e360.
3. Bergethon K, Ju C, DeVore A, Hardy NC, Fonarow GC, Yancy CW, Heidenreich PA, Bhatt DL, Peterson ED, Hernandez AF. Trends in 30-day readmission rates for patients hospitalized with heart failure. Circulation. 2016;9:e002594. originally published June 14, 2016. doi: https://doi.org/10.1161/CIRCHEARTFAILURE.115.002594
4. "The Hospital Readmissions Reduction (HRR) Program." *Centers for Medicare & Medicaid Services*, 24 Apr. 2017, https://www.cms.gov/Medicare/Quality-Initiatives-Patient-Assessment-Instruments/Value-Based-Programs/HRRP/Hospital-Readmission-Reduction-Program.html. Accessed 4 June 2018.
5. Wasfy JH, Zigler CM, Choirat C, Wang Y, Dominici F, Yeh RW. Readmission rates after passage of the hospital readmissions reduction program: a pre–post analysis. Ann Intern Med. 2017;166:324–31. https://doi.org/10.7326/M16-0185.
6. Fingar, K, Washington, R. Trends in Hospital Readmissions for Four High-Volume Conditions, 2009–2013: Statistical Brief #196. Healthcare Cost and Utilization Project (HCUP) Statistical Briefs [Internet]. Rockville (MD): Agency for Healthcare Research and Quality (US); 2006-2015 Nov.
7. Zolfaghar K, Meadem N, Teredesai A, Roy SB, Chin SC, Muckian B. Big data solutions for predicting risk-of-readmission for congestive heart failure patients. In Big Data, 2013 IEEE International Conference on 2013 Oct 6 (pp. 64-71). IEEE. https://doi.org/10.1109/BigData.2013.6691760.
8. Rumsfeld JS, Joynt KE, Maddox TM. Big data analytics to improve cardiovascular care: promise and challenges. Nat Rev Cardiol. 2016 Jun;13(6):350–9. https://doi.org/10.1038/nrcardio.2016.42.
9. Zhou H, Della PR, Roberts P, et al. Utility of models to predict 28-day or 30-day unplanned hospital readmissions: an updated systematic review. BMJ Open. 2016;6:e011060. https://doi.org/10.1136/bmjopen-2016-011060.
10. Ouwerkerk W, Voors AA, Zwinderman AH. Factors influencing the predictive power of models for predicting mortality and/or heart failure hospitalization in patients with heart failure. JACC Heart Fail. 2014;2:429–36. https://doi.org/10.1016/j.jchf.2014.04.006.
11. Bayati M, Braverman M, Gillam M, Mack KM, Ruiz G, Smith MS, Horvitz E. Data-driven decisions for reducing readmissions for heart failure: general methodology and case study. PLoS One. 2014;9:e109264. https://doi.org/10.1371/journal.pone.0109264.
12. Hon CP, et al. Risk Stratification for Hospital Readmission of Heart Failure Patients: A Machine Learning Approach. Proceedings of the 7th ACM International Conference on Bioinformatics, Computational Biology, and Health Informatics. Seattle, WA, USA, ACM: 491-492. 2016. doi: https://doi.org/10.1145/2975167.2985648.
13. Shameer K, et al. Predictive modeling of hospital readmission rates using electronic medical record-wide machine learning: a case study using Mount Sinai heart failure cohort. Pac Symp Biocomput. 2016;22:276–87.
14. Frizzell JD, et al. Prediction of 30-day all-cause readmissions in patients hospitalized for heart failure: comparison of machine learning and other statistical approaches. JAMA Cardiol. 2017;2(2):204–9.
15. Bergstra J, Yamins D, Cox DD. Hyperopt: a python library for optimizing the hyperparameters of machine learning algorithms. In: Proceedings of the 12th Python in science conference (pp. 13-20); 2013.
16. Yancy, Clyde W., et al. 2013 ACCF/AHA guideline for the management of heart failure: a report of the American College of Cardiology Foundation/American Heart Association task force on practice guidelines. Circulation 2014; 129(25 Suppl 2):S49-S73. doi: https://doi.org/10.1161/01.cir.0000437741.48606.98.
17. Sun J, Hu J, Luo D, Markatou M, Wang F, Edabollahi S, Steinhubl SE, Daar Z, Stewart WF. Combining knowledge and data driven insights for identifying risk factors using electronic health records. AMIA Annu Symp Proc. 2012; 2012:901–10.
18. Friedman J, Trevor H, Robert T. The elements of statistical learning. Second edition Vol. 1. New York: springer series in. statistics. 2001;
19. Dagan, I, Lillian L, Fernando P. Similarity-based methods for word sense disambiguation. Proceedings of the Thirty-Fifth Annual Meeting of the Association for Computational Linguistics and Eighth Conference of the European Chapter of the Association for Computational Linguistics. 1997: 56–63. doi:https://doi.org/10.3115/979617.979625. Retrieved 2008-03-09.
20. Ravì, Daniele, et al: Deep learning for health informatics. IEEE journal of biomedical and health informatics 21.1: 4-21. 2017.
21. Futoma, Joseph, Jonathan Morris, and Joseph Lucas: a comparison of models for predicting early hospital readmissions. J Biomed Inform 56: 229-238. 2015.
22. Yang, C., Delcher, C., Shenkman, E., & Ranka, S: Predicting 30-day all-cause readmissions from hospital inpatient discharge data." e-Health Networking, Applications and Services (Healthcom), 2016 IEEE 18th International Conference on. IEEE, 2016.
23. Chen, T., & Guestrin, C. Xgboost: A scalable tree boosting system. In: Proceedings of the 22nd acm sigkdd international conference on knowledge discovery and data mining (pp. 785-794). San Fransicso: ACM; 2016. https://dl.acm.org/citation.cfm?id=2939785.
24. Goodfellow, I. J., Warde-Farley, D., Mirza, M., Courville, A., & Bengio, Y. Maxout networks. arXiv preprint arXiv:1302.4389. 2013.
25. Broderick A. Partners HealthCare: Connecting Heart Failure Patients to Providers Through Remote Monitoring. New York: The Commonwealth Fund; 2013.
26. Agboola S, Jethwani K, Khateeb K, Moore S, Kvedar J. Heart failure remote monitoring: evidence from the retrospective evaluation of a real-world remote monitoring program. J Med Internet Res. 2015;17(4):e101. https://doi.org/10.2196/jmir.4417.
27. Lang CC, Mancini DM. Non-cardiac comorbidities in chronic heart failure. Heart. 2007 Jun;93(6):665–71. https://doi.org/10.1136/hrt.2005.068296.
28. Widmer F. [comorbidity in heart failure]. Translated from German. Ther Umsch. 2011;68(2):103–6. https://doi.org/10.1024/0040-5930/a000127.
29. Ather S, Chan W, Bozkurt B, Aguilar D, Ramasubbu K, Zachariah AA, Wehrens XHT, Deswal A. Impact of non-cardiac comorbidities on morbidity and mortality in a predominantly male population with heart failure and preserved versus reduced ejection fraction. J Am Coll Cardiol. 2012 Mar 13; 59(11):998–1005. https://doi.org/10.1016/j.jacc.2011.11.040.
30. Saczynski JS, Go AS, Magid DJ, Smith DH, McManus DD, Allen L, Ogarek J, Goldberg RJ, Gurwitz JH. Patterns of comorbidity in older patients with heart failure: the cardiovascular research network PRESERVE study. J Am Geriatr Soc. 2013 Jan;61(1):26–33. https://doi.org/10.1111/jgs.12062.
31. Lee CS, Chien CV, Bidwell JT, Gelow JM, Denfeld QE, Creber RM, Buck HG, Mudd JO. Comorbidity profiles and inpatient outcomes during hospitalization for heart failure: an analysis of the U.S. Nationwide inpatient sample. BMC Cardiovasc Disord. 2014;14:73. https://doi.org/10.1186/1471-2261-14-73.
32. Mentz RJ, Kelly JP, von Lueder TG, Voors AA, Lam CSP, Cowie MR, Kjeldsen K, Jankowska EA, Atar D, Butler J, Fiuzat M, Zannad F, Pitt B, O'Connor CM. Noncardiac comorbidities in heart failure with reduced versus preserved ejection fraction. J Am Coll Cardiol. 2014 Dec 2;64(21):2281–93. https://doi.org/10.1016/j.jacc.2014.08.036.
33. Rushton CA, Satchithananda DK, Jones PW, Kadama UT. Non-cardiovascular comorbidity, severity and prognosis in non-selected heart failure populations: a systematic review and meta-analysis. Int J Cardiol. 2015 Oct 1;196:98–106. https://doi.org/10.1016/j.ijcard.2015.05.180.
34. HCUP Clinical Classifications Software (CCS). Healthcare Cost and Utilization Project (HCUP). U.S. Agency for Healthcare Research and Quality, Rockville, MD. Updated April 2014.
35. Jencks SF, et al. Rehospitalizations among patients in the Medicare fee-for-service program. N Engl J Med. 2009;360(14):1418–28. https://doi.org/10.1056/NEJMsa0803563.
36. Dharmarajan K, et al. Diagnoses and timing of 30-day readmissions after hospitalization for heart failure, acute myocardial infarction, or pneumonia. JAMA. 2013;309(4):355–63.
37. Gunning D. Explainable artificial intelligence (xai). Defense Advanced Research Projects Agency (DARPA), Arlington County, VA. 2017. https://www.darpa.mil/attachments/XAIProgramUpdate.pdf. Accessed 3 Oct 2017.

SwissMTB: establishing comprehensive molecular cancer diagnostics in Swiss clinics

Franziska Singer[1,2†], Anja Irmisch[3†], Nora C. Toussaint[1,2], Linda Grob[1,2], Jochen Singer[2,4], Thomas Thurnherr[2,4], Niko Beerenwinkel[2,4], Mitchell P. Levesque[3], Reinhard Dummer[3], Luca Quagliata[6], Sacha I. Rothschild[5], Andreas Wicki[5], Christian Beisel[4] and Daniel J. Stekhoven[1,2*]

Abstract

Background: Molecular precision oncology is an emerging practice to improve cancer therapy by decreasing the risk of choosing treatments that lack efficacy or cause adverse events. However, the challenges of integrating molecular profiling into routine clinical care are manifold. From a computational perspective these include the importance of a short analysis turnaround time, the interpretation of complex drug-gene and gene-gene interactions, and the necessity of standardized high-quality workflows. In addition, difficulties faced when integrating molecular diagnostics into clinical practice are ethical concerns, legal requirements, and limited availability of treatment options beyond standard of care as well as the overall lack of awareness of their existence.

Methods: To the best of our knowledge, we are the first group in Switzerland that established a workflow for personalized diagnostics based on comprehensive high-throughput sequencing of tumors at the clinic. Our workflow, named SwissMTB (Swiss Molecular Tumor Board), links genetic tumor alterations and gene expression to therapeutic options and clinical trial opportunities. The resulting treatment recommendations are summarized in a clinical report and discussed in a molecular tumor board at the clinic to support therapy decisions.

Results: Here we present results from an observational pilot study including 22 late-stage cancer patients. In this study we were able to identify actionable variants and corresponding therapies for 19 patients. Half of the patients were analyzed retrospectively. In two patients we identified resistance-associated variants explaining lack of therapy response. For five out of eleven patients analyzed before treatment the SwissMTB diagnostic influenced treatment decision.

Conclusions: SwissMTB enables the analysis and clinical interpretation of large numbers of potentially actionable molecular targets. Thus, our workflow paves the way towards a more frequent use of comprehensive molecular diagnostics in Swiss hospitals.

Keywords: Molecular diagnostics, NGS, Personalized medicine, Cancer diagnostics, Molecular tumor board

Background

In recent years, molecular profiling based on high-throughput techniques has become an emerging practice in hospitals all over the world [1]. Decreased sequencing costs shifted the focus from traditional Sanger sequencing of a few specific genomic loci [2] to gene panels targeting a broader set of genes [3–5] and more comprehensive approaches, including whole-exome sequencing (WES) and whole-genome sequencing (WGS) [6, 7].

These emerging technologies hold great promise, in particular in regard to the identification of therapies for cancer patients [8]. Cancer is one of the leading causes of death in developed countries [9]. Despite decades of research the mechanisms underlying carcinogenesis are not fully understood and suitable treatment is not always available. Therapies are typically active only in a limited number of patients. Further, they are only successful for a short period of time before the tumor develops resistance mechanisms that lead to further disease progression [10–12]. Since

* Correspondence: stekhoven@nexus.ethz.ch
†Franziska Singer and Anja Irmisch contributed equally to this work.
[1]NEXUS Personalized Health Technologies, ETH Zurich, Otto-Stern-Weg 7, 8093 Zurich, Switzerland
[2]SIB Swiss Institute of Bioinformatics, 4058 Basel, Switzerland
Full list of author information is available at the end of the article

tumors evolve via complex genetic changes [13], genomic profiling of a tumor allows the prediction of targeted therapies that are more likely to be active [6].

In recent years, an increasing number of molecular targets and corresponding drugs have been identified. Prominent examples are BRAF mutations in metastatic melanoma [14] and HER2 overexpression in breast cancer, which can be targeted by specific kinase inhibitors or monoclonal antibodies, e.g. vemurafenib and trastuzumab, respectively [15, 16]. Consequently, the first molecular diagnostics initiatives using comprehensive next-generation sequencing (NGS) were launched 3–4 years ago [17], initially mainly in the US (MD Anderson [18], Mayo Clinic [19], Weill Cornell [20]), but recently also in Europe (DKFZ/NCT [21]). In these initiatives, WES is used to comprehensively analyze the protein-coding genes of the tumor genome. This allows us to detect not only cancer type specific alterations, but also mutations common in other cancer types, or mutations with associated therapies that are currently in clinical development. These efforts personalize cancer treatment with a focus on suggesting therapy options for late-stage patients for whom standard treatment is no longer effective. In this setting, reported success rates of proposing therapies are at approximately 30% [19, 21]. When standard therapy options are also included (for instance when applied as part of routine diagnostics), therapy recommendations can be made for approximately 60% of the patients [22]. At first glance, these numbers appear low; however, there are multiple factors influencing the actual success rate when using personalized molecular diagnostics. First of all, it can be expected that with more known targets these numbers will increase. In addition, one major hurdle for precision medicine is drug access [19], as therapies beyond standard of care are often not available, i.e., not approved or not covered by health insurances, and access to clinical trials is limited. Furthermore, currently comprehensive molecular diagnostics is mainly applied to end-stage cancer patients progressive on standard therapies. This limits the number of therapies left for suggestion. Also, rapid health deterioration or death is the main reason for these patients not receiving molecular diagnostics-based therapy. Finally, patient drop-out as well as limited awareness of therapy options are a major issue impeding the measurable success of molecular diagnostics [23].

In Swiss hospitals, targeted deep amplicon sequencing mainly based on the Ion Torrent sequencing platform [24] is currently the established standard for molecular diagnostics. In targeted sequencing, not the complete exome but rather an a priori defined set of genes is analyzed in order to reduce sequencing costs and analytical complexity [3–5]. Gene panels need to be updated regularly to follow the discovery of new targeted therapies. In the last 2 years, 20 new oncological therapies have been approved by regulatory authorities in Switzerland [25]. However, by design gene panels used in the clinic (e.g. the different Ion Torrent Oncomine gene panels [26]) only include the most common targetable genes matching approved therapies. Thus, to identify therapy options beyond standard of care more comprehensive sequencing technologies such as WES or WGS may be beneficial.

Regardless of the sequencing technology, high-throughput sequencing-based molecular diagnostics need a reliable framework for annotation and clinical interpretation of genetic variants [27, 28]. Currently, clinical interpretation is mainly performed manually and thus very time-consuming. Also, it is prone to miss very recent or less well-known treatment options. In addition, available databases for drug-gene interactions are either lacking the level of manual curation necessary for reliable variant interpretation [29–31] or are manually curated but cover only a subset of available targets and therapies (e.g. the current build of mycancergenome.org contains information on 823 genes and 24 cancer types [32]). While the major focus of molecular diagnostics is to propose a suitable therapy, the amount of time used to reach such a proposition is of importance as well. For instance, patients that showed progressive disease on all standard therapy lines usually have only limited survival prospective. Currently, the turnaround time of comprehensive molecular diagnostics workflows is typically about 3–12 weeks [20, 33]. This needs to be reduced considerably in order to make routine clinical application feasible, particularly for end-of-treatment line patients.

Clinical interpretation has to be based on an accurate picture of the genetic landscape of the tumor and its origin. Thus, reliable variant calling is an important part of each molecular profiling workflow. Benchmarks on existing variant calling pipelines indicate that the performance of variant detection methods can vary significantly [34–36]. Each tumor presents a unique set of genetic alterations that were involved in carcinogenesis. Moreover, tumors do not evolve homogeneously, but as subclonal populations. Each subclone has certain variants not shared with other clones of the same tumor, which is challenging for the accurate variant identification. As a result, choosing the right set of tools and parameters for a particular analysis is difficult. These multifaceted challenges, which reach across different fields of expertise, require an interdisciplinary approach that combines different areas of knowledge and experience to advance the treatment of cancer patients [17, 28]. Clinical staff and bioinformaticians need to collaborate to identify common criteria and goals to enable a meaningful analysis and interpretation of genetic variants. In addition, a definition of general rules for data sharing between hospitals and computational groups is required to enable a smooth and secure data exchange.

With the aforementioned challenges in mind, over the last 2 years we combined the bioinformatics expertise of the ETH technology platform NEXUS Personalized Health Technologies (NEXUS) with the clinical expertise of the University Hospitals in Zurich and Basel to design and implement a workflow for molecular diagnostics of cancer patients. We aimed at supporting treatment decisions by comprehensively analyzing the genetic landscape of tumors to link actionable genetic variants with therapy recommendations. Tumor biopsies were collected at the hospitals and then underwent high-throughput sequencing by WES, WGS, RNA sequencing (RNA-seq), or gene panels. The tumor samples were analyzed to identify targetable genetic variants, which were further prioritized based on their clinical significance. All findings were summarized in a concise clinical report and discussed in a multidisciplinary molecular tumor board with the goal to recommend treatment options to the treating clinician.

Methods

As depicted in Fig. 1, SwissMTB is a collaborative effort of clinicians and bioinformaticians. A tumor biopsy and preferably a matched normal control sample (e.g., blood) undergoes DNA and possibly RNA extraction, followed by sequencing. Afterwards, the samples are analyzed with regard to somatic alterations, i.e., genetic changes that appear in the tumor, but not in the normal tissue. If tumor RNA-seq data is available, gene expression levels are determined and compared to a suitable reference cohort, e.g. TCGA Skin Cutaneous Melanoma [37], to identify over- and underexpressed genes. Both genetic and transcriptomic changes are then associated with possible therapy options. Relevant therapies are summarized in a clinical report that is discussed in an interdisciplinary tumor board.

In our pilot study, we included patients from University Hospital Zurich and University Hospital Basel. In Zurich, samples from stage IV melanoma patients progressive on standard therapy were analyzed using WES, WGS, and, when feasible, RNA-seq. In Basel, samples of various cancer types were analyzed using different Ion Torrent amplicon panels. Our main objective is to identify targetable aberrations and to recommend new therapy options for patients. Therefore, somatic variants such as single nucleotide variants (SNVs), small insertions and deletions (InDels), and copy number variants (CNVs) were of particular interest. In addition, the overall mutational burden as an indicator of response to immunotherapy in melanoma [38] is determined based on WES. Furthermore, WES enables inference of the patient's HLA-I type as a treatment co-determining factor, which is required for certain vaccination trials [39, 40]. RNA-seq is used to determine differentially expressed genes as well as to validate targetable genomic variants, in particular copy number changes.

A: Sample extraction and sequencing

Tumor tissue and, if possible, a normal control sample (blood) of the patient are collected at the hospital. For the SwissMTB pilot study fresh frozen samples (WES/WGS/RNA-seq) as well as formalin-fixed paraffin embedded (FFPE) samples (gene panels) were used. Integrated quality control steps ensure that genetic aberrations and potential therapies are only inferred for samples and regions passing previously defined quality thresholds.

DNA was extracted from the samples and prepared according to the respective sequencing protocols. Panel sequencing was performed directly at the pathology department of the University Hospital Basel. WES and WGS sequencing were performed in external sequencing facilities, either the Genomics Facility Basel or the Functional Genomics Center Zurich. To save costs, in our pilot study we performed a combined analysis of deep coverage WES (approx. 120x-230x tumor coverage) for somatic variant calling and low coverage (approx. 4x-13x tumor coverage) WGS for CNV calling. For technical details such as used panel type refer to Section "Results".

B: Bioinformatics analysis

After sequencing, the resulting short DNA and RNA fragments (called *reads*) were analyzed in order to identify

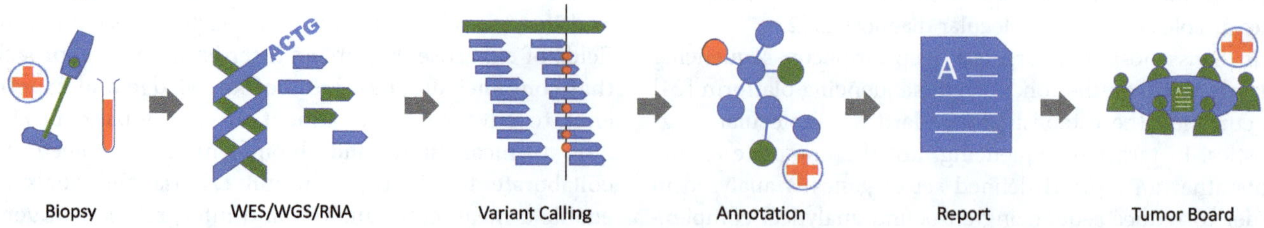

Fig. 1 SwissMTB molecular diagnostics workflow. DNA (and RNA) is extracted from a tumor biopsy (and paired control tissue, e.g., blood) and sequenced. The resulting data is analyzed to detect genetic alterations (only in the tumor sample), which are associated with potential therapy options. Suitable therapies and clinical trial options are summarized in a clinical report, which is returned to the clinician and discussed in the molecular tumor board

genomic and transcriptomic aberrations. In the following, we briefly describe the bioinformatics analysis (Fig. 2).

DNA analysis

WES, WGS, and panel analysis mainly differ in their pre-processing steps. The annotation and clinical interpretation of variants is independent of the sequencing type. First, the short DNA reads generated by the sequencing machine are mapped to the human reference genome. The resulting mapping is post-processed and used as the basis for somatic variant (SNPs and InDels) and CNV calling (based on WGS). The pipeline for WES/WGS analysis from reads to unannotated variant calls is based on the framework described in [41], employing the Snakemake workflow environment [42]. Briefly, we follow the GATK best practices for variant calling [43]. Instead of using a single somatic variant caller we use a combination of three callers, namely MuTect [44], VarScan2 [45], and Strelka [46]. Only variants reported by at least two callers are considered, in order to identify variants with greater confidence and to reduce the number of false positive calls. For CNV calling on WGS data we use BIC-seq2 [47]. If WGS is not available, we use EXCAVATOR [48] on WES data. Variant calling on panel data depends on the sequencing platform. For Ion Torrent data we rely on variants called by Ion Reporter [26], the software suite accompanying Ion Torrent. For Illumina data, we use the variant callers mentioned above, i.e., MuTect, VarScan2, and Strelka.

RNA analysis

If available, RNA-seq data is processed based on the TCGA mRNA-seq Pipeline for UNC data [49], using STAR [50] to align RNA reads to the human reference genome. Typically, RNA-seq is only performed on tumor tissue, since it is often infeasible to obtain an RNA sample extracted from corresponding normal tissue. In order to determine if the expression of a gene is altered, we compare it to the gene's expression in the most appropriate publicly available reference cohort. In our pilot study, we used either the TCGA Skin Cutaneous Melanoma [37] (SKCM) or the TCGA Uveal Melanoma [51] (UVM) cohort. Normalized gene expression values for those cohorts were downloaded from the Broad Institute TCGA GDAC Firehose website [52]. Targetable genes are considered for inclusion in the clinical report if they are either over- or underexpressed. Furthermore, gene expression is also used in the prioritization of genomic variants. For instance, a gene deletion detected by WGS or WES would be supported by RNA-seq if the observed gene expression is low or the gene is not expressed at all.

Annotation and prioritization

The number of observed somatic variants differs greatly depending on the tumor type [53]. However, the number of potentially interesting variants for a patient is usually too large to be processed manually, particularly within the desired short time-frame for generating a clinical report. Thus, the identified variants are annotated with information from databases such as COSMIC [54], dbSNP [55, 56], and ClinVar [57]. Additionally, we query cBioPortal [58, 59] to inform on the incidence of each variant across cancer types. Further, we annotate overall mutation type (e.g., missense or nonsense mutation, splice site mutation etc.), likely functional impact, and associated pathways. These types of information help to prioritize variants with respect to their significance for

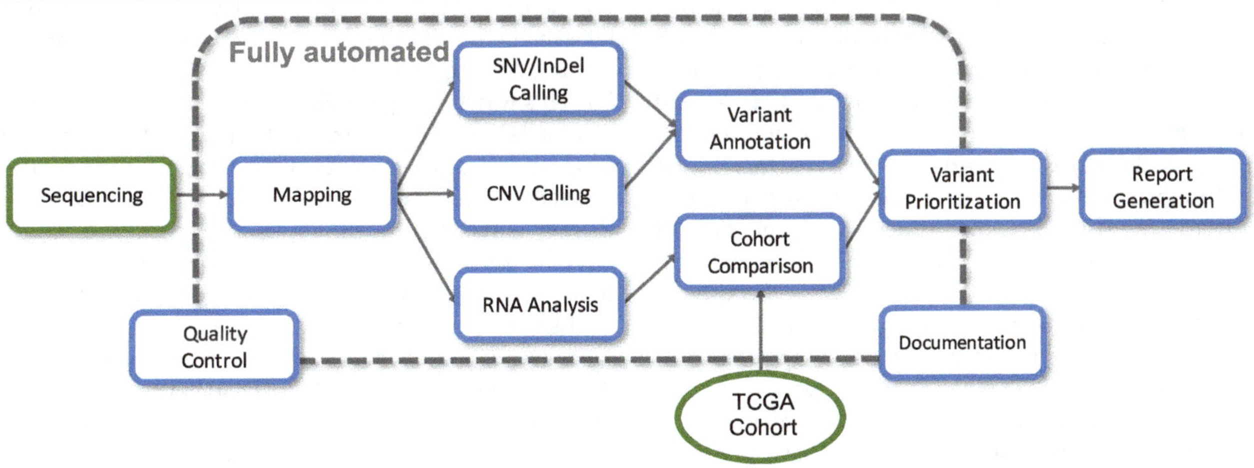

Fig. 2 Overview of the SwissMTB bioinformatics analysis workflow. The reads generated by the sequencer are first mapped to the human reference genome. Afterwards, somatic variant and copy number variant calling is performed. Variants are annotated and then prioritized according to clinical relevance. RNA-seq based gene expression levels are compared to publicly available tumor sample cohorts. The findings are summarized in a clinical report. All steps from mapping to prioritization are fully automatized using a Snakemake-based pipeline. Selecting variants and therapies for the report is currently mainly manual work. All steps are documented and quality controlled, partly based on built-in routines in the analysis pipelines

tumor development or treatment resistance. For instance, in colorectal cancer new mutations in the MAPK signaling pathway can confer resistance against combined RAF/ MEK therapy by sustaining the activity of the pathway [60].

Furthermore, we query DGIdb [29, 61, 62] to get the drug-gene interactions reported in a collection of 30 databases, of which several are expert-curated (e.g. MyCancerGenome [63]). The more databases support an interaction, the higher the priority of the drug. In addition, we query all possible drugs at Swissmedic [25], the Swiss regulatory authority for drugs and medical products. Of highest priority are drugs that are available in Switzerland. Finally, based on drug-gene interactions identified in DGIdb we collect associated clinical trials at ClinicalTrials.gov. Clinical trials are important in two regards: First, completed trials inform on the suitability of a therapy and its confidence level in the report. Second, open clinical trials make therapies available to the patient, if the patient is eligible for the trial. Trials that explicitly require the observed variant for therapy eligibility are of particular interest.

The combination of the aforementioned information is essential for the generation of a clinical report reliably summarizing all relevant therapies for the treating clinician. Until this point, all steps are automated, and depending on sequencing depth the bioinformatics analyses takes approximately six hours. The main bottleneck regarding turnaround time is the manual generation of the clinical report, which is described in the following section.

C: Clinical report

The clinical report is a concise summary of relevant therapies identified based on the genetic and transcriptomic landscape of the tumor. It is the basis for discussion in a molecular tumor board and informs on therapy options arising from the molecular alterations present in the tumor. Each recommended therapy is associated with an identified variant, and the relevance and reliability of each therapy is assessed based on evidence in the literature, such as previous preclinical studies and clinical trials. The clinical report is intended to only present the relevant subset of variants found in a tumor. This subset is derived based on the knowledge at the time of analysis and is thus likely to change over time, for instance if new targets are identified or therapies become Swissmedic approved. Therefore, each report is accompanied by an addendum listing all identified aberrations.

The clinical report is structured such that the results are communicated to the tumor board as purposeful as possible [64]. It has an overview page, presenting the most important information regarding therapy recommendations, accompanied by various sections with relevant details (Additional file 1).

The overview page (Fig. 3) contains basic data on the patient, the tumor sample, and the treating clinician. It further summarizes the proposed therapy options, and presents results on mutational burden and HLA-I type. In addition, it gives an overview of the mutational status of genes frequently described as mutated in the given cancer, to allow the clinician to easily assess whether important genes are mutated or not. For instance, the status of BRAF in melanoma (mutations prevalent in 40–50% of all cases [14]) or ALK in lung cancer (rearrangements prevalent in 4–5% of all non-small cell lung cancers [65]) influences eligibility for clinical trials. The list of important genes is derived either by personal communication with the responsible clinician or based on MyCancerGenome [63] and relevant literature.

In addition to therapy recommendations, also indicating possible drug resistances is of interest. For instance, various TP53 mutations have been reported to confer resistance to platinum-based chemotherapy in ovarian cancer [66]. Such findings are reported in a separate section (entitled "Therapies potentially lacking benefit") and are also highlighted on the overview page. In our example, the low mutational burden indicates only limited benefit of Anti-CTLA4 therapy (Fig. 4) [38].

We categorize findings into different levels of confidence that are used to assess the relevance of the potential therapy. For categorization, we follow the guidelines in [67] (refer to Fig. 5 for the confidence level overview).

Recommended drugs that are Swissmedic approved have the highest confidence level (level A), followed by those that have proven successful for treatment in several well-powered clinical studies (preferably phase 3). Drug targets that are Swissmedic approved for a different type of cancer or have been tested in smaller studies for the cancer type at hand have lesser confidence (level C). Finally, targets that have only been tested in preclinical studies are in the lowest confidence category (level D). This way the applicability of a recommended therapy can be assessed easily. In addition, we list the literature support for each included drug-gene interaction to allow a detailed assessment of the reasons why this particular therapy is recommended.

In the report, therapies are grouped into different sections (Fig. 6), namely "cancer type specific therapies" (Swissmedic approved for the given indication), "non cancer type specific therapies" (Swissmedic approved for a different indication), and "investigational therapies" (not Swissmedic approved). The different sections contain the most relevant information for each recommendation: gene and drug name, observed variant, variant frequency or copy number, associated pathway, variant effect (if known, for instance gain-of-function or loss-of-function as indicated in OncoKB [68]), confidence level, and literature support. Further, as exemplified in Fig. 6, the relative gene

MOLECULAR TUMOR REPORT

Patient	Specimen	Customer
Gender: xxx **YOB:** xxx **Case number:** xxx **Diagnosis:** Melanoma	**Tumor specimen site:** Subcutaneous metastasis, thoracic **Normal specimen site:** Blood **WES Tumor/Normal coverage:** 187.3x/128.1x **WGS Tumor/Normal coverage:** 6.0x/5.8x **Sequenced:** WES/WGS/RNA **Platform:** Illumina HiSeq	xxx

Mutation summary

Mutational burden[1]

19 SNVs (16 non-synonymous -> 0.27/Mb), 14 CNVs (affecting 3357 genes)

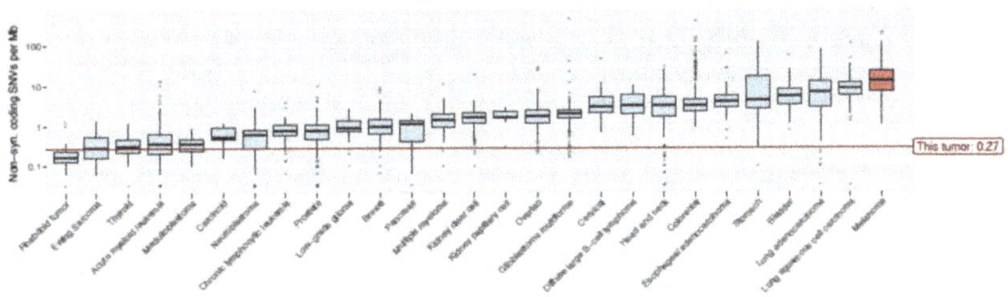

Genes commonly mutated in melanoma

Mutated: BRAF 38.1% p.Val600Glu | CTNNB1 0.5x Hemizygous deletion | CDKN2A 0.5x Hemizygous deletion

Not mutated: CDK4/6, GNAQ, EGFR, EIF1AX, KIT, MEK1, MET, NF1, NRAS, PIK3CA, PTEN, SF3B1

Therapy summary

Cancer type specific: Dabrafenib, Vemurafenib

Non cancer type specific: Nintedanib, Palbociclib, Ponatinib

Investigational: LTT462, LXH254, MSC2490484, LY3076226

Reduced efficacy: Anti-CTLA4 therapy

HLA type

A*26:01 A*02:01 B*38:01 B*27:05 C*12:03 C*02:02 (inferred using OptiType [2])

Fig. 3 The overview page of an example clinical report including the categorization of therapies into cancer type specific, off-label (non cancer type specific), investigational, and possibly contraindicated therapies. We indicate the mutation status of commonly mutated genes, visualize the mutational burden of the patient, and inform on the patient's HLA type

Therapies potentially lacking benefit

Gene	Variant	Frequency or Copy number	Relative gene expression[19]	Therapy	Description	References
Low mutational burden		-	-	Anti-CTLA4 therapy	Low mutational burden associated with limited or no clinical benefit	[18]

Fig. 4 Report section for therapies potentially lacking benefit. Gene name and variant type, as well as observed frequency, copy number, or gene expression are presented to indicate resistance-causing events. Furthermore, details on the affected therapy, as well as a brief description of the finding and literature support are provided

Confidence levels [20]	
A	Biomarkers that predict response or resistance to swissmedic-approved therapies for a specific type of tumor or have been included in professional guidelines as therapeutic, diagnostic, and/or prognostic biomarkers for specific types of tumors.
B	Biomarkers that predict response or resistance to a therapy based on well-powered studies with consensus from experts in the field, or have diagnostic and/or prognostic significance of certain diseases based on well-powered studies with expert consensus.
C	Biomarkers that predict response or resistance to therapies approved by swissmedic or professional societies for a different tumor type (ie, off-label use of a drug), serve as inclusion criteria for clinical trials, or have diagnostic and/or prognostic significance based on the results of multiple small studies.
D	Biomarkers that show plausible therapeutic significance based on preclinical studies, or may assist disease diagnosis and/or prognosis themselves or along with other biomarkers based on small studies or multiple case reports with no consensus.
-	The cited references do not fit into any of the above categories. Confidence is very low.

Fig. 5 Therapy recommendation confidence levels, based on categorization by the Association for Molecular Pathology, American Society of Clinical Oncology, and College of American Pathologists [67]

Cancer type specific therapies

Swissmedic-approved for the given indication.

Gene	Variant	Frequency or Copy number	Relative gene expression[19]	Pathway/ Function	Therapy	Confidence	References
BRAF	p.Val600Glu	38.1%		MAPK signaling	Dabrafenib	A	[3,4,6]
					Vemurafenib	A	[3,4,5]

Non cancer type specific therapies

Swissmedic-approved for a different indication.

Gene	Variant	Frequency or Copy number	Relative gene expression[19]	Pathway/ Function	Therapy	Confidence	References
CDKN2A	Deletion	0.5		Cell cycle	Palbociclib	B	[7,8,9,10]
					Ribociclib	D	[23,24]
FGFR3	Amplification	4.2		MAPK, PI3K and PKC signaling	Ponatinib	D	[11,21,22]
					Nintedanib	D	[12,22]
FGFR4[a]	Over expression	-		Growth factor signaling	Ponatinib	D	[11,21,22]

[a] An FGFR4 amplification is detected confidently in WES data but only with low confidence (below threshold) in WGS data.

Investigational therapies

Not Swissmedic-approved.

Gene	Variant	Frequency or Copy number	Relative gene expression[19]	Pathway/ Function	Therapy	Confidence	References
BRAF	p.Val600Glu	38.1%		MAPK signaling	LTT462	-	[17,25]
					LXH254	C	[13]
PRKDC	Amplification	5.9		Non-homologous end-joining	MSC2490484A	-	[15,16]
FGFR3	Amplification	4.2		MAPK, PI3k and PKC signaling	LY3076226	-	[14,26]

Fig. 6 Example for therapy categories for a melanoma patient presenting (among other mutations) several copy number mutations, an FGFR4 overexpression, and a BRAF V600E point mutation, identified based on WES, WGS, and RNA-seq data. Each table is structured as follows: Column "Gene" shows the name of the affected gene. Column "Variant" either contains the exact amino acid change resulting from a point mutation, or states the copy number change (amplification or deletion), or presents the change observed by the RNA-seq analysis (e.g. overexpression). Column "Frequency or Copy number" presents the variant frequency of point mutations (in percent), or presents the copy number observed for the affected gene. Column "Relative gene expression" includes the boxplot that shows the expression of the particular gene in comparison to the TCGA cohort of the same cancer type. For ease of interpretation, the different types of boxplot are explained in the "Guide section" of the clinical report, Additional file 1. Column "Pathway/Function" gives details on the functions of a gene. Column "Therapy" shows the name of the drug with a potential drug-gene interaction, while columns "Confidence" and "References" present the confidence level and the literature support of the drug-gene interaction, respectively

expression of the mutated gene in comparison to the TCGA cohort of the same cancer type is shown in a separate column (the gene expression plots are explained in the report glossary, Additional file 1).

Finally, not only therapies are recommended to the treating clinician, but also potentially relevant open clinical trials (refer to Fig. 7 for an example table). We prefer trials of higher phase and located in or near Switzerland, and give a brief overview of each trial by including study title, trial phase, and location. Ultimately, suitability of a trial has to be decided by the clinician, because we do not have access to all information necessary to assess a patient's eligibility.

The BRAF mutation observed in our example patient illustrates how the clinical report can be utilized to facilitate clinical decision making. BRAF V600E is a well-known therapy target in melanoma and thus assigned the highest confidence. As shown in Fig. 6 in the green table, Swissmedic approved therapies are available (dabrafenib and vemurafenib). However, also investigational therapies targeting BRAF are possible, namely LTT462 and LXH254. Both compounds are not yet Swissmedic approved and have only been tested in a few studies, but they might become relevant therapy options if the patient has already received (and progressed on) other therapies. As shown in Fig. 7, for both LTT462 and LXH452 clinical trials are recruiting in Switzerland, such that the compounds might indeed be accessible to the patient. This example shows the tight link between the different sections of the clinical report: at first glance investigational therapies might seem rather irrelevant and hardly accessible, but the clinical trials section directly shows whether the drug might nevertheless be available. It also highlights the advantages of comprehensive sequencing: only focusing on well-known targets cannot provide information on newer and less known therapy targets. Since tumors often become resistant to the applied therapies, pointing out alternatives that might work on these resistant tumors may be important for pre-treated patients.

Results

Up to now, 22 patients progressive on standard treatments have been included in the SwissMTB study. From the dermatology department at the University Hospital Zurich we prospectively analyzed eleven patients with metastatic cutaneous, uveal, and mucosal melanoma (Table 1). These patients were sequenced based on WES accompanied by WGS (except for the first patient for whom only WES was performed). For five of the most recent patients we also performed RNA-seq to identify transcriptomic aberrations. In three of these patients, gene expression results affected therapy recommendations. From the University Hospital Basel, we analyzed eleven patients with various cancer types (Table 2). These samples were analyzed in retrospect, after the actual therapy had been applied.

The SwissMTB analyses for the University Hospital Zurich were performed before treatment. Thus, for some patients the molecular findings could influence treatment

Selected clinical trial opportunities

Gene	Therapy	Trial ID	Title	Phase	Country
BRAF	LXH254	NCT02607813	Phase I Study of LXH254 in Patients With Advanced Solid Tumors Haboring MAPK Pathway Alterations	1	CH, DE
BRAF	LTT462	NCT02711345	A Phase I Clinical Study With Investigational Compound LTT462 in Adult Patients With Specific Advanced Cancers	1	CH, DE
BRAF	Dabrafenib + Trametinib + Pembrolizumab	NCT02625337	Study Comparing Pembrolizumab With Dual MAPK Pathway Inhibition Plus Pembrolizumab in Melanoma Patients (IMPemBra)	2	NL
BRAF	Dabrafenib + Trametinib + Pembrolizumab	NCT03149029	Abbreviated MAPK Targeted Therapy Plus Pembrolizumab in Melanoma	2	US
BRAF	Dabrafenib + Trametinib + Nivolumab	NCT02910700	Study of the Anti-PD-1 Antibody Nivolumab in Combination With Dabrafenib and/or Trametinib in Patients With BRAF or NRAS-Mutated Metastatic Melanoma	2	US
CDKN2A	Palbociclib	NCT02202200	Phase I-II Study With Tumor Molecular Pharmacodynamic (MPD) Evaluation and Pharmacokinetics of PD-0332991 in Patients Suffering Metastatic Melanoma (OPTIMUM)	1/2	F
CDKN2A	Palbociclib	NCT01037790	Phase II Trial oft he Cyclin-dependent Kinase Inhibitor PD-0332991 in Patients with Cancer	2	US
FGFR3	LY3076226	NCT02529553	A Study of LY3076226 in Participants With Advanced or Metastatic Cancer	1	US
PRKDC	MSC2490484A	NCT02516813	Phase 1 Trial of MSC2490484A, an Inhibitor of a DNA-dependent Protein Kinase, in Combination With Radiotherapy	1	US

Fig. 7 Example for clinical trial options presented in a clinical report

Table 1 Overview of patients analyzed based on comprehensive sequencing

Patient	Cancer Type	Sequen-cing	No. of actionable variants	No. of therapies (cancer-type specific, off-label, investigational)	No. of therapies lacking benefit	Comments
1	Cutaneous Melanoma	WES	13	12 (2,4,6)	NA (not yet part of workflow)	Patient died before the report could be delivered. Based on an observed PTCH1 amplification reported in the SwissMTB analysis, vismodegib would have been considered as treatment.
2	Cutaneous Melanoma	WES	13	19 (2,12,5)	5	Based on the high mutational load of this tumor anti-CTLA4 treatment was recommended. The patient was treated accordingly and showed a complete response.
3	Cutaneous Melanoma	WES/WGS	6	12 (3,4,5)	5	NRAS Q61K resistance variant identified and trametinib treatment recommended.
4	Uveal Melanoma	WES/WGS	3	7 (0,4,3)	5	Based on a PXR loss Taxol treatment was recommended. The patient was treated accordingly, but progressed after 2 months of therapy.
5	Cutaneous Melanoma	WES/WGS	5	8 (2,5,1)	3	Based on the high mutational load anti-CTLA4 treatment was recommended. The patient was treated accordingly with a combination of anti-CTLA4 and anti-PD1 therapy and showed partial response.
6	Mucosal Melanoma	WES/WGS/ RNA-seq	3	7 (0,4,3)	3	At the time of report delivery, the condition of the patient did not allow any treatment.
7	Mucosal Melanoma	WES/WGS/ RNA-seq	6	12 (0,7,5)	1	Patient died before the report could be delivered.
8	Uveal Melanoma	WES/WGS	4	10 (0,4,6)	1	Based on GNA11 Q209L variant treatment with sorafenib was decided but insurance did not cover drug costs.
9	Uveal Melanoma	WES/WGS/ RNA-seq	4	10 (0,4,6)	1	Patient died before the report could be delivered.
10	Uveal Melanoma	WES/WGS/ RNA-seq	5	11 (0,5,6)	1	Based on observed FGFR4 overexpression, ponatinib was recommended as off-label treatment. However, the patient died before the report could be discussed in the molecular tumor board.
11	Cutaneous Melanoma	WES/WGS/ RNA-Seq	4	6 (0,4,2)	0	Based on observed MET overexpression the patient received crizotinib as off-label treatment.
Summary: median (IQR)			5 (2)	10 (4.5)	2 (3.5)	

Abbreviations: *IQR* Interquartile range

decisions. Unfortunately, similar as in other molecular tumor board approaches (e.g. [19, 69]), half of the patients experienced rapid health deterioration, such that for only six patients SwissMTB treatment recommendations could be discussed in the molecular tumor board. Namely, from the eleven patients presented in Table 1, patients 1, 6, 7, 9, and 10 died or were too far declined in health before the findings could be presented to the clinicians. Results from the six remaining patients have been discussed, and for five patients, namely patients 2, 4, 5, 8, and 11, the SwissMTB findings indeed influenced the treatment decision.

To be more specific, for patient 2 (refer to Table 1) the WES analysis showed that the sequenced tumor material had a very high mutational load with 826 non-synonymous protein-coding mutations. A high mutational load above 100 non-synonymous coding mutations has been shown to be predictive of positive response to ipilimumab therapy in melanoma [38]. Based on this finding and the recent approval of the combined checkpoint blockade of anti-CTLA4 and anti-PD1 therapy that results in higher response rates than single anti-CTLA4 treatment [70], combination treatment with ipilimumab and nivolumab was started. The patient experienced complete tumor regression after 2 months and continued on immunotherapy treatment, where he stayed tumor-free for 8 months. Furthermore, the patient's tumor harbored amplifications of BRAF, EGFR, MET, and CDK6, which provides a rationale for this tumor's acquired resistance to the triple BRAF/MEK/CDK4&6 inhibitor treatment applied before sequencing [71, 72].

For patient 3 (Table 1) the results showed an NRAS Q61K activation resistance variant, which leads to reactivation of the MAPK pathway in the presence of BRAF inhibitors. Trametinib, which inhibits the downstream MEK kinase, was therefore suggested as a matching drug on the report. However, it is known that the in vitro response of double NRAS and BRAF mutated cells to MEK inhibitors is heterogeneous [73]. The tumor board therefore decided on the newly approved combination

Table 2 Overview of patients analyzed based on panel data, only tumor samples were sequenced

Patient	Cancer Type	Panel type	No. of actionable variants	No. of therapies (cancer-type specific, off-label, investigational)	No. of therapies lacking benefit	Comments
12	Fibroblastic osteosarcoma	Oncomine Comprehensive Panel	0	0	0	Only germline variants detected in sample.
13	Head and Neck Squamous cell carcinoma	Cancer HotSpot Panel 2.0	12	12 (6,6,0)	0	Various damaging variants in genes of MAPK signaling pathway detected. Tyrosine kinase inhibitor treatment recommended.
14	Lung neuroendocrine carcinoma	Cancer HotSpot Panel 2.0	1	1 (0,1,0)	0	Based on FBXW7 D440Y variant mTOR inhibitor treatment recommended.
15	Ovarian serous carcinoma	Cancer HotSpot Panel 2.0	1	1 (1,0,0)	1	Based on observed TP53 V173 L resistance variant doxorubicin treatment recommended and platinum-based treatment discouraged. As indicated in SwissMTB analysis, progressive disease under carboplatin treatment.
16	Cutaneous melanoma	Cancer HotSpot Panel 2.0	2	3 (2,1,0)	0	Based on CDKN2A R80* loss-of-function variant off-label treatment with palbociclib recommended.
17	Chondrosarcoma	Oncomine Solid Tumor DNA Panel	10	9 (0,9,0)	3	Tyrosine kinase inhibitor treatment recommended. Patient was treated with pazopanib, response status unknown. Four resistance-associated variants found: ALK G1202R, KRAS S65 N, TP53 C275Y, and TP53 G245D.
18	Lung adenocarcinoma	Liquid Biopsy, Oncomine Solid Tumor DNA Panel	0	0	0	No tumor DNA contained in sample.
19	Lung adenocarcinoma	Liquid Biopsy, Oncomine Solid Tumor DNA Panel	1	0	1	Use of ALK inhibitors discouraged because of ALK G1202R resistance variant. As indicated in SwissMTB analysis, progressive disease under crizotinib treatment.
20	Lung squamous cell carcinoma	Oncomine Solid Tumor DNA Panel	1	1 (1,0,0)	1	Paclitaxel recommended based on observed TP53 R342* variant.Contradictive case, as a second TP53 R248Q variant is associated with increased chemotherapy resistance.
21	Neuroectodermal sarcoma	Cancer HotSpot Panel 2.0	0	0	0	No variants identified.
22	Cutaneous melanoma	Cancer HotSpot Panel 2.0	5	11 (1,9,1)	1	Multi-kinase inhibitor treatment recommended, cisplatin treatment discouraged based on TP53 R273S resistance variant.
Summary: median (IQR)			1 (3)	1 (6)	0 (1)	

Note that the SwissMTB analysis of these samples was performed retrospectively. *Abbreviations*: *IQR* Interquartile range

therapy of the checkpoint inhibitors ipilimumab with nivolumab. The patient progressed on this therapy, which is in concordance with the low mutation rate reported by WES analysis and the associated contraindication of immunotherapy indicated in the report. At the time of manuscript submission, it was not yet decided whether the therapy will be switched to the alternatively proposed drug trametinib.

For patient 4 (refer to Table 1), who has a rare uveal melanoma, we reported the loss of the pregnane X receptor (PXR) as an actionable variant. This receptor binds chemotherapy agents such as taxanes and regulates drug metabolizing enzymes. PXR knockdown in cancer cells induces increased paclitaxel sensitivity and apoptotic cell death [74]. Also, in uveal melanoma paclitaxel treatment is known to induce stable disease in one third of patients [75]. The tumor board therefore decided to initiate treatment with paclitaxel. However, the patient progressed with new metastases after 2 months of treatment.

For patient 5 (Table 1) the report indicated a high mutational load. Therefore, the patient was treated with combined immune checkpoint blockade, which resulted in a partial response with most metastases regressing.

In patient 6 an amplification of the Src kinase LYN was detected in the WGS analysis. This indicates benefit of the LYN kinase inhibitors masitinib and bosutinib, which have been shown to be effective in cancer therapy [76, 77]. However, RNA-seq analysis showed that LYN expression is comparatively low with respect to the TCGA SKCM cohort [37]. Therefore, therapy with bosutinib and masitinib would likely have lacked benefit in this patient. This finding was included in the report. However, at the time of report delivery, the condition of the patient did not allow any treatment.

Based on the variant GNA11 Q209L identified in the uveal melanoma of patient 8 off-label treatment with sorafenib was decided by the tumor board. However, the insurance did not cover the therapy costs. Up to the time of manuscript submission no alternative treatment decision has been made.

For patient 10 FGFR4 overexpression was determined by comparing the patient's gene expression to the TCGA UVM cohort [51]. Ponatinib and other pan-FGFR inhibitors are currently being investigated in clinical trials to determine their potential in treating FGFR aberrant cancers [78]. These treatments were included in the report. However, patient 10 died before report delivery, and thus these findings were not discussed in the tumor board. For patient 11 we reported a significant MET overexpression with respect to the TCGA SKCM [37] cohort. In a recent study, Yang et al. [79] reported tumor shrinkage and clinical benefit in gastric cancer patients with MET overexpression on crizotinib treatment. Based on these findings, off-label treatment with crizotinib was started. Unfortunately, the patient progressed on this treatment and died after a few weeks.

In Basel, the SwissMTB workflow was applied retrospectively to samples of patients who had already been treated. Thus, the SwissMTB findings did not influence treatment decision, but we can compare recommended and discouraged therapies with the actual therapy choice. Table 2 summarizes the results of the SwissMTB analysis for the panel-based analysis of patients 12 to 22. Since patients 12, 18, and 21 presented no actionable variants we did not recommend any therapies. For all of the remaining eight patients we found variants with possible treatment relevance. Only patient 20 presented inconclusive results that would need further investigation. In four of the patients, namely patients 15, 17, 19, and 22, resistance mutations were identified. Notably, in two of these cases (patients 15 and 19) the patients had received therapies for which we found resistance mutations, and indeed the clinical follow-up showed lack of response to these therapies.

For patient 13 several damaging variants were identified in genes associated with the MAPK signaling pathway. Thus, in the report use of tyrosine kinase inhibitors was recommended, e.g. pazopanib or lenvatinib. However, at the time of treatment decision information on these molecular targets was not available to the clinician, and thus a targeted therapy was not considered. The patient instead received and progressed on three lines of therapy including carboplatin+paclitaxel chemotherapy and immunotherapy with nivolumab.

For patient 14 the SwissMTB molecular diagnostic identified a variant in the WD40 domain of the tumor suppressor gene FBXW7. We recommended mTOR inhibitor treatment, for instance with everolimus [80]. Mixed responses to this treatment have been reported in the literature [81]. However, low response was shown in particular in the presence of other simultaneous variants, for instance in KRAS. Since in the panel-based analysis the observed FBXW7 variant appeared as the only mutation, a therapy with mTOR inhibitors such as everolimus might be justified. For this patient no clinical follow-up data was available.

Patient 15, who had ovarian cancer, showed a TP53 V173 L mutation that is associated with a higher likelihood of platinum treatment resistance [66, 82]. The patient received the platinum-based chemotherapy carboplatin, and indeed the therapy lacked efficacy. In the SwissMTB report we instead recommended doxorubicin treatment, which was reported to be effective in in the presence of platinum resistance [83, 84].

Patient 16 received anti-CTLA4 immunotherapy, which resulted in a stable disease. In case of disease progression the SwissMTB report recommends off-label treatment with palbociclib to target the observed loss-of-function variant R80* in CDKN2A [85, 86].

Patient 17 presented four different resistance mutations, namely ALK G1202R, KRAS S65 N, TP53 C275Y, and TP53 G245D. Thus, in the SwissMTB report we discouraged the use of ALK inhibitors, cetuximab, and cisplatin treatment. Instead, we recommended treatment with tyrosine kinase and mTOR inhibitors such as pazopanib and everolimus based on several variants in genes associated to the MAPK signaling pathway and mTOR signaling pathway. The patient was treated with pazopanib; however, at the time of writing no information on treatment response was available.

Patient 19 presented a lung adenocarcinoma with an ALK G1202R variant, a mutation associated with general resistance against ALK inhibition [87–89]. As predicted based on the observed variant, the patient showed a progressive disease when treated with the ALK kinase inhibitor crizotinib.

The SwissMTB analysis of the lung squamous cell carcinoma of patient 20 presents an example of inconclusive results. Here, the only two identified variants were TP53 R342* and TP53 R248Q. Contradicting results are reported regarding the sensitivity or resistance to paclitaxel treatment in the presence of these variants [90, 91]. Thus, paclitaxel is indicated in the clinical report as possible therapy option that needs further investigation.

For patient 22 we identified TP53 R273S, a variant associated to cisplatin therapy resistance in a variety of cancer types [82, 92]. The patient showed a progressive disease under anti-CTLA4 and anti-PD1 immunotherapy. According to the SwissMTB molecular diagnostic other therapy options would have been off-label tyrosine kinase inhibition, e.g. with sunitinib or regorafenib, based on multiple variants in the MAPK signaling pathway and a KIT exon11 variant [93, 94].

Discussion

The conducted pilot project only comprises a small number of patients and can thus only serve as a proof-of-concept to show the feasibility of the SwissMTB workflow in a clinical setting. Larger clinical trials including a control group are required to determine whether approaches based on comprehensive molecular tumor analysis offer significant clinical benefit to late stage cancer patients. Nonetheless, single patients showed clinical benefit from our SwissMTB approach.

In summary, we were able to recommend therapies for 19 out of 22 patients (86%), which exceeds the recommendation success rate of 60% generally reported in the literature [22]. As clinicians were directly involved in the SwissMTB workflow, our study did not suffer from limitations such as lack of awareness of available therapies. Thus, when the influence of factors like limited awareness of therapeutic options and patient drop-out is reduced, the actual benefit of molecular diagnostics might be higher than visible from numbers reported in the literature. For five out of eleven patients analyzed before treatment, the SwissMTB diagnostics influenced the treatment decision. Four of them received the recommended therapy (in one case the insurance did not cover the treatment costs), and two of these patients responded well. In addition, we identified clinically relevant variants in eight of eleven cases in the retrospective analysis based on panels. For six of these patients, SwissMTB proposed promising actionable targets and possible targeted treatments. Since most patients included in the pilot cohort progressed on their received standard therapy, these findings would have been relevant treatment alternatives or follow-up treatment options. Importantly, we also identified resistance variants for treatments that indeed proved ineffective in the clinical follow-up. Thus, for two patients analysed retrospectively, our analysis likely would have prevented a non-beneficial therapy. Overall, the results of this pilot cohort, despite being small and preliminary, indicate the benefit of the SwissMTB workflow. Further, the pilot study suggests an added value of integrating RNA-seq information, as gene expression results affected therapy recommendations in three out of the five cases with available RNA.

In Switzerland, SwissMTB is the first workflow for a molecular tumor board based on comprehensive sequencing techniques like WES, WGS, and RNA-seq. Other initiatives, e.g. at the Weill Cornell Cancer Center in New York [20], or at the DKFZ in Heidelberg [21], also implement comprehensive molecular diagnostics, although typically they are based on WES only [19, 20]. Only few cohort studies published so far include RNAseq-based analysis for direct treatment prediction [95, 96]. Importantly, since Swiss regulations differ from regulations in other countries, e.g. the US or Germany, molecular tumor board workflows from other countries cannot be applied straightforwardly in Switzerland. In contrast, SwissMTB was specifically designed to be used in Swiss clinical practice, and thus it adheres to the guidelines of the Swiss authorities.

Already today, many hospitals have implemented molecular tumor boards to discuss treatment decisions. However, these tumor boards almost exclusively look at NGS results from gene panel sequencing. In contrast, SwissMTB targets not only a limited set of genes, but offers a comprehensive view on the genomic and, additionally, transcriptional landscape of the tumor. Thus, it goes beyond the workflows currently implemented in the hospitals. Reasons why in Swiss hospitals gene panels are the de facto standard for NGS-based analyses are mostly the lower sequencing costs and straightforward variant interpretation. However, WES and WGS are more comprehensive and can provide a clearer picture of the mutational landscape of the tumor. For instance, important features such as the HLA type cannot be assessed with commonly used panels, but only with more comprehensive approaches. Similarly, tumor mutational burden, an important predictor of immune checkpoint therapy response, cannot be analyzed by most smaller routine panels. Routine diagnostics often lack the computational methods to filter and prioritize the often large number of variants identified in WES/WGS. Since SwissMTB provides the means to analyze and perform drug-matching of a large numbers of variants, our workflow paves the way towards a more frequent use of comprehensive molecular diagnostics in Swiss hospitals.

Another advantage of SwissMTB is its support of the simultaneous analysis of tumor and matched control samples. In Swiss hospitals NGS-based diagnostics is almost exclusively performed on tumor-only samples. However, we strongly encourage the use of a matched normal sample in order to directly call somatic aberrations and to decrease the risk of identifying germline variants. Recently, a study by Sun et al. [97] showed that clinically reliably somatic variant calling is also possible without a matched normal. However, the approach has various constraints such as requiring high sequencing depths of more than 500x, and thus is currently infeasible for WES and WGS in clinical practice. However, particularly for WES and WGS sequencing the number of germline variants would impede the search for tumor-relevant variants. Furthermore, investigating germline variants of a patient requires special ethical consideration. For panel sequencing the use of a matched normal control is advisable for the same reason. However, it is not yet common practice – and sometimes not even possible – to obtain such a sample. In our study, a matched normal sample was used for WES and WGS. In contrast, both panel-based analysis and RNA-seq were exclusively performed on tumor samples. As discussed below, this led to germline variant identification in one of the patients.

When we compare the overall results of the analysis based on comprehensive sequencing versus panel sequencing, we see that with panels generally less actionable variants are found, resulting in less therapy options and less insight into drug resistance and clinical trials. This effect can be observed independently of the panel type used, and further underlines the benefit of using comprehensive sequencing instead of targeted panels. Notably, the patients from University Hospital Basel presented various cancer types. Thus, compared to melanoma there might be less actionable variants and therapies available. For better comparability we only considered the patients with melanoma (two patients) or lung cancer (four patients) for a less biased second comparison. However, even on this limited number of patients overall less actionable variants and corresponding treatments were identified, namely a median number of one variant and one therapy, including standard therapies.

Notably, the patients from our cohort had already received a number of therapies before they entered our study. Even when excluding these therapies, still off-label and investigational therapies were recommended for all eleven patients analyzed with WES/WGS, and only for six patients analyzed based on panels. Each report based on comprehensive sequencing proposes a median number of ten such therapies linked to a median number of six trials per patient. Note that this number already represents a selected set of preferable trials (e.g. trials conducted in or near Switzerland, if those were available).

In the panel-based analysis, we identified actionable variants in eight of the eleven patients. For these eight patients, a median of two therapies was recommended per patient with a median of one off-label or investigational therapy linked to a median number of 2.5 clinical trials. There are several possible reasons for the lack of actionable variants in three of the eleven patients. In case of patient 18 (refer to Table 2) the amount of tumor DNA in the sample was not sufficient. This sample was taken by liquid biopsy, a technique that extracts cell-free circulating tumor DNA from the blood. Here, wild-type DNA is much more abundant than tumor DNA. Thus, the sequencing and bioinformatics analysis of liquid biopsy samples is even more challenging compared to tumor biopsy samples [98]. For patients 12 and 21 (Table 2) no variants could be identified, except for germline variants in patient 12. On the one hand, this shows the importance of a normal control sample to decrease the risk of identifying germline variants. On the other hand, both patient 12 and 21 presented rare tumor types (fibroblastic osteosarcoma and neuroectodermal sarcoma, respectively) for which few therapy targets are known. Patients with such rare tumor types might benefit from an analysis based on comprehensive WES/WGS, since panels might not contain the required targets.

In general, it would be advantageous to perform molecular diagnostics directly at the entry point in the clinic. This is particularly true for panel-based analyses. Patients at later stages that already received a number of standard therapies might need off-label and investigational therapy recommendations. The gene panel might not cover the relevant therapy targets and thus could fail to inform on additional therapy options, as can be observed in our study where for only six of the patients analyzed based on panels therapies beyond standard of care could be identified. However, Table 1 shows that also molecular diagnostics based on comprehensive sequencing would benefit from an earlier time of sequencing. To speed up the report delivery, we implemented a two-step procedure. A so-called level-1 report that includes unfiltered actionable variants and corresponding treatments is generated automatically without manual inspection. Thus, it is delivered to the clinicians and oncologists within one day after the sequencing has finished. The level-2 report, namely the clinical report including the filtered and manually inspected variants and treatments, is reported after approximately 4 weeks. However, even with this two-step procedure five of the ten dermatology patients died or presented a too severe health condition to allow starting new therapies before the report could be delivered. This stresses the importance of decreasing the analysis turnaround time. It also shows that patients can benefit most from molecular diagnostics if tumors are sequenced at diagnosis or before entering the last standard treatment line.

Conclusions

In conclusion, molecular profiling based on high-throughput technologies is an emerging practice in hospitals all over the world that allows for the detection of genomic aberrations involved in carcinogenesis and therapy resistance. To the best of our knowledge, we introduced the first comprehensive high-throughput sequencing based molecular profiling workflow in Swiss clinics. In a collaboration of the NEXUS Clinical Bioinformatics Unit of ETH Zurich and the University Hospitals Zurich and Basel a workflow for tumor sample extraction, bioinformatics analysis, and clinical reporting has been implemented and tested in a pilot project involving 22 patients. We identified actionable targets in 86% of the patients, and in addition identified several resistance-causing variants. In five of eleven patients sequenced before treatment, SwissMTB findings influenced treatment decisions, which demonstrates the benefit of comprehensive sequencing based molecular diagnostics. We have shown that the close collaboration of clinicians and bioinformaticians enables the identification of new therapy options for end-of-treatment line patients. The wealth of information accessible with comprehensive high-throughput sequencing requires sophisticated analysis workflows, but allows for generating novel treatment suggestions. Thus, already today traditional Sanger sequencing-based diagnostic methods are being replaced by high-throughput NGS-based techniques.

Once decreasing sequencing costs will make reimbursement from Swiss health insurances for WES and WGS feasible, these methods likely will become standard diagnostic tools, not only for patients that have progressed on standard therapies but for every cancer patient entering the clinic. Our molecular diagnostics workflow provides a prototype that can form the basis for streamlined profiling and reporting required to enable such routine clinical use in Switzerland.

Possible extensions of the SwissMTB workflow include the integration of other molecular profiling technologies, such as proteomics and single cell sequencing [99, 100]. Proteomic analysis would provide information on the translated proteins in the tumor, thereby verifying variants identified on the genomic and transcriptomic level and additionally detecting post-translational modifications. Post-translational modifications, such as phosphorylation or histone modifications, have been shown to play a critical role in the development of a variety of cancer types [101, 102] and in drug resistance development. Their analysis would thus open a new window for therapy possibilities [103]. Single-cell sequencing provides more detailed information on the genetic makeup of the whole tumor tissue and its heterogeneous subclones [100, 104]. Currently, treatments target actionable variants that might be present in the majority, but not all tumor cells. Cells without the variant can survive and over time the tumor regrows. Single-cell sequencing could inform on treatments necessary to target all subclones of the tumor.

With declining sequencing costs, high coverage WGS will become feasible not only for research, but also in the clinics. This will enable the analysis of larger structural variants and eventually eliminate the need for WES or panel sequencing. Already today, for instance the 100,000 genomes project in the UK performs WGS of each sample at depths sufficient for variant calling [105]. In Swiss clinics currently panel sequencing is the standard diagnostic high-throughput technique as it is the least cost- and analysis-intensive, and covered by health insurances. However, decreasing costs for WES and WGS will enable reimbursement also for these techniques and shift the focus in routine diagnostics from panel sequencing to whole exome and ultimately whole genome analysis. Simultaneously, molecular diagnostics based on high-throughput techniques will become the tool of choice also for early diagnostics, not only to find last therapy options for patients that have progressed on all standard treatments. Applying comprehensive molecular cancer diagnostics already at the clinical entry point also has benefits for patients with unknown primary tumor. The genetic makeup of the the tumor can predict the tumor type, which improves the choice of suitable therapies [106].

One of the greatest challenges in the SwissMTB is the prioritization and clinical interpretation of genomic aberrations. This task is not yet fully automated and requires manual inspection of sometimes large numbers of drug-target combinations. Given the aspired short turnaround time, further work is needed to automate the literature search for prioritization of targetable variants. Here, one possible approach is the integration of text mining methods to pre-filter variants with respect to their importance and occurrence in the literature. Reducing the list of possible targets to only promising ones will greatly reduce the time and effort necessary to formulate a concise clinical report.

In addition to these technical developments, also the management and communication within the SwissMTB is a constant learning process. Bridging the gap between clinic and research and making the application of cutting edge technologies feasible for clinical use requires that experts from both clinical and bioinformatics world come together and discuss their needs for sufficient sample analysis. This involves the required analysis types and results, as well as the way findings are reported. Consequently, our clinical reports have evolved over time and will probably continue to evolve, based both on new technologies and on feedback from the treating clinician regarding the interpretability of analysis results. This iterative integration of new technologies and feedback into SwissMTB will also introduce new challenges. Various sources of information need to be summarized and presented in a concise and easily interpretable report to be useful for discussion in a tumor board. In the near future, the increasing number of profiling sources will require an interactive report rather than the traditional pdf document to prioritize information, to allow focussing on the most promising, and to access details on demand [64].

Because our workflow exclusively proposes therapies by summarizing the evidence seen in the genomic and transcriptomic landscape of the tumor, it is a new diagnostic tool for the clinician. Therefore, there is no need for a research-related patient consent. However, using such a consent form (as is common practice in Swiss hospitals) has the benefit to ensure that potential future research projects can access these data. For instance, with a growing number of sequenced patients a new valuable resource to interpret results develops. Given the appropriate consent, variants found in a certain tumor type, as well as chosen therapies and their outcomes, can form a resource which facilitates and improves therapy recommendations for new patients. This was for instance shown for acute myeloid leukemia in [107]. Naturally, also here the feedback from clinicians is essential, and data has to be handled carefully in order to ensure patient privacy.

Finally, approaching cancer therapy from a molecular perspective demands a new design for clinical trials. In recent years, so called basket trials emerged that stratify patients not by their disease but rather based on their genetic variants [69, 108]. These trials will be invaluable to assess the actual therapy potential of specific actionable variants across different cancer types. In addition, as was for instance shown in [109], they can serve to identify new molecular targets and thus broaden our understanding of tumor development and therapy.

Abbreviations

CNV: Copy number variant; DKFZ: Deutsches Krebsforschungszentrum; DNA: Deoxyribonucleic acid; FFPE: Formalin-fixed paraffin embedded; HLA: Human leukocyte antigen; InDel: Insertion and deletion; IRB: Institutional review board; NCT: Nationales Centrum für Tumorerkrankungen; NGS: Next-generation sequencing; RNA: Ribonucleic acid; RNA-seq: RNA sequencing; SKCM: Skin cutaneous melanoma; SNV: Single nucleotide variant; SwissMTB: Swiss Molecular Tumor Board; TCGA: The Cancer Genome Atlas; UNC: Uniform naming convention; UVM: Uveal melanoma; WES: Whole exome sequencing; WGS: Whole genome sequening

Acknowledgements

The authors gratefully acknowledge employers of the University Hospitals Zurich and Basel for preparing tumor biopsies and blood samples. We thank the members of the Genomics Facility Basel and the Functional Genomics Center Zurich for their great efforts to timely deliver high-quality sequences.

Funding

Sequencing and SwissMTB prototype implementation was funded by ETH Zurich and the USZ innovation grants INOV00006 and INOV00017. The funding did not influence the overall design of the study or the analysis and interpretation of the data.

Authors' contributions

FS developed the WES/WGS pipeline, contributed to report design, and analyzed patient samples. AI prepared patient samples, contributed to report design, and performed clinical interpretation. NCT and LG developed the RNA-seq analysis pipeline, contributed to the WES/WGS pipeline and reporting, and analyzed patient samples. JS and TT implemented parts of the analysis pipeline. NB contributed to pipeline design. MPL and RD contributed to report design, provided patient samples, and performed clinical interpretation. LQ, SIR, and AW provided patient samples and contributed to report design. CB was responsible for sequencing some of the samples. DJS contributed to pipeline and report design. All authors were involved in writing the manuscript. All authors read and approved the manuscript.

Competing interests

SIR: Research support: AbbVie, AstraZeneca, BMS, Merck; Honoraria for advisory boards (to the institution): Abbvie, AstraZeneca, BMS, Eisai, Merck, MSD, Novartis, Pfizer, Roche, Takeda.

DJS: Honoraria for scientific advisory board at BC Platforms.

All other authors declare that they have no competing interests.

Author details

[1]NEXUS Personalized Health Technologies, ETH Zurich, Otto-Stern-Weg 7, 8093 Zurich, Switzerland. [2]SIB Swiss Institute of Bioinformatics, 4058 Basel, Switzerland. [3]Department of Dermatology, University Hospital Zurich, 8091 Zurich, Switzerland. [4]Department of Biosystems Science and Engineering, ETH Zurich, 4058 Basel, Switzerland. [5]Division of Oncology, Department of Biomedicine, University Hospital Basel, Petersgraben 4, 4031 Basel, Switzerland. [6]Department of Pathology, University Hospital Basel, Schönbeinstrasse 40, 4056 Basel, Switzerland.

References

1. Shin SH, Bode AM, Dong Z. Addressing the challenges of applying precision oncology. NPJ Precision Onc. 2017;1:28. https://doi.org/10.1038/s41698-017-0032-z.
2. Rehm HL. Disease-targeted sequencing: a cornerstone in the clinic. Nat Rev Genet. 2013;14:295–300. https://doi.org/10.1038/nrg3463.
3. Hovelson DH, McDaniel AS, Cani AK, Johnson B, Rhodes K, Williams PD, et al. Development and validation of a scalable next-generation sequencing system for assessing relevant somatic variants in solid tumors. Neoplasia. 2015;17:385–99. https://doi.org/10.1016/j.neo.2015.03.004.
4. Hamblin A, Wordsworth S, Fermont JM, Page S, Kaur K, Camps C, et al. Clinical applicability and cost of a 46-gene panel for genomic analysis of solid tumours: retrospective validation and prospective audit in the UK National Health Service. PLoS Med. 2017;14:e1002230. https://doi.org/10.1371/journal.pmed.1002230.
5. Tsongalis GJ, Peterson JD, de Abreu FB, Tunkey CD, Gallagher TL, Strausbaugh LD, et al. Routine use of the ion torrent AmpliSeq™ Cancer Hotspot panel for identification of clinically actionable somatic mutations. Clin Chem Lab Med. 2014;52:707–14. https://doi.org/10.1515/cclm-2013-0883.
6. Beltran H, Eng K, Mosquera JM, Sigaras A, Romanel A, Rennert H, et al. Whole-exome sequencing of metastatic Cancer and biomarkers of treatment response. JAMA Oncol. 2015;1:466–74. https://doi.org/10.1001/jamaoncol.2015.1313.
7. Strom SP, Lee H, Das K, Vilain E, Nelson SF, Grody WW, et al. Assessing the necessity of confirmatory testing for exome-sequencing results in a clinical molecular diagnostic laboratory. Genet Med. 2014;16:510–5. https://doi.org/10.1038/gim.2013.183.
8. Hyman DM, Taylor BS, Baselga J. Implementing genome-driven oncology. Cell. 2017;168:584–99. https://doi.org/10.1016/j.cell.2016.12.015.
9. Stewart BW, Wild CP. World Cancer Report 2014. Lyon, France: International Agency for Research on Cancer. World Health Organization; 2014:630.
10. Zahreddine H, Borden KLB. Mechanisms and insights into drug resistance in cancer. Front Pharmacol. 2013;4:28. https://doi.org/10.3389/fphar.2013.00028.
11. Housman G, Byler S, Heerboth S, Lapinska K, Longacre M, Snyder N, et al. Drug resistance in cancer: an overview. Cancers (Basel). 2014;6:1769–92. https://doi.org/10.3390/cancers6031769.
12. Lackner MR, Wilson TR, Settleman J. Mechanisms of acquired resistance to targeted cancer therapies. Future Oncol. 2012;8:999–1014. https://doi.org/10.2217/fon.12.86.
13. Sabarinathan R, Pich O, Martincorena I, Rubio-Perez C, Juul M, Wala J, et al. The whole-genome panorama of cancer drivers. BioRxiv. 2017. https://doi.org/10.1101/190330.
14. Cancer Genome Atlas Network. Genomic classification of cutaneous melanoma. Cell. 2015;161:1681–96. https://doi.org/10.1016/j.cell.2015.05.044.
15. Chapman PB, Hauschild A, Robert C, Haanen JB, Ascierto P, Larkin J, et al. Improved survival with vemurafenib in melanoma with BRAF V600E mutation. N Engl J Med. 2011;364:2507–16. https://doi.org/10.1056/NEJMoa1103782.
16. Cuello M, Ettenberg SA, Clark AS, Keane MM, Posner RH, Nau MM, et al. Down-regulation of the erbB-2 receptor by trastuzumab (herceptin)

enhances tumor necrosis factor-related apoptosis-inducing ligand-mediated apoptosis in breast and ovarian cancer cell lines that overexpress erbB-2. Cancer Res. 2001;61:4892–900.
17. Gómez-López G, Dopazo J, Cigudosa JC, Valencia A, Al-Shahrour F. Precision medicine needs pioneering clinical bioinformaticians. Brief Bioinformatics. 2017. https://doi.org/10.1093/bib/bbx144.
18. MD Anderson. MD Anderson Cancer Center. https://www.mdanderson.org/. Accessed 6 Apr 2018.
19. Bryce AH, Egan JB, Borad MJ, Stewart AK, Nowakowski GS, Chanan-Khan A, et al. Experience with precision genomics and tumor board, indicates frequent target identification, but barriers to delivery. Oncotarget. 2017;8: 27145–54. https://doi.org/10.18632/oncotarget.16057.
20. Rennert H, Eng K, Zhang T, Tan A, Xiang J, Romanel A, et al. Development and validation of a whole-exome sequencing test for simultaneous detection of point mutations, indels and copy-number alterations for precision cancer care. NPJ Genomic Med. 2016;1. https://doi.org/10.1038/npjgenmed.2016.19.
21. NCT Heidelberg. NCT MASTER. http://www.nct-heidelberg.de/forschung/nct-master/clinical-translation.html. Accessed 6 Apr 2018.
22. Britschgi C, Diehl C, Rechsteiner M, Valtcheva N, Freiberger S, Wong C, et al. 38Implications of routine NGS testing for daily clinical practice--the Zurich experience with the OFA panel. Annals of Oncology. 2017;28(7).
23. Meric-Bernstam F, Brusco L, Shaw K, Horombe C, Kopetz S, Davies MA, et al. Feasibility of large-scale genomic testing to facilitate enrollment onto Genomically matched clinical trials. J Clin Oncol. 2015;33:2753–62. https://doi.org/10.1200/JCO.2014.60.4165.
24. Merriman B, Ion Torrent R&D Team, Rothberg JM. Progress in ion torrent semiconductor chip based sequencing. Electrophoresis. 2012;33:3397–417. https://doi.org/10.1002/elps.201200424.
25. Swissmedic. Swissmedic. https://www.swissmedic.ch/swissmedic/de/home/ueber-uns/publikationen/swissmedic-journal.html. Accessed 6 Apr 2018.
26. ThermoFisher. Oncomine Assays. http://www.thermofisher.com/ch/en/home/clinical/preclinical-companion-diagnostic-development/oncomine-oncology.html. Accessed 6 Apr 2018.
27. Singer J, Irmisch A, Ruscheweyh H-J, Singer F, Toussaint NC, Levesque MP, et al. Bioinformatics for precision oncology. Brief Bioinformatics. 2017. https://doi.org/10.1093/bib/bbx143.
28. Roychowdhury S, Chinnaiyan AM. Translating cancer genomes and transcriptomes for precision oncology. CA Cancer J Clin. 2016;66:75–88. https://doi.org/10.3322/caac.21329.
29. Wagner AH, Coffman AC, Ainscough BJ, Spies NC, Skidmore ZL, Campbell KM, et al. DGIdb 2.0: mining clinically relevant drug-gene interactions. Nucleic Acids Res. 2016;44:D1036–44. https://doi.org/10.1093/nar/gkv1165.
30. Griffith M, Griffith OL, Coffman AC, Weible JV, McMichael JF, Spies NC, et al. DGIdb: mining the druggable genome. Nat Methods. 2013;10:1209–10. https://doi.org/10.1038/nmeth.2689.
31. Wishart DS, Knox C, Guo AC, Shrivastava S, Hassanali M, Stothard P, et al. DrugBank: a comprehensive resource for in silico drug discovery and exploration. Nucleic Acids Res. 2006;34(Database issue):D668–72. https://doi.org/10.1093/nar/gkj067.
32. Abrahamson R. Overview of targeted therapies for Cancer. My Cancer Genome. 2017. https://www.mycancergenome.org/content/molecular-medicine/overview-of-targeted-therapies-for-cancer/. Accessed 20 Mar 2018.
33. Roychowdhury S, Iyer MK, Robinson DR, Lonigro RJ, Wu Y-M, Cao X, et al. Personalized oncology through integrative high-throughput sequencing: a pilot study. Sci Transl Med. 2011;3:111ra121. https://doi.org/10.1126/scitranslmed.3003161.
34. O'Rawe J, Jiang T, Sun G, Wu Y, Wang W, Hu J, et al. Low concordance of multiple variant-calling pipelines: practical implications for exome and genome sequencing. Genome Med. 2013;5:28. https://doi.org/10.1186/gm432.
35. Hofmann AL, Behr J, Singer J, Kuipers J, Beisel C, Schraml P, et al. Detailed simulation of cancer exome sequencing data reveals differences and common limitations of variant callers. BMC Bioinformatics. 2017;18:8. https://doi.org/10.1186/s12859-016-1417-7.
36. Ewing AD, Houlahan KE, Hu Y, Ellrott K, Caloian C, Yamaguchi TN, et al. Combining tumor genome simulation with crowdsourcing to benchmark somatic single-nucleotide-variant detection. Nat Methods. 2015;12:623–30. https://doi.org/10.1038/nmeth.3407.
37. TCGA. TCGA-SKCM. https://portal.gdc.cancer.gov/projects/TCGA-SKCM. Accessed 6 Apr 2018.
38. Snyder A, Makarov V, Merghoub T, Yuan J, Zaretsky JM, Desrichard A, et al. Genetic basis for clinical response to CTLA-4 blockade in melanoma. N Engl J Med. 2014;371:2189–99. https://doi.org/10.1056/NEJMoa1406498.
39. Legat A, Maby-El Hajjami H, Baumgaertner P, Cagnon L, Abed Maillard S, Geldhof C, et al. Vaccination with LAG-3Ig (IMP321) and peptides induces specific CD4 and CD8 T-cell responses in metastatic melanoma patients--report of a phase I/IIa clinical trial. Clin Cancer Res. 2016;22:1330–40. https://doi.org/10.1158/1078-0432.CCR-15-1212.
40. Nagorsen D, Thiel E. HLA typing demands for peptide-based anti-cancer vaccine. Cancer Immunol Immunother. 2008;57:1903–10. https://doi.org/10.1007/s00262-008-0493-6.
41. Singer J, Ruscheweyh H-J, Hofmann AL, Thurnherr T, Singer F, Toussaint NC, et al. NGS-pipe: a flexible, easily extendable and highly configurable framework for NGS analysis. Bioinformatics. 2018;34:107–8. https://doi.org/10.1093/bioinformatics/btx540.
42. Köster J, Rahmann S. Snakemake--a scalable bioinformatics workflow engine. Bioinformatics. 2012;28:2520–2. https://doi.org/10.1093/bioinformatics/bts480.
43. Van der Auwera GA, Carneiro MO, Hartl C, Poplin R, Del Angel G, Levy-Moonshine A, et al. From FastQ data to high confidence variant calls: the genome analysis toolkit best practices pipeline. Curr Protoc Bioinformatics. 2013;11:11.10.1–11.10.33. https://doi.org/10.1002/0471250953.bi1110s43.
44. Cibulskis K, Lawrence MS, Carter SL, Sivachenko A, Jaffe D, Sougnez C, et al. Sensitive detection of somatic point mutations in impure and heterogeneous cancer samples. Nat Biotechnol. 2013;31:213–9. https://doi.org/10.1038/nbt.2514.
45. Koboldt DC, Zhang Q, Larson DE, Shen D, McLellan MD, Lin L, et al. VarScan 2: somatic mutation and copy number alteration discovery in cancer by exome sequencing. Genome Res. 2012;22:568–76. https://doi.org/10.1101/gr.129684.111.
46. Saunders CT, Wong WSW, Swamy S, Becq J, Murray LJ, Cheetham RK. Strelka: accurate somatic small-variant calling from sequenced tumor-normal sample pairs. Bioinformatics. 2012;28:1811–7. https://doi.org/10.1093/bioinformatics/bts271.
47. Xi R, Lee S, Xia Y, Kim T-M, Park PJ. Copy number analysis of whole-genome data using BIC-seq2 and its application to detection of cancer susceptibility variants. Nucleic Acids Res. 2016;44:6274–86. https://doi.org/10.1093/nar/gkw491.
48. Magi A, Tattini L, Cifola I, D'Aurizio R, Benelli M, Mangano E, et al. EXCAVATOR: detecting copy number variants from whole-exome sequencing data. Genome Biol. 2013;14:R120. https://doi.org/10.1186/gb-2013-14-10-r120.
49. TCGA. UNC mRNAseq summary. 2013. https://webshare.bioinf.unc.edu/public/mRNAseq_TCGA/UNC_mRNAseq_summary.pdf. Accessed 6 Apr 2018.
50. Dobin A, Davis CA, Schlesinger F, Drenkow J, Zaleski C, Jha S, et al. STAR: ultrafast universal RNA-seq aligner. Bioinformatics. 2013;29:15–21. https://doi.org/10.1093/bioinformatics/bts635.
51. TCGA. TCGA-UVM. https://portal.gdc.cancer.gov/projects/TCGA-UVM. Accessed 6 Apr 2018.
52. GDAC. GDAC Firehose. 2016. https://gdac.broadinstitute.org/. Accessed 6 Apr 2018.
53. Alexandrov LB, Nik-Zainal S, Wedge DC, Aparicio SAJR, Behjati S, Biankin AV, et al. Signatures of mutational processes in human cancer. Nature. 2013;500: 415–21. https://doi.org/10.1038/nature12477.
54. Forbes SA, Beare D, Gunasekaran P, Leung K, Bindal N, Boutselakis H, et al. COSMIC: exploring the world's knowledge of somatic mutations in human cancer. Nucleic Acids Res. 2015;43(Database issue):D805–11. https://doi.org/10.1093/nar/gku1075.
55. Sherry ST, Ward M, Sirotkin K. dbSNP-database for single nucleotide polymorphisms and other classes of minor genetic variation. Genome Res. 1999;9:677–9.
56. Sherry ST, Ward MH, Kholodov M, Baker J, Phan L, Smigielski EM, et al. dbSNP: the NCBI database of genetic variation. Nucleic Acids Res. 2001;29:308–11. https://doi.org/10.1093/nar/29.1.308.
57. Landrum MJ, Lee JM, Riley GR, Jang W, Rubinstein WS, Church DM, et al. ClinVar: public archive of relationships among sequence variation and human phenotype. Nucleic Acids Res. 2014;42(Database issue):D980–5. https://doi.org/10.1093/nar/gkt1113.
58. Gao J, Aksoy BA, Dogrusoz U, Dresdner G, Gross B, Sumer SO, et al. Integrative analysis of complex cancer genomics and clinical profiles using the cBioPortal. Sci Signal. 2013;6:pl1. https://doi.org/10.1126/scisignal.2004088.
59. Cerami E, Gao J, Dogrusoz U, Gross BE, Sumer SO, Aksoy BA, et al. The cBio cancer genomics portal: an open platform for exploring multidimensional cancer genomics data. Cancer Discov. 2012;2:401–4. https://doi.org/10.1158/2159-8290.CD-12-0095.

60. Ahronian LG, Sennott EM, Van Allen EM, Wagle N, Kwak EL, Faris JE, et al. Clinical acquired resistance to RAF inhibitor combinations in BRAF-mutant colorectal Cancer through MAPK pathway alterations. Cancer Discov. 2015;5: 358–67. https://doi.org/10.1158/2159-8290.CD-14-1518.
61. Cotto KC, Wagner AH, Feng Y-Y, Kiwala S, Coffman AC, Spies G, et al. DGIdb 3.0: a redesign and expansion of the drug-gene interaction database. Nucleic Acids Res. 2017. https://doi.org/10.1093/nar/gkx1143.
62. Thurnherr T, Singer F, Stekhoven DJ, Beerenwinkel N. Genomic variant annotation workflow for clinical applications. F1000Research. 2016;5:1963.
63. MyCancerGenome. MyCancerGenome. 2018. https://www.mycancergenome.org/. Accessed 6 Apr 2018.
64. Shneiderman B. The eyes have it: a task by data type taxonomy for information visualizations. In: Proceedings 1996 IEEE Symposium on Visual Languages: IEEE Comput. Soc. Press; 1996. p. 336–43. https://doi.org/10.1109/VL.1996.545307.
65. Chia PL, Mitchell P, Dobrovic A, John T. Prevalence and natural history of ALK positive non-small-cell lung cancer and the clinical impact of targeted therapy with ALK inhibitors. Clin Epidemiol. 2014;6:423–32. https://doi.org/10.2147/CLEP.S69718.
66. Kang HJ, Chun S-M, Kim K-R, Sohn I, Sung CO. Clinical relevance of gain-of-function mutations of p53 in high-grade serous ovarian carcinoma. PLoS One. 2013;8:e72609. https://doi.org/10.1371/journal.pone.0072609.
67. Li MM, Datto M, Duncavage EJ, Kulkarni S, Lindeman NI, Roy S, et al. Standards and guidelines for the interpretation and reporting of sequence variants in cancer: a joint consensus recommendation of the association for molecular pathology, american society of clinical oncology, and college of american pathologists. J Mol Diagn. 2017;19:4–23. https://doi.org/10.1016/j.jmoldx.2016.10.002.
68. Chakravarty D, Gao J, Phillips S, Kundra R, Zhang H, Wang J, et al. OncoKB: A Precision Oncology Knowledge Base. JCO Precis Oncol. 2017:1–16.
69. Massard C, Michiels S, Ferté C, Le Deley M-C, Lacroix L, Hollebecque A, et al. High-throughput genomics and clinical outcome in hard-to-treat advanced cancers: results of the MOSCATO 01 trial. Cancer Discov. 2017;7:586–95. https://doi.org/10.1158/2159-8290.CD-16-1396.
70. Larkin J, Chiarion-Sileni V, Gonzalez R, Grob JJ, Cowey CL, Lao CD, et al. Combined nivolumab and ipilimumab or monotherapy in untreated melanoma. N Engl J Med. 2015;373:23–34. https://doi.org/10.1056/NEJMoa1504030.
71. Della Corte CM, Fasano M, Papaccio F, Ciardiello F, Morgillo F. Role of HGF-MET signaling in primary and acquired resistance to targeted therapies in Cancer. Biomedicine. 2014;2:345–58. https://doi.org/10.3390/biomedicines2040345.
72. Sun C, Wang L, Huang S, Heynen GJJE, Prahallad A, Robert C, et al. Reversible and adaptive resistance to BRAF(V600E) inhibition in melanoma. Nature. 2014;508:118–22. https://doi.org/10.1038/nature13121.
73. Raaijmakers MIG, Widmer DS, Narechania A, Eichhoff O, Freiberger SN, Wenzina J, et al. Co-existence of BRAF and NRAS driver mutations in the same melanoma cells results in heterogeneity of targeted therapy resistance. Oncotarget. 2016;7:77163–74. https://doi.org/10.18632/oncotarget.12848.
74. Masuyama H, Nakatsukasa H, Takamoto N, Hiramatsu Y. Down-regulation of pregnane X receptor contributes to cell growth inhibition and apoptosis by anticancer agents in endometrial cancer cells. Mol Pharmacol. 2007;72: 1045–53. https://doi.org/10.1124/mol.107.037937.
75. Homsi J, Bedikian AY, Papadopoulos NE, Kim KB, Hwu W-J, Mahoney SL, et al. Phase 2 open-label study of weekly docosahexaenoic acid-paclitaxel in patients with metastatic uveal melanoma. Melanoma Res. 2010;20:507–10. https://doi.org/10.1097/CMR.0b013e3283403ce9.
76. Isakoff SJ, Wang D, Campone M, Calles A, Leip E, Turnbull K, et al. Bosutinib plus capecitabine for selected advanced solid tumours: results of a phase 1 dose-escalation study. Br J Cancer. 2014;111:2058–66. https://doi.org/10.1038/bjc.2014.508.
77. Soria JC, Massard C, Magné N, Bader T, Mansfield CD, Blay JY, et al. Phase 1 dose-escalation study of oral tyrosine kinase inhibitor masitinib in advanced and/or metastatic solid cancers. Eur J Cancer. 2009;45:2333–41. https://doi.org/10.1016/j.ejca.2009.05.010.
78. Babina IS, Turner NC. Advances and challenges in targeting FGFR signalling in cancer. Nat Rev Cancer. 2017;17:318–32. https://doi.org/10.1038/nrc.2017.8.
79. Yang Y, Wu N, Shen J, Teixido C, Sun X, Lin Z, et al. MET overexpression and amplification define a distinct molecular subgroup for targeted therapies in gastric cancer. Gastric Cancer. 2015;19:778–88. https://doi.org/10.1007/s10120-015-0545-5.
80. Yao JC, Fazio N, Singh S, Buzzoni R, Carnaghi C, Wolin E, et al. Everolimus for the treatment of advanced, non-functional neuroendocrine tumours of the lung or gastrointestinal tract (RADIANT-4): a randomised, placebo-controlled, phase 3 study. Lancet. 2016;387:968–77. https://doi.org/10.1016/S0140-6736(15)00817-X.
81. Jardim DL, Wheler JJ, Hess K, Tsimberidou AM, Zinner R, Janku F, et al. FBXW7 mutations in patients with advanced cancers: clinical and molecular characteristics and outcomes with mTOR inhibitors. PLoS One. 2014;9: e89388. https://doi.org/10.1371/journal.pone.0089388.
82. Brachova P, Thiel KW, Leslie KK. The consequence of oncomorphic TP53 mutations in ovarian cancer. Int J Mol Sci. 2013;14:19257–75. https://doi.org/10.3390/ijms140919257.
83. Lawrie TA, Bryant A, Cameron A, Gray E, Morrison J. Pegylated liposomal doxorubicin for relapsed epithelial ovarian cancer. Cochrane Database Syst Rev. 2013:CD006910. https://doi.org/10.1002/14651858.CD006910.pub2.
84. Pisano C, Cecere SC, Di Napoli M, Cavaliere C, Tambaro R, Facchini G, et al. Clinical trials with pegylated liposomal doxorubicin in the treatment of ovarian cancer. J Drug Deliv. 2013;2013:898146. https://doi.org/10.1155/2013/898146.
85. González-Cao M, Rodón J, Karachaliou N, Sánchez J, Santarpia M, Viteri S, et al. Other targeted drugs in melanoma. Ann Transl Med. 2015;3:266. https://doi.org/10.3978/j.issn.2305-5839.2015.08.12.
86. Kim ES, Scott LJ. Palbociclib: a review in HR-positive, HER2-negative, advanced or metastatic breast Cancer. Target Oncol. 2017;12:373–83. https://doi.org/10.1007/s11523-017-0492-7.
87. Fontana D, Ceccon M, Gambacorti-Passerini C, Mologni L. Activity of second-generation ALK inhibitors against crizotinib-resistant mutants in an NPM-ALK model compared to EML4-ALK. Cancer Med. 2015;4:953–65. https://doi.org/10.1002/cam4.413.
88. Lovly CM, Pao W. Escaping ALK inhibition: mechanisms of and strategies to overcome resistance. Sci Transl Med. 2012;4:120ps2. https://doi.org/10.1126/scitranslmed.3003728.
89. Friboulet L, Li N, Katayama R, Lee CC, Gainor JF, Crystal AS, et al. The ALK inhibitor ceritinib overcomes crizotinib resistance in non-small cell lung cancer. Cancer Discov. 2014;4:662–73. https://doi.org/10.1158/2159-8290.CD-13-0846.
90. King TC, Akerley W, Fan AC, Moore T, Mangray S, Hsiu Chen M, et al. p53 mutations do not predict response to paclitaxel in metastatic nonsmall cell lung carcinoma. Cancer. 2000;89:769–73. https://doi.org/10.1002/1097-0142(20000815)89:4<769::AID-CNCR8>3.0.CO;2-6.
91. Muller PAJ, Vousden KH. Mutant p53 in cancer: new functions and therapeutic opportunities. Cancer Cell. 2014;25:304–17. https://doi.org/10.1016/j.ccr.2014.01.021.
92. Chang FL, Lai MD. Various forms of mutant p53 confer sensitivity to cisplatin and doxorubicin in bladder cancer cells. J Urol. 2001;166:304–10. https://doi.org/10.1016/S0022-5347(05)66150-2.
93. Minor DR, Kashani-Sabet M, Garrido M, O'Day SJ, Hamid O, Bastian BC. Sunitinib therapy for melanoma patients with KIT mutations. Clin Cancer Res. 2012;18:1457–63. https://doi.org/10.1158/1078-0432.CCR-11-1987.
94. Clinical trial. Phase II clinical trial NCT02307500: Regorafenib in Patients With Metastatic Solid Tumors Who Have Progressed After Standard Therapy (RESOUND) . clinicaltrials.gov. 2014. https://clinicaltrials.gov/ct2/show/NCT02307500?term=NCT02307500&rank=1. Accessed 23 Mar 2018.
95. Oberg JA, Glade Bender JL, Sulis ML, Pendrick D, Sireci AN, Hsiao SJ, et al. Implementation of next generation sequencing into pediatric hematology-oncology practice: moving beyond actionable alterations. Genome Med. 2016;8:133. https://doi.org/10.1186/s13073-016-0389-6.
96. Mody RJ, Wu Y-M, Lonigro RJ, Cao X, Roychowdhury S, Vats P, et al. Integrative clinical sequencing in the management of refractory or relapsed cancer in youth. JAMA. 2015;314:913–25. https://doi.org/10.1001/jama.2015.10080.
97. Sun JX, He Y, Sanford E, Montesion M, Frampton GM, Vignot S, et al. A computational approach to distinguish somatic vs germline origin of genomic alterations from deep sequencing of cancer specimens without a matched normal. PLoS Comput Biol. 2018;14:e1005965. https://doi.org/10.1371/journal.pcbi.1005965.
98. Macías M, Alegre E, Díaz-Lagares A, Patiño A, Pérez-Gracia JL, Sanmamed M, et al. Liquid biopsy: from basic research to clinical practice. Adv Clin Chem. 2018;83:73–119. https://doi.org/10.1016/bs.acc.2017.10.003.
99. Senft D, Leiserson MDM, Ruppin E, Ronai ZA. Precision oncology: the road ahead. Trends Mol Med. 2017;23:874–98. https://doi.org/10.1016/j.molmed.2017.08.003.
100. Wang Y, Navin NE. Advances and applications of single-cell sequencing technologies. Mol Cell. 2015;58:598–609. https://doi.org/10.1016/j.molcel.2015.05.005.

101. Lu H, Li G, Zhou C, Jin W, Qian X, Wang Z, et al. Regulation and role of post-translational modifications of enhancer of zeste homologue 2 in cancer development. Am J Cancer Res. 2016;6:2737–54.
102. Khan SA, Reddy D, Gupta S. Global histone post-translational modifications and cancer: biomarkers for diagnosis, prognosis and treatment? World J Biol Chem. 2015;6:333–45. https://doi.org/10.4331/wjbc.v6.i4.333.
103. Casado P, Hijazi M, Britton D, Cutillas PR. Impact of phosphoproteomics in the translation of kinase-targeted therapies. Proteomics. 2017;17. https://doi.org/10.1002/pmic.201600235.
104. Bedard PL, Hansen AR, Ratain MJ, Siu LL. Tumour heterogeneity in the clinic. Nature. 2013;501:355–64. https://doi.org/10.1038/nature12627.
105. Genomics England. Genomics England. https://www.genomicsengland.co.uk/the-100000-genomes-project/. Accessed 6 Apr 2018.
106. Soh KP, Szczurek E, Sakoparnig T, Beerenwinkel N. Predicting cancer type from tumour DNA signatures. Genome Med. 2017;9:104. https://doi.org/10.1186/s13073-017-0493-2.
107. Gerstung M, Papaemmanuil E, Martincorena I, Bullinger L, Gaidzik VI, Paschka P, et al. Precision oncology for acute myeloid leukemia using a knowledge bank approach. Nat Genet. 2017;49:332–40. https://doi.org/10.1038/ng.3756.
108. Coyne GO, Takebe N, Chen AP. Defining precision: the precision medicine initiative trials NCI-MPACT and NCI-MATCH. Curr Probl Cancer. 2017;41:182–93. https://doi.org/10.1016/j.currproblcancer.2017.02.001.
109. Hyman DM, Piha-Paul SA, Won H, Rodon J, Saura C, Shapiro GI, et al. HER kinase inhibition in patients with HER2- and HER3-mutant cancers. Nature. 2018;554:189–94. https://doi.org/10.1038/nature25475.

Sharing longitudinal, non-biological birth cohort data

Kiran Pohar Manhas[1,3,8*], Shawn X. Dodd[3], Stacey Page[1,4], Nicole Letourneau[5], Carol E. Adair[1], Xinjie Cui[6] and Suzanne C. Tough[2,7]

Abstract

Background: Mandates abound to share publicly-funded research data for reuse, while data platforms continue to emerge to facilitate such reuse. Birth cohorts (BC) involve longitudinal designs, significant sample sizes and rich and deep datasets. Data sharing benefits include more analyses, greater research complexity, increased opportunities for collaboration, amplification of public contributions, and reduced respondent burdens. Sharing BC data involves significant challenges including consent, privacy, access policies, communication, and vulnerability of the child. Research on these issues is available for biological data, but these findings may not extend to BC data. We lack consensus on how best to approach these challenges in consent, privacy, communication and autonomy when sharing BC data. We require more stakeholder engagement to understand perspectives and generate consensus.

Methods: Parents participating in longitudinal birth cohorts completed a web-based survey investigating consent preferences for sharing their, and their child's, non-biological research data. Results from a previous qualitative inquiry informed survey development, and cognitive interviewing methods ($n = 9$) were used to improve the question quality and comprehension. Recruitment was via personalized email, with email and phone reminders during the 14-day window for survey completion.

Results: Three hundred and forty-six of 569 parents completed the survey in September 2014 (60.8%). Participants preferred consent processes for data sharing in future independent research that were less-active (i.e. no consent or opt-out). Parents' consent preferences are associated with their communication preferences. Twenty percent (20.2%) of parents generally agreed that their child should provide consent to continue participating in research at age 12, while 25.6% felt decision-making on sharing non-biological research data should begin at age 18.

Conclusions: These finding reflect the parenting population's preference for less project-specific permission when research data is non-biological and de-identified and when governance practices are highly detailed and rigourous. Parents recognize that children should become involved in consent for secondary data use, but there is variability regarding when and how involvement occurs. These findings emphasize governance processes and participant notification rather than project-specific consent for secondary use of de-identified, non-biological data. Ultimately, parents prefer general consent processes for sharing de-identified, non-biological research data with ultimate involvement of the child.

Keywords: Consent, Data sharing, Non-biological data, Parent, Pediatric, Data repository

* Correspondence: kpmanhas@ucalgary.ca
[1]Community Health Sciences, University of Calgary, Calgary, Canada
[3]University of Alberta, Edmonton, Canada
Full list of author information is available at the end of the article

Background

Data platforms, such as biobanks and secondary data repositories, are proliferating and facilitating innovation via large-scale data mobilization. Internationally, the funders and custodians of public research encourage or mandate, the sharing and re-use of research data, especially via data platforms [1–6]. The benefits of secondary research data use include (a) further analyses, replications, and verifications [1]; (b) increased diversity, novelty and complexity of research opportunities [5]; (c) decreased risk of "failure to discover" [7]; (d) more intra- and inter- disciplinary collaborations; (e) cost savings benefiting the public, funders, researchers and trainees [1]; (f) timely information for policy and practice; and, (g) maximized participant contributions and conservation of research resources. There are challenges to both privacy and consent when data are stored for such secondary use.

Privacy and consent are related: while privacy represents a right "to be let alone," [8], consent transforms what may be a privacy violation into a permissible act [9]. In health research, informed consent allows individuals to exercise control over who may collect, view, use, disclose and store their personal information [10–12]. Only in exceptional circumstances can personal information be used without consent, with level of identifiability and research ethics board approval as key determinants of such exceptions [10–14]. Valid consent must be voluntary, informed, and provided by individuals with decision-making capacity [13, 15, 16]. Traditionally, in research, consent is operationalized through discussions between participants and researchers about the known research intent, including risks benefits and privacy considerations. In secondary data use, research intents cannot be fully, specifically known at the time of data collection.

Longitudinal cohort studies initiated prior to birth can be particularly rich as sources of secondary data [17]. Such studies involve large samples, multiple data collection points, and a wealth of information, including physical, emotional, developmental, social, and demographic data. Access to such data may permit strong study designs, greater statistical power and increased opportunities to examine diverse issues and relationships in the health, development, and well-being of children, mothers and families [17–20].

The benefits of secondary data use come with significant ethico-legal challenges including security and privacy protections, consent, governance, access and communication strategies [15, 21–30]. Pediatric populations add a dimension around consent and vulnerability [18–20, 31–36]. Very young children lack decision-making capacity, so parents or guardians act as surrogate decision-makers. As the child matures, decision-making capacity evolves and the applicability of parental consent becomes questionable. Risks of privacy breaches, discrimination or stigma noted for genomic studies introduce long-term risks when children are involved [18]. Longitudinal cohort data involving genetic information are, thus, flagged as requiring detailed consideration of ethical and legal safeguards for the child participants [18, 22, 37, 38]. However, biobank and epidemiologic data differ and standards originally developed for biological data may be overly restrictive, inappropriate, or may disregard unique concerns when applied to non-biological data [39]. For example, the risks of re-identification and familial implication can be better redressed with epidemiologic, compared to biological, data [39].

The appropriate consent process for secondary use is unclear. Because the intent of future research is unknown at the point of primary collection, project-specific consent is impossible. Cost and feasibility issues hinder re-contacting participants for each secondary use within large-scale data platforms. Consensus is lacking on (a) the most appropriate form of consent for biobanks and repositories; (b) if/how participants can withdraw their data from repositories; (c) how best to communicate between repositories, researchers and participants about re-use and findings; (d) how child age or experience influences child assent and dissent; (e) how consent is influenced by parent-child disagreement; and (f) the feasibility issues for pediatric biobanks and repositories [15, 16, 36, 40, 41]. This lack of consensus produces logistical, ethical and legal obstacles for data repositories.

Currently, Canadian research ethics policy (TCPS2) permits secondary use of research data to proceed without consent, if data are de-identified and research ethics approval is gained (Article 5.5B, TCPS2) [13]. This balances the risks to individuals against the benefits to society from data use and knowledge advancement. Secondary use of identifiable, or potentially identifiable, data hinges on consent. Waiver of consent is possible, if several, specific criteria are met including the importance of the research question outweighing the potential harms of the individuals and the infeasibility of garnering consent (Article 5.5A, TCPS2) [13]. For children, the TCPS2 has moved from age-based restrictions on consent to capacity, so that children under the age of majority may consent when deemed capable [13]. Capacity is generally considered on a case-by-case basis, which introduces feasibility and cost hurdles for secondary data repositories and researchers.

Consent processes can vary based on level of engagement. The five most commonly-considered consent processes span high to low levels of engagement: (1) the traditional consent model; (2) broad, periodic consent model; (3) broad, one-time consent model; (4) tiered (or conditional) consent model; and, (5) opt-out consent model (Fig. 1). It should be noted that opt-out consent is a model discussed in the bioethics literature but is not a consent mode recognized by law, or the TCPS2, in

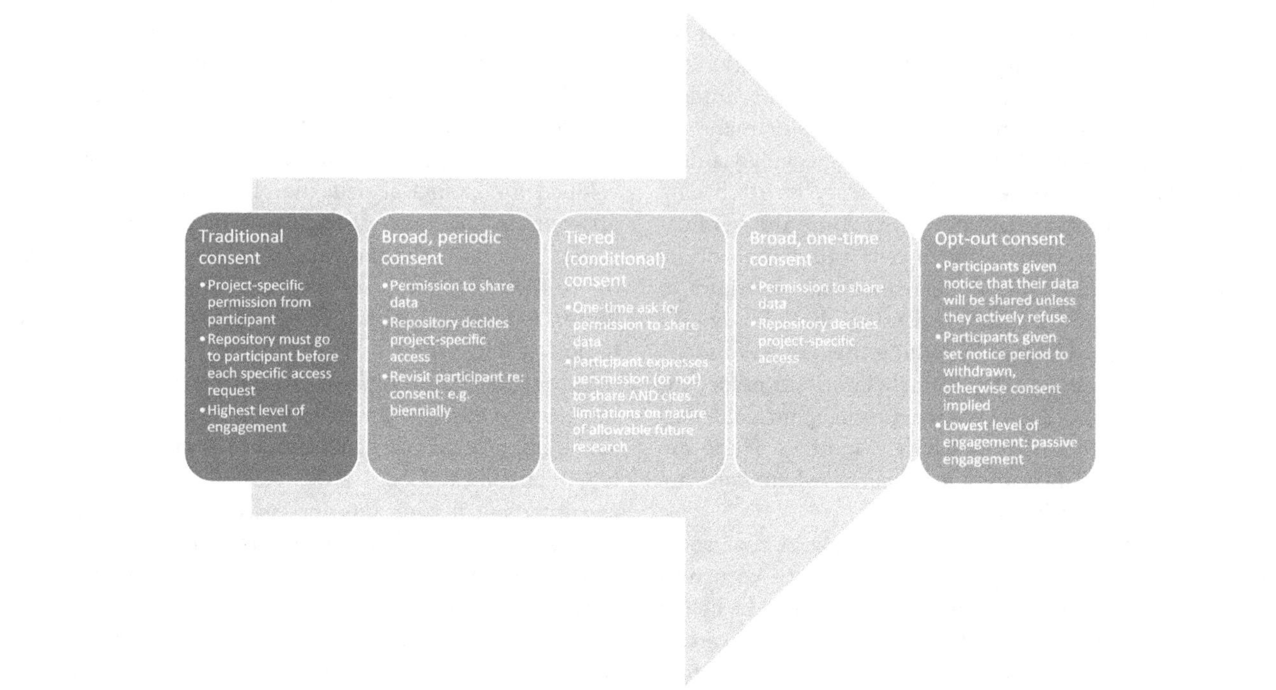

Fig. 1 Definitions of the five consent models examined in this survey (from highest to lowest level of engagement)

Canada. The traditional consent model is project-specific and involves high-level engagement; the three broad- or tiered- consent models are focused on enabling secondary use broadly, while the final, opt-out consent model utilizes passive engagement with consent implied if permission is not actively withdrawn.

TCPS2 advocates engagement with relevant populations to seek input on ethical issues and appropriate privacy protection [13]. Parents are critical stakeholders, as they are the gatekeepers to data. Parent perspectives have been solicited about biobank participation for their children [42–45] and for themselves [43, 46]. Parent concerns impacting agreement to repository participation include lack of information about future uses; risks of stigma; privacy or consent issues; researcher credibility questions; and inability to be re-contacted for results [43, 44, 46]. Ethnicity appears to impact biobank participation in the US, with minorities more reticent than Caucasians [46, 47].

Few studies have specifically examined parent consent preferences. In a structured-interview-based study, 84 parents in hospital-based pediatric clinics were asked their opinion on the layout of a draft biorepository opt-out consent form [42]. Only one parent explicitly stated he preferred opt-in consent and eight parents wished for more information [42]. Because parents were not asked to compare or even consider other consent processes, this perceived acceptability of opt-out consent for biobanking is incomplete. In another study, 166 parents of children in pediatric wards were surveyed about consent preferences for hypothetical observational research [48]. Fifty-two percent chose an opt-in consent approach, 33% selected opt-out, and about 15% felt that consent was unnecessary [48]. The generalizability of consent preferences for observational research compared to consent for secondary data use is unclear as the latter is characterized by greater diversity and uncertainty.

Another recent study compared parent ($n = 113$) and adult ($n = 196$) participants from six genomic studies on data sharing consent [45]. While adults and parents are not mutually exclusive, this study investigated the perspective of parents (mostly mothers) versus that of adults who do not have children for whom surrogate decision-making is required. Parents and adult participants were randomly assigned to one of three experimental consent forms (traditional, broad and tiered), and asked whether they would release their child's data publicly and openly, with restrictions and access processes, or not release at all [45]. This study looked more at parents versus adults and the access level permitted for sharing, rather than preference amongst consent processes. Parents were found to be significantly more restrictive in data release decisions than adults because of autonomy and control preferences, not understanding or perceived benefits; parents also always selected the more restrictive data sharing option when such option was available to them for sharing their child's data [45]. No studies were found of parent's willingness to enrol themselves or their children in a data repository or their preferences for future consent for use of their or their child's data, or on preferred consent models for this circumstance.

A few studies have solicited child and adolescent preferences directly. A study of five focus groups with adolescents yielded their concerns with biobanking as including parental involvement, growing autonomy, information needs, benefits and burdens [49]. Adolescents trusted their parents, but requested engagement in decision-making as they aged [49]. A qualitative study of 21 seven-year-olds elicited their general experience participating in a longitudinal birth cohort [50]. Children involved in longitudinal research enjoyed active participation (e.g. involving moving, running, or playing with a computer), but disapproved of venipunctures, some to the point of refusal [70]. Minors generally felt that researchers should re-contact children upon reaching majority for consent, although this was not considered mandatory with best-efforts requested [49].

A recent qualitative study with 55 adolescents aged 17–19 years who were involved in a birth cohort, from before their birth, examined views around data sharing via data linkage of cohort data [51]. This study found that although different consent processes were explained, participants viewed consent generally as 'opt-in' consent where project-specific permission was requested [51]. Participants raising similar concerns (e.g. social sensitivity of research question, questionable effectiveness of anonymization, ownership of personal information) came to different conclusions on whether consent was needed [51]. Adolescent views changed when presented with alternative scenarios and were somewhat inconsistent [51]. The authors of this study questioned "... the validity of 'informed consent' as a cornerstone of good governance, and the extent to which potential research participants understand different types of consent and what they are consenting, or not consenting, to" [51]. This dearth of child and adolescent perspectives on consent for data sharing whether biological or non-biological data calls for further empirical understanding of stakeholder perspectives on consent preferences when sharing non-biological research data of parents and children in longitudinal research.

To fill these gaps, this study was conducted to address "what are parents preferences amongst alternatives in the secondary use of their and their child's non-biological, de-identified birth cohort data?"

Methods

A cross-sectional, online survey was used to assess consent preferences of parents enrolled in two Alberta birth cohorts for the secondary use of adult and child non-biological, de-identified cohort data via a non-biological data repository. This survey represents the final stage of a mixed-methods study examining parental views on privacy, consent and governance in secondary data use; the qualitative findings that preceded and informed survey development are published elsewhere [52–54].

Study sample

Participants were recruited from two provincial longitudinal birth cohorts, All Our Families (AOF) [15] and Alberta Pregnancy Outcomes and Nutrition (APrON) [16]. These two cohorts began in 2007 and are prospective, community-based birth cohorts, situated in Alberta, Canada. Together these cohorts include approximately 5200 mother-baby pairs and 1200 fathers. Detailed overviews of the cohorts' methods and design, are described elsewhere [55, 56].

Of the participants who consented to re-contact for future research, cohort research assistants contacted a randomly-generated list of participants to obtain permission to share contact information for this survey's recruitment. Those who agreed received a personalized, email invitation to complete the survey. Pre-notification of the survey and its purpose was provided. Participants from earlier phases of the study were excluded from the online survey.

Online survey development

The online survey was administered via the University of Alberta's Electronic Patient Reported Outcomes (ePRO) platform. Survey design was based on previous qualitative findings, a literature review of participant and public and parent perspectives on data sharing, and pre-testing using cognitive interviewing (CI) [53, 54].

The CI pre-test involved one-on-one interviews ($n = 9$) [57]. CI recruitment followed the qualitative study [53, 54]. During CI interviews, participants completed the draft survey on ePRO (or on paper as needed), while receiving verbal probes from the CI interviewer [57]. Questions explored respondents' understanding and preferences around survey layout, questions, and choices [57]. Specifically, item content, construction, comprehension, confidence judgment, and possible participant reactions were addressed [32, 57]. Concurrent analyses of CI findings involved text-based and thematic analysis. The survey was revised after every other CI; revisions were then discussed in subsequent CIs.

The final survey contained five sections: (a) parents' motivations and reservations surrounding research, data and data repositories; (b) protective and organizational approaches for data repositories; (c) consent preferences; (d) sensitivity of pediatric data and secondary research using this data; and (e) preferences for modes of communication between data repository administrators and parent participants. The survey used fixed-choice response options and Likert scales. Previous qualitative work suggested that the survey topic was not commonly discussed in this population [53, 54]. Background information, particularly on repository governance, was thus provided to promote shared understanding (summarized in Additional file 1).

In this survey, child involvement in research consent discussions and in secondary data use was innovatively presented as three phases: tell, talk and decide. The 'tell' phase encompassed when parents informed their child of their participation. The 'talk' phase considered when parents involved their child in two-way discussions, including child's expression of opinions and preferences. In both the 'tell' and 'talk' phases, parents decided the child's participation. The final 'decide' phase encompassed when parents allowed their child to decide their own participation. When a parent respondent agreed with the utility of any phase, they were to indicate the child's age to start that phase.

The initial, personalized email invitation requested survey completion within 2 weeks. Reminders were emailed on days 3 and 11 [58]. The AOB participants received a follow-up call on day 7 to ensure receipt of the invitation and to answer questions [58]. Upon survey completion, participants could submit their e-mail for a lottery (prize: iPod Touch); this information was segregated from survey data. The study was approved by the Conjoint Health Research Ethics Board at the University of Calgary.

Data analysis

The data were summarized using frequency distributions. Chi-squares and Fisher's exact tests were used to test for associations between participant motivations and reservations towards data sharing, communication preferences and consent preferences. Missing responses varied by question. Reported percentages are item-specific (denominator varies).

The relationship between desired level of engagement and preferred consent model was examined. Consent models were collapsed into three groups: traditional consent, broad consents, and opt-out consent. The broad-consents category included broad, one-time consent; broad, periodic consent; and tiered consent. When comparing parent's level of agreement to involving their child in decision-making, the five-point scale was collapsed. The response options "strongly agree" and "agree" were collapsed into "agree"; "strongly disagree" and "disagree" were collapsed into "disagree." STATA for Mac version 14.1 was used and a significance level of $p < 0.05$ set.

Results

Three hundred and forty-six participants completed the survey from 569 personalized invitations sent in September 2014 (response rate = 60.8%). This included 106 AOB participants, 190 APrON participants, and 50 participants who were members of both cohorts (Table 1). Amongst the survey respondents, 86.7% were Canadian; 98.0% were female; 69.1% were over the age of 35. Most (96.2%) had some post-secondary education.

Preferred engagement for consent process

This survey queried participants on the five most commonly considered consent processes: traditional consent; broad, periodic consent; broad, one-time consent; tiered consent; and, opt-out consent (Fig. 1). All questions around consent centred on the research best practice of using de-identified data, which cannot completely anonymize a dataset especially when opportunities exist to combine data from multiple sources or perspectives.

About 55.8% of respondents felt that their consent should be obtained before their de-identified, non-biological data is provided to a data repository for future, secondary use. These respondents were then asked their preferred process for contributing their data to a repository for secondary use (Table 2). The near-majority preferred the least-engaging opt-out consent process

Table 1 Participant demographics

Characteristic	n (%)
Longitudinal Birth Cohort	
All Our Babies	105 (30.3)
Alberta Pregnancy Outcomes and Nutrition	188 (54.3)
Both	50 (14.5)
Missing	3 (0.8)
Sex	
Male	5 (1.4)
Female	339 (98.0)
Missing	2 (0.5)
Age (years of age)	
$\leq$ 35	110 (31.8)
> 35	208 (69.1)
Missing	28 (8.1)
Education	
High School (Completed)	9 (2.6)
Business, Trade, Technical School (Incomplete or completed)	51 (14.7)
Bachelor's Degree (Incomplete or completed)	190 (54.9)
Graduate School (Incomplete or completed)	92 (26.6)
Missing	4 (1.2)
Country of Origin	
Canada	300 (86.7)
Other	34 (9.8)
Missing	12 (3.4)

Table 2 Participant consent preferences for secondary use

	Preferred consent model if asked to share data from their original cohort n(%)	Preferred consent model if participating in a new study n(%)
Traditional, Opt-In Consent (Participant asked each time dataset shared)	75 (21.9)	78 (22.8)
Broad, One-Time Consent (Participant is asked permission one-time at beginning for all future uses)	33 (9.6)	35 (10.2)
Broad, Periodic Consent (Participant is asked every two years for permission to continue sharing data)	33 (9.6)	25 (7.3)
Tiered (or Conditional) Consent (Participant identifies allowable uses of their data when granting permission)	40 (11.7)	41 (12.0)
Opt-Out Consent (Participant must declare withdrawal within 3 months or permission is assumed)	162 (47.2)	163 (47.7)

(47.2%), while the next most favourable process was the highly-engaging traditional consent (21.9%).

Respondents were asked to rank each consent process on six domains including respectfulness, cost, convenience, informative-ness, feasibility, and control before selecting their preference. Previous qualitative findings in this population suggested that such focussed consideration might better-inform consent preferences (Additional file 2), [53, 54]. Most respondents rated traditional opt-in consent as the most expensive (89.0%), most informative (75.8%), and most affording of control to participants (79.3%). Opt-out consent was ranked lowest on cost (1.6%), informative-ness (2.2%), respectfulness (2.6%), and, tied with broad one-time consent, on control (3.2%). Considering respect and convenience, respondent perceptions were divided. The three processes most often cited as respectful were traditional opt-in (54.5%), tiered (18.3%), and broad-periodic consent (14.7%). The three processes most often cited as convenient were broad, one-time (40.4%), tiered (23.4%) and opt-out consent (23.4%).

Respondents indicated that their preferred means to communicate consent was by email (71.0%), with a password-protected online account (16.1%) being the second-most preferred option. Telephone was the least preferred communication mode (5.7%).

Respondents considered consent processes for a hypothetical new research study that anticipated the to-be-collected data would be shared upon study completion (Table 2). Again, respondents were most supportive of the opt-out consent model (47.7%) followed by the traditional consent model (22.8%).

Future communication preferences vs. consent preferences

Respondents were asked what information would most interest them from a research data repository that housed and shared their or their child's data. The majority of respondents were interested in information pertaining to specific projects that used their dataset (86.7%) and general findings from their dataset (87.9%). Respondents were less interested in general findings arising from the repository's full complement of datasets (35.5%) and information about administrative changes (40.2%). Respondents indicated preferences with the frequency and mode of communication with repositories. Respondents most frequently wanted to hear from the repository once a year (39.2%) through a personalized email (50.1%) or a general newsletter (39.4%).

Statistically significant associations were detected between consent preference and communication frequency and information type (Table 3). Respondents who preferred more engaging models of consent (traditional or broad consent models), were more interested in receiving information pertaining to projects that arose from their dataset ($p = 0.004$), general findings from the repository ($p = 0.033$) and changes to the repository ($p = 0.035$). Respondents preferring engaging consent also wished for more frequent communication ($p = 0.003$).

Consent preferences for Child's data

Parents generally agreed (79.0%) that, at some point, they would tell their child of their involvement in a longitudinal research project (Table 4). This sentiment was shared in both the 'talk' (74.6%) and 'decide' (89.2%) phases. Despite this widespread agreement to involve children, the age at which to begin each phase varied substantially. For the 'talk' and 'tell' phases, parent's felt most frequently comfortable involving children at 12 years of age (19.5%) with a median age of 10 (Fig. 2). Twelve years of age represented the mode (20.2%) and median age for parents feeling comfortable to let children act as primary decision-maker.

Parents provided input on involving children in decision-making for secondary data use. Wide support by respondents for child involvement was expressed for the 'talk' and 'tell' phases (82.0% and 81.0%, respectively) when discussing data sharing (Table 4). Although the majority of respondents were supportive of the 'decide'

Table 3 Relationships between consent preferences, communication frequency and information type

	Preferred consent model if asked to share their data from their original cohort. Consent should be reviewed…			
	Each time dataset is shared n(row/column%)	Periodically n(row/column%)	Never n(row/column%)	p-value
Are you interested in receiving information about projects that arise from the study you participated in?				
Yes	73 (24.58/97.33)	92 (30.98/86.79)	132 (44.44/81.48)	0.004
No	2 (4.35/2.67)	14 (30.43/13.21)	30 (65.22/18.52)	
Are you interested in receiving information about the general findings from the dataset you contributed to?				
Yes	68 (22.59/90.67)	92 (30.56/86.79)	141 (46.84/87.04)	0.684
No	7 (16.67/9.33)	14 (33.33/13.21)	21 (50.00/12.96)	
Are you interested in receiving information about the general findings from all the data at the data repository?				
Yes	36 (29.75/48.00)	34 (28.10/32.08)	51 (42.15/31.48)	0.033
No	39 (17.57/52.00)	72 (32.43/67.92)	111 (50.00/68.52)	
Are you interested in receiving information about any changes made to the data repository?				
Yes	35 (25.55/46.67)	49 (35.77/46.23)	53 (38.69/32.72)	0.035
No	40 (19.42/53.33)	57 (27.67/53.77)	109 (52.91/67.28)	
Based on the information you would like to receive, how often would you most like to hear from the data repository?				
Anytime new information arises	30 (34.09/41.10)	17 (19.32/16.04)	41 (46.59/26.11)	0.003
Every 6 months	23 (23.71/31.51)	33 (34.02/31.13)	41 (42.27/26.11)	
Once a year	18 (13.43/24.66)	52 (38.81/49.06)	64 (47.76/40.76)	
Every other year	2 (11.76/2.74)	4 (23.53/3.77)	11 (64.71/7.01)	
Please indicate your most preferred method of contact.				
A personalized email	41 (23.98/55.41)	60 (35.09/57.14)	70 (40.94/43.75)	0.060
A general newsletter	21 (15.67/28.38)	39 (29.10/37.14)	74 (55.22/46.25)	
A secure, regularly-updated website only open to participants	9 (33.33/12.16)	5 (18.52/4.76)	13 (48.15/8.12)	
A secure, regularly-updated website open to the public	3 (42.86/4.05)	1 (14.29/0.95)	3 (42.86/1.88)	

phase (64.9%), there was a decrease in support for secondary use compared to the 'decide' phase for research participation.

When asked the appropriate age to begin child involvement in data sharing decisions, respondents expressed similar preferences to those for research participation. Twelve years of age represented both the mode (21.5% and 22.9%) and the median age for telling and talking (respectively) with their child about data sharing (Fig. 2). The age increased for when respondents felt comfortable allowing their child to act as primary decision-maker. Most respondents preferred 18 years (25.6%), whereas the median age was 16 years old. Finally, the majority of respondents (63.8%) favoured the repository informing parents of the child's decision regarding data sharing.

Table 4 Parent preferences on child involvement in decision-making for longitudinal research participation

	Level of agreement with child involvement in RESEARCH STUDIES			Level of agreement with child involvement in DATA SHARING		
	Disagree	Neutral	Agree	Disagree	Neutral	Agree
Tell - My child will be informed that they are part of a research study/their non-biological, de-identified data is being shared. As their parent. I decide the availability of their participation.	36 (10.5)	39 (11.3)	271 (79.0)	26 (7.5)	36 (10.4)	283 (82.1)
Talk - My child will be involved in discussions about their participation in the research study/sharing their non-biological, de-identified data. They can express their opinion and preferences. As their parent, I will decide their participation.	39 (11.4)	51 (14.8)	255 (74.6)	28 (8.2)	37 (10.8)	277 (81.0)
Decide - My child will decide whether or not, and how, they participate in the research study/share their non-biological, de-identified data.	21 (6.1)	19 (5.5)	305 (89.2)	75 (21.8)	46 (13.3)	224 (64.9)

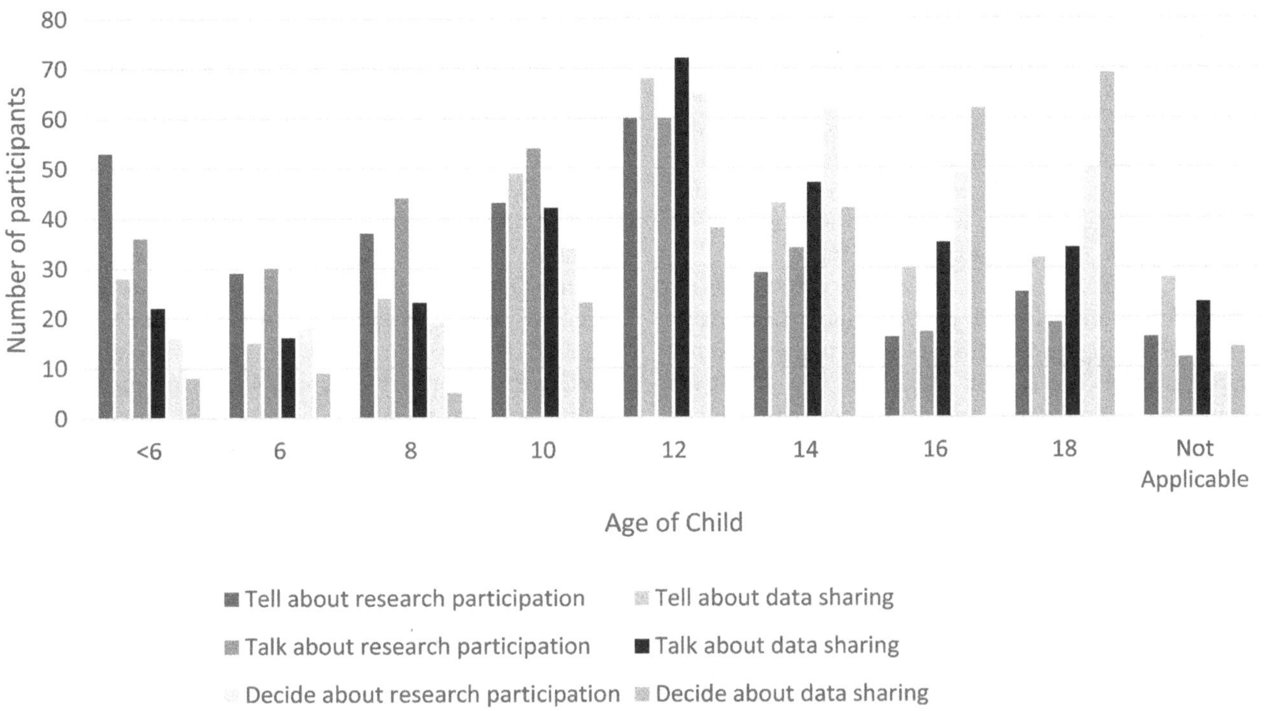

Fig. 2 Parent views on appropriate child ages to "tell", "talk" and "decide" about research participation and data sharing

Discussion

This survey reveals that the majority of parents prefer less-engaging consent processes when discussing secondary data use of de-identified, cohort data for themselves and their children. Parents' consent preferences are associated with their communication preferences. Parents also recognize that children should become gradually involved in consent decision-making around research and secondary data use participation. However, parents vary greatly on when and how that involvement should arise.

When compared to local and provincial data sources, the cohort participants are generally representative of the pregnant and parenting population in Calgary and Alberta, [59]. This study provides evidence of parent perspectives on data sharing, with certain limitations. First, this study population may be more supportive of research than the general population which may overestimate the support of the general population towards data sharing. Secondly, topic complexity may have influenced understanding and preferences. Detailed background information was provided to participants for each section of the survey, which may have altered participants' perspectives.

When longitudinal birth cohort data are first collected, parental permission is sought for the secondary use of both parent and child data. In this study, it appears that parent-respondents are interested in fairly low levels of engagement in being asked for permission to share de-identified cohort data. About 44% of respondents did not feel consent was needed before a dataset including their and their child's de-identified data were shared, consistent with the TCPS2 standard. Those participants were therefore excluded from the questions on consent preferences. Thereafter, a modest majority of parents preferred that they be asked for their consent generally. Nearly half of those consent-preferring parents specifically chose the least-engaging opt-out consent process. This intimates that the majority of respondents overall want no to low levels of engagement in consent for sharing their de-identified non-biological data.

In selections of the most preferred consent process, the remaining 55.8% of respondents were divided: about half preferred the least engaging opt-out model, which they also considered the least expensive, least informative, least controlling, and least respectful. Only 23.4% of respondents considered opt-out consent to be most convenient of the five consents presented. Participants were not different, from a practical standpoint, when considering consent for first-time primary research participation versus secondary data use. When the three broad consents were collapsed, respondent preference did not differ between broad consents and traditional, project-specific consent.

There did not appear to be any consensus in the ranking of consent model preferences; but there was a clear trend that requests for consent are not the highest priority for this parent population. Parents seem to recognize the implications of not asking for consent or going with a low-engagement model: less information, less control, less cost, and less respect. These findings support previous research that identified parent preference of opt-out consent in biobanking [42]. This survey moves beyond another to note that parents preferred opt-out (or no consent) over other processes, rather than simply not voicing an objection, [48]. This coincides with a recent systematic review that suggested that no consensus exists on the most appropriate consent for biobanks [16].

Parents were asked specifically about sharing de-identified, non-biological cohort data, which distinguishes the findings greatly from other parent engagement research around consent and biobanking [42–47]. It may be somewhat inappropriate and unduly restrictive to consider consent preferences for biological data as synonymous for those with non-biological data. There may be differences, particularly more comfort, in sharing de-identified non-biological data versus de-identified biological data: either because there is greater confidence in the ability to truly divest identifiable information from non-biological data versus biological data, or because there is greater trust in researchers and research involved with this parent population. In the latter case, survey respondents came from a long-term cohort study and previously consented to consider additional research. They may be more supportive of, and trusting in, research than other parent populations. The survey also elaborated the governance mechanisms involved in regulating data access, and participants provided input on such mechanisms. It is unclear how influential this discussion and questioning were on consent preferences. Our findings on governance (discussed elsewhere [60]), suggest that governance elements were more important to parents than privacy issues. These elements include the criteria and processes required for gaining access to data; the monitoring of data access; and, the bodies involved in governance of secondary use. Further research is required to determine the role, if any, of governance features on participants' consent preferences for secondary data use.

Communication preferences largely mirrored consent preferences. Respondents most wanted limited engagement: yearly contact through one-way communications such as email or newsletter. There were corresponding increases in communication specificity and frequency desired among respondents preferring more engaging consent processes. This relationship makes sense and is consistent with a perspective that less interaction is necessary when long-term research participants share non-biological, de-identified data. Less desired interaction signalled greater trust in researchers, research and repositories. These findings may not be generalizable to all secondary use instances, but only to those with structured governance and data access processes including scientific review, qualification criteria, research ethics board approval, formal approval by the governing privacy authority, up-to-date information technology, a non-profit and research-focused agenda, and, sharing de-identified, non-biological datasets.

The majority of parent respondents supported gradual inclusion of children in decision-making for research and secondary data use. Amongst great variability, 12 years seemed the age at which most parents would inform children of, and begin discussions around, their information being used in research and secondary use. Decision-making for specific research would transition to children from parents around 12 years old. Decision-making for secondary data use, which has greater uncertainty on the specifics, logistics and implications of information use, fell more in line with legal definitions of majority at 18 years which contrasts current Canadian standards that demarcate capacity not age as the threshold for research decision-making. Parent views coincide with the scant literature on adolescent perspectives on data sharing [49–51], in that there is great variability but a general favouring of re-consent at the age of majority. Previous research with adolescents favoured a renewed focus on governance rather than consent when approaching secondary use of longitudinal cohort data [51].

Conclusions

Both parents and youth involved in cohorts recognize the value of their data for secondary use and knowledge advancement. The consent conversation may not be crucial to garner access to that valuable data resource. Flexible, trustworthy approaches to the governance of data sharing are necessary to ensure long-term access to these data assets and safeguard public trust in research. Ensuring data storage is highly secure and up-to-date is crucial, as is confirming data access is restricted to approved researchers and entities and monitoring access and its outputs. Trust in institutions seems to move the conversation and responsibility away from parents and child participants to the researchers and repositories for de-identified, non-biological data [40]. This movement may be appropriate because parents and children lack the experience and capacity to assess and monitor the appropriateness and security of all future secondary data users.

Additional files

Additional file 1: Overview of background material provided for each section of the survey. This table overviews the background information provided to participants in each section of the survey, given the findings 635 in the qualitative work that this population required some background 636 information to inform their preferences. (DOCX 17 kb)

Additional file 2: Parents' perspectives on ranking consent models. This table reveals how parent respondents' ranked each consent model on 639 features such as respectfulness, cost, convenience, and informativeness. (DOCX 16 kb)

Abbreviations
AOF: All our families; APrON: Alberta pregnancy outcomes and nutrition; CI: Cognitive interviewing; ePRO: Electronic patient reported outcomes

Acknowledgements
We would like to acknowledge and thank the participants for this research project for their time and insight. We are grateful for the AOF and APrON research teams, especially with their support in recruitment. We are grateful to Laurence Richer, Rick Watts, and the ePRO team at the Women & Children's Health Research Institute at the University of Alberta for their significant support in the administration of the online survey. We are grateful to PolicyWise for Children & Families, which provided the external grant funding for the study and salary support for a principal investigator (KPM).

Funding
The author(s) disclosed receipt of the following financial support for the research, authorship, and/or publication of this article: This research was completed with project funding support from the Alberta Children's Hospital Research Institute and PolicyWise for Children & Families (13SM-Tough, Manhas). Post-doctoral fellowship funding for the lead researcher was supported by PolicyWise for Children & Families.

Authors' contributions
KPM led the study design and drafted the manuscript. SD led the data analysis, drafted tables, and contributed drafts of methods-related sections of the manuscript. All authors (KPM, SD, SP, NL, CA, XC, and ST) provided significant input into the original research proposal; provided significant input into the design and implementation of the survey; provided significant input into the data analysis and manuscripts drafts; and have read and approved this manuscript.

Competing interests
The authors declare that they have no competing interests.

Author details
[1]Community Health Sciences, University of Calgary, Calgary, Canada. [2]PolicyWise for Children & Families, Calgary, Canada. [3]University of Alberta, Edmonton, Canada. [4]Conjoint Health Research Ethics Board, University of Calgary, Calgary, Canada. [5]University of Calgary, Calgary, Canada. [6]PolicyWise for Children & Families, Edmonton, AB, Canada. [7]Pediatrics & Community Health Sciences, University of Calgary, Calgary, Canada. [8]Alberta Health Services, Calgary, Canada.

References

1. Organization for Economic Cooperation and Development. OECD principles and guidelines for access to research data from public funding. 2007. https://www.oecd.org/sti/sci-tech/38500813.pdf. Accessed 15 May 2017.
2. Social Sciences and Humanities Research Council. Research data archiving policy. 2012. http://www.sshrc-crsh.gc.ca/about-au_sujet/policies-politiques/statements-enonces/edata-donnees_electroniques-eng.aspx. Accessed 13 Oct 2013.
3. Canadian Institutes of Health Research. CIHR open access policy. 2013. http://www.cihr-irsc.gc.ca/e/46068.html. Accessed 13 Oct 2013.
4. Canadian Institutes of Health Research. CIHR response and action plan - 2011 international review panel recommendations. Ottawa: Government of Canada; 2011.
5. Medical Research Council. MRC policy and guidance on sharing of research data from population and patient studies. 2011 https://www.mrc.ac.uk/publications/browse/mrc-policy-and-guidance-on-sharing-of-research-data-from-population-and-patient-studies/. Accessed 15 Oct 2013.
6. National Institutes of Health. NIH data sharing policy and implementation guidance. 2003. https://grants.nih.gov/grants/policy/data_sharing/data_sharing_guidance.htm. Accessed 15 Oct 2013.
7. Office of the Information and Privacy Commissioner for British Columbia. Report of the roundtable discussion on access to data for health research. 2012. https://www.oipc.bc.ca/special-reports/1483. Accessed 15 Oct 2013.
8. Warren SD, Brandeis LD. The right to privacy. Harv Law Rev. 1890;4(5):193–220.
9. Solove DJ. A taxonomy of privacy. Univ Pa Law Rev. 2006;154(3):477–560.
10. Solove DJ. A Brief History of Information Privacy Law. In: Mathews KJ, editor. Proskauer on Privacy: A Guide to Privacy and Data Secruity Law in the Information Age. New York: Practising Law Institute; 2006.
11. Solove DJ. HIPAA turns 10: analyzing the past, present, and future impact. J Am Health Inf Manag Assoc. 2013;84:22–8.
12. Service Alberta and the Office of the Information and Privacy Commissioner. A Guide for Businesses and Organizations on the Personal Information and Privacy Act. Edmonton: Service Alberta; 2008.
13. Canadian Institutes of Health Research, National Sciences and engineering research council, and Social Sciences and Humanities Research Council of Canada. Tri-Council policy statement: ethical conduct of research involving humans. 2010.
14. Stoddart J, Chan B, Joly Y. The European Union's adequacy approach to privacy and international data sharing in Health Research. J Law Med Ethics. 2016;44(1):143–55.
15. Caulfield T. Consent, privacy & research biobanks. GenEdit. 2010;1:10–6.
16. Master Z, Nelson E, Murdoch B, Caulfield T. Biobanks, consent and claims of consensus. Nat Methods. 2012;9(9):885–8.
17. Golding J, Jones R, Brune MN, Pronczuk J. Why carry out a longitudinal birth survey? Paediatr Perinat Epidemiol. 2009;23(Suppl 1):1–14.
18. Ries NM. Growing up as a research subject: ethical and legal issues in birth cohort studies involving genetic research. Health Law J. 2007;15:1–42.
19. Ries NM, LeGrandeur J, Caulfield T. Handling ethical, legal and social issues in birth cohort studies involving genetic research: responses from studies in six countries. BMC Med Ethics. 2010;11:4.
20. Samuel J, Ries NM, Malkin D, Knoppers BM. Biobanks and longitudinal studies: where are the children? GenEdit. 2008;6(3):1–8.
21. Cambon-Thomsen A, Rial-Sebbag E, Knoppers BM. Trends in ethical and legal frameworks for the use of human biobanks. Eur Respir J. 2007;30(2):373–82.
22. Laurie G. Reflexive governance in biobanking: on the value of policy led approaches and the need to recognise the limits of law. Hum Genet. 2011; 130(3):347–56.
23. Knoppers BM, Avard D, Cardinal G, Glass KC. Science and society: children and incompetent adults in genetic research: consent and safeguards. Nat Rev Genet. 2002;3(3):221–5.
24. Knoppers BM, Saginur M. The babel of genetic data terminology. Nat Biotechnol. 2005;23(8):925–7.
25. Kosseim P, Dove ES, Baggaley C, Meslin EM, Cate FH, Kaye J, Harris JR, Knoppers BM. Building a data sharing model for global genomic research. Genome Biol. 2014;15(8):430.
26. Bertier G, Carrot-Zhang J, Ragoussis V, Joly Y. Integrating precision cancer medicine into healthcare-policy, practice, and research challenges. Genome Med. 2016;8(1):108.
27. Caulfield T, Chandrasekharan S, Joly Y, Cook-Deegan R. Harm, hype and evidence: ELSI research and policy guidance. Genome Med. 2013;5(3):21.
28. Joly Y, Dove ES, Knoppers BM, Bobrow M, Chalmers D. Data sharing in the post-genomic world: the experience of the international Cancer genome consortium (ICGC) data access compliance office (DACO). PLoS Comput Biol. 2012;8(7):e1002549.
29. Joly Y, Dyke SO, Knoppers BM, Pastinen T. Are data sharing and privacy protection mutually exclusive? Cell. 2016;167(5):1150–4.
30. McGuire AL, Basford M, Dressler LG, Fullerton SM, Koenig BA, Li R, McCarty CA, Ramos E, Smith ME, Somkin CP, et al. Ethical and practical challenges of sharing data from genome-wide association studies: the eMERGE consortium experience. Genome Res. 2011;21(7):1001–7.
31. Gurwitz D, Fortier I, Lunshof JE, Knoppers BM. Research ethics. Children and population biobanks. Science (New York, N.Y.). 2009;325(5942):818–9.
32. Adair CE, Holland AC, Patterson ML, Mason KS, Goering PN, Hwang SW. Cognitive interviewing methods for questionnaire pre-testing in homeless persons with mental disorders. J Urban Health. 2012;89(1):36–52.
33. Hens K, Cassiman JJ, Nys H, Dierickx K. Children, biobanks and the scope of parental consent. Eur J Hum Genet. 2011;19(7):735–9.
34. Hens K, Levesque E, Dierickx K. Children and biobanks: a review of the ethical and legal discussion. Hum Genet. 2011;130(3):403–13.

35. Hens K, Nys H, Cassiman JJ, Dierickx K. The return of individual research findings in paediatric genetic research. J Med Ethics. 2011;37(3):179–83.
36. El Emam K, Buckeridge D, Tamblyn R, Neisa A, Jonker E, Verma A. The re-identification risk of Canadians from longitudinal demographics. BMC Med Inform Decis Mak. 2011;11:46.
37. Samuel J, Knoppers BM, Avard D. Paediatric biobanks: what makes them so unique? J Paediatr Child Health. 2012;48(2):E1–3.
38. Dove ES, Black E, Avard D, Knoppers BM. Charting the privacy landscape in Canadian Paediatric biobanks. Health Law J. 2013;20:1–46.
39. Brakewood B, Poldrack RA. The ethics of secondary data analysis: considering the application of Belmont principles to the sharing of neuroimaging data. NeuroImage. 2013;82:671–6.
40. O'Doherty KC, Burgess MM, Edwards K, Gallagher RP, Hawkins AK, Kaye J, McCaffrey V, Winickoff DE. From consent to institutions: designing adaptive governance for genomic biobanks. Soc Sci Med. 2011;73(3):367–74.
41. Godard B, Schmidtke J, Cassiman JJ, Ayme S. Data storage and DNA banking for biomedical research: informed consent, confidentiality, quality issues, ownership, return of benefits. A professional perspective. Eur J Hum Genet. 2003;11(Suppl 2):S88–122.
42. Brothers KB, Clayton EW. Parental perspectives on a pediatric human non-subjects biobank. AJOB Prim Res. 2012;3(3):21–9.
43. Joseph JW, Neidich AB, Ober C, Ross LF. Empirical data about women's attitudes toward a biobank focused on pregnancy outcomes. Am J Med Genet A. 2008;146a(3):305–11.
44. Neidich AB, Joseph JW, Ober C, Ross LF. Empirical data about women's attitudes towards a hypothetical pediatric biobank. Am J Med Genet A. 2008;146a(3):297–304.
45. Burstein MD, Robinson JO, Hilsenbeck SG, McGuire AL, Lau CC. Pediatric data sharing in genomic research: attitudes and preferences of parents. Pediatrics. 2014;133(4):690–7.
46. Jenkins MM, Reed-Gross E, Rasmussen SA, Barfield WD, Prue CE, Gallagher ML, Honein MA. Maternal attitudes toward DNA collection for gene-environment studies: a qualitative research study. Am J Med Genet A. 2009; 149a(11):2378–86.
47. Halverson CM, Ross LF. Attitudes of African-American parents about biobank participation and return of results for themselves and their children. J Med Ethics. 2012;38(9):561–6.
48. Fernandes DM, Roland AP, Morris MC. Parental opinions regarding an opt-out consent process for inpatient pediatric prospective observational research in the US. Pragmat Obs Res. 2017;8:1–8.
49. Hens K, Nys H, Cassiman JJ, Dierickx K. The storage and use of biological tissue samples from minors for research: a focus group study. Public Health Genomics. 2011;14(2):68–76.
50. Gammelgaard A, Knudsen LE, Bisgaard H. Perceptions of parents on the participation of their infants in clinical research. Arch Dis Child. 2006;91(12): 977–80.
51. Audrey S, Brown L, Campbell R, Boyd A, Macleod J. Young people's views about consenting to data linkage: findings from the PEARL qualitative study. BMC Med Res Methodol. 2016;16:34.
52. Manhas KP, Mitchell I. (dis)-trust in transitioning ventilator-dependent children from hospital to homecare. Nurs Ethics. 2015;22(8):913–27.
53. Manhas KP, Page S, Dodd SX, Letourneau N, Ambrose A, Cui X, Tough SC. Parent perspectives on privacy and governance for a pediatric repository of non-biological, research data. J Empir Res Hum Res Ethics. 2015;10(1):88–99.
54. Manhas KP, Page S, Dodd SX, Letourneau N, Ambrose A, Cui X, Tough SC. Parental perspectives on consent for participation in large-scale, non-biological data repositories. Life Sci Soc Policy. 2016;12:1.
55. McDonald SW, Lyon AW, Benzies KM, McNeil DA, Lye SJ, Dolan SM, Pennell CE, Bocking AD, Tough SC. The all our babies pregnancy cohort: design, methods, and participant characteristics. BMC Pregnancy Childbirth. 2013; 13(Suppl 1):S2.
56. Kaplan BJ, Giesbrecht GF, Leung BM, Field CJ, Dewey D, Bell RC, Manca DP, O'Beirne M, Johnston DW, Pop VJ, et al. The Alberta pregnancy outcomes and nutrition (APrON) cohort study: rationale and methods. Matern Child Nutr. 2014;10(1):44–60.
57. Willis GB: Cognitive interviewing: A "how to" guide. 1999.
58. De Leeuw ED, Hox JJ, Dillman DA (eds). International Handbook of Survey Methodology. New York: Taylor & Francis Group; 2008.
59. Leung BM, McDonald SW, Kaplan BJ, Giesbrecht GF, Tough SC. Comparison of sample characteristics in two pregnancy cohorts: community-based versus population-based recruitment methods. BMC Med Res Methodol. 2013;13:149.
60. Dodd SXM, K. P, Page S, Letourneau N, Cui X, Tough SC. Governance and privacy in a provincial data repository: a cross-sectional analysis of longitudinal birth cohort parent Participants' perspectives on sharing adult vs. child research data. Madrid: DATA 2017: 6th international conference on data science, technology and applications conference and proceedings; 2017. p. 1–8. http://www.scitepress.org/Papers/2017/64308/64308.pdf.

19

Patients' perception of the information security management in health centers: the role of organizational and human factors

Hamid Reza Peikari[1], Ramayah T.[2], Mahmood Hussain Shah[3] and May Chiun Lo[4*]

Abstract

Background: Researchers paid little attention to understanding the association of organizational and human factors with patients' perceived security in the context of health organizations. This study aims to address numerous gaps in this context. Patients' perceptions about employees' training on security issues, monitoring on security issues, ethics, physical & technical protection and trust in hospitals were identified as organizational and human factors.

Methods: After the development of 12 hypotheses, a quantitative, cross-sectional, self-administered survey method was applied to collect data in 9 hospitals in Iran. After the collection of 382 usable questionnaires, the partial least square structural modeling was applied to examine the hypotheses and it was found that 11 hypotheses were empirically supported.

Results: The results suggest that patients' trust in hospitals can significantly predict their perceived security but no significant associations were found between patients' physical protection mechanisms in the hospital and their perceived information security in a hospital. We also found that patients' perceptions about the physical protection mechanism of a hospital can significantly predict their trust in hospitals which is a novel finding by this research.

Conclusions: The findings imply that hospitals should formulate policies to improve patients' perception about such factors, which ultimately lead to their perceived security.

Keywords: Security, Trust, Technical and physical protection, Monitoring, Training, Ethics

Background

Information security breaches result in an average of $7 Billion worth of losses every year in the healthcare industry [1]. This has motivated many researchers to conduct research from different perspectives with an aim to reduce the likelihood of security breaches and the costs associated with it. While the researchers in the field of computer science have explored the phenomenon of information security, most of them have studied the issue from the engineering perspective and focused on the development of technical solutions and neglected to study security from a behavioral approach [2]. Behavioral approach refers to studying the factors which shape individuals' perception and behavior towards the practice of information security in organizations. Therefore, this research intends to answer the following question: what are the anticipating factors of individuals' perceived security?

Investigating the antecedents of information security from the behavioral perspective is important because it plays an important role in evaluating and ensuring the level of information security. Indeed, since most individuals lack technical knowledge of the security technologies implemented, they assess the data protection levels of the organization based on some cues. This phenomenon is called perceived security. Therefore, in order to reduce individuals' concerns about the security of their information, the factors that play a significant role in shaping their perceived security should be enhanced.

* Correspondence: mclo@unimas.my
[4]Research & Innovation Management Centre (UNIMAS INNOVATION), Universiti Malaysia Sarawak (UNIMAS), 94300 Kota Samarahan, Sarawak, Malaysia
Full list of author information is available at the end of the article

Although some studies related to behavioral security have been conducted, there are some gaps associated with such research. Some studies in this field, have focused on perceived security in online environment [3–8], and have emphasized only the role of technical factors and ignored the role of organizational and human factors in influencing individuals' perceived security. Organizational factors in this context refer to the managerial and organizational policies practiced (such as monitoring and training the employees, or the deployment of technical and physical protection equipment) to address the information security issues in the organization. Human factors, on the other hand, refer to individual employees' behaviors and practices (such as employees' ethics), which can strengthen or weaken information security situations in the organization. The lack of sufficient research in this field has led to the emergence of a new research stream, which has highlighted the role of organizational and human factors, besides the technical factors, in studying perceived security [1, 8–12].

While most of the past research on the perceived security is in the field of e-commerce or employees' perceived security, studying the factors that enhance patients' perceived security (in the field of health information) is crucial. Over time, a patients' medical and health record accumulates sensitive individual information, which may be misused by unauthorized parties [9]. This makes patients concerned with regards to the potential unauthorized disclosure and misuse of their information. Patients have to provide information to the health service providers to help them better diagnose and prescribe, leading to facilitating the provision of healthcare services. However, patients may refuse to share sensitive, private and important information where there are potentially embarrassing health problems such as HIV or psychological disorders, due to their concern regarding the disclosure of such information to non-authorized parties and people [9]. This is because they may feel that disclosure will result in social shame and discrimination. Consequently, such concerns and non-disclosure of sensitive information may worsen the patients' health conditions, exposing their lives to risk. Hence, studying the factors which contribute in the patients' perceived security of their sensitive information is an important factor for ultimately providing effective health services to them. Despite the importance of the issue, limited studies have focused on health sector, which calls upon models different from other sectors [9]. The violation of patients' information security is the second highest reported breach [9], implying that patients are concerned of such violations and threats. Appendix illustrates the factors and contexts studied in the past research related to the behavioral security. As shown, all the papers illustrated in Appendix have focused on employees' perceptions and the factors preventing employees from a security breach in organizations and none of them have examined the factors leading to behavioral information security in the context of health sector and from the view point of patients. In other words, the models and findings presented by the past research cannot be applied to the context of health information security from the patients' perspective and this field lacks a thorough understanding of what makes patients perceive that their information is protected against security threats.

Another research gap in the context of perceived information security is regarding the antecedents of perceived security in the past research. As shown in Appendix, most of the past research has examined perceived certainty and severity of penalties (sanctions/penalties), normative belief, attitude and self-efficacy. Most of the past studies in this field have used general deterrence theory to study the antecedents of perceived security. However, more factors other than those examined in the past research have been suggested as the antecedents of perceived security by some researchers. For instance, perceived employees' training [1, 2, 11, 13–16], monitoring [11, 15, 17], physical and technical protection [18, 19], and ethics [15, 17, 20–22]. The researchers however neglected to empirically examine the association of the mentioned factors with perceived security. Hence, it is essential to study the association of such factors in the model. Moreover, the dominant theory in behavioral security studies is the general deterrence theory, which has made our knowledge and understanding limited and hence, more theories should be used in this field to enrich the knowledge available in this field.

Considering the above research gaps, this research aims to develop and validate a model which predicts patients' perceived information security. Therefore, as discussed earlier, six factors, namely technical protections, physical protection, trust in hospital, monitoring employees, security training and security were identified as the less-studied factors in the past research. Therefore, the mentioned factors were considered as the potential antecedent of perceived security and this research intends to examine their relation with patient perceived security. The findings and implications of this paper will contribute in the academic front by posing and examining a new theoretical model to understand the interrelations that exist between the determinants of patients' perceived security. This can enrich the existing theories and knowledge regarding the determinant factors of individuals' perceived security. The findings can also help managers and practitioners in the healthcare industry gain a better knowledge and understanding of the patients' perceived security which in turn enables them to provide effective and efficient provisions designed to address and improve patients' perceived security. This can lead to the patients' disclosure of critical, sensitive information which ultimately helps improve the delivery of higher quality health services to the patients.

Literature review and hypotheses development

Chellappa and Pavlou [3] refer to perceived security as the individuals' belief of the subjective probability that their sensitive information will not be accessed, by inappropriate parties, and in accordance with their confident expectations. According to [15], security has an impact on organizational technology, processes and the employees' manner in processing information. While some researchers have studied the role of technical factors and solutions in the protection of information security [4, 6, 8], some others have highlighted the role of human factors with regards to information security threats in organizations [1, 9–11, 13]. Hence, both factors should be considered in the evaluation of information security in organizations.

According to [10], health organizations' success in protecting information security is rooted in two factors: i-technical aspects and ii-organizational and human factors. Therefore, this research categorizes threats to patients' information security into two main areas:

1- Technical threats, rooted in the technical vulnerabilities of the information systems; and
2- Organizational and human threats, rooted in inappropriate/unauthorized access of patients' information by internal parties, abusing their privileges.

The first form of threat can be managed by utilizing robust technical solutions to deal with the technical threats to penetrate the system and access sensitive data with no authorization. On the other hand, the second type of threat can be managed by organizational policies such as training the personnel to protect sensitive data, monitoring them to make sure they do not violate any rules and communicating the principles of ethics amongst personnel to encourage ethical working practices. Hence, in this research, the technical and physical protection variables are considered as the technical aspect of information security while employees' training, ethics and monitoring are considered as the organizational determinants of perceived security. Moreover, since there is an association between trust and security [23, 24], we propose and consider trust in hospital as an antecedent of security.

This research refers to cue utilization theory, cue consistency theory and environmental psychology to develop its theoretical foundation. According to cue utilization theory, the quality of a product or service can be assessed by two different cues: (1) extrinsic cues, and (2) intrinsic cues. The former refers to alterable product/service attributes and the latter are related to non-alterable, inherent product/service features and characteristics [8, 25]. This holds true for information security protection as a service to be offered and ensured for patients in hospitals. When patients refer to a hospital, they evaluate the services offered by the hospital by using intrinsic cues; and extrinsic cues such as security policy, monitoring, training, or operating policy statements of the hospital. When numerous cues are consistent, a synergic interaction is created among them and the presence of each cue strengthens the association of the other cues, which is called the Cue Consistency Theory [25]. Therefore, patients use their perception regarding different factors and evidences as cues to make judgments about the unknown [26]. According to the environmental psychology, a place's atmosphere can influence individuals' beliefs about that place [8]. Therefore, if an organization (including a hospital) has an atmosphere to assist clients to find it trustworthy, they will perceive it as a reliable organization that does not intend to violate its clients' interests, including the security of their information [27]. Clients may look for organizational factors and features to judge the confidentiality measures and security of their information [28]. Moreover, a well-managed organization might influence clients' perceptions that their information will be safe and secured [8]. Hence, organizational factors can predict perceptions regarding the security of information.

Physical protection, employees' monitoring, and training lead to security

Colwill [13] argues that employees' training is the greatest non-technical tool to protect the information security in organizations. Health organizations do not usually employ security trained staff, which leads to vulnerabilities in their information security [1]. Training staff to improve their knowledge and awareness on security issues and threats is one of the best non-technical solutions, which prevents insiders from disclosing the sensitive information to unauthorized parties [11, 13]. Good training and effective and efficient policies to deal with security threats are good sources of preventing security breaches in health organizations [1, 14, 16]. Training can increase staff knowledge and awareness about the threats and consequences of a security breach, leading to the prevention of such incidents [21]. Likewise, [15] speculate that employees' training and monitoring can influence the security of information in organizations. Personnel monitoring is used by organizations to ensure that their employees adhere to their rules and regulations. According to [11], employee monitoring and surveillance reduces the likelihood of an employee related security breach by increasing their perceived certainty and severity of punishments and the potential consequences for such behaviors. According to [17], monitoring employees to find and correct their unacceptable behavior can lead to the deterrence of problematic behaviors, including security breaches. Monitored employees are very unlikely to take risks with regards to disclosing sensitive information and take care of their responsibilities in relation to information security. Hence, it is suggested that:

H1. Patients' perceptions about the training of employees on information security have a positive relationship with their overall perceived information security.

H2. Patients' perceptions about the monitoring of employees on information security have a positive relationship with their overall perceived information security.

Moreover, physical protection aids information security by deploying measures that are too difficult to defeat [19]. Physical protection is the third stream of security management in conjunction with policies and personnel countermeasures [18]. A physical protection mechanism integrates procedures, people, and tools to protect the assets against sabotage, theft, and terrorist attacks [19]. Indeed, when an intruder intends to access the information, one way is to personally and physically access the data storage/transition instruments. Hence, when an organization deploys robust physical protection mechanisms (such as locks, CCTV, etc), the intruders cannot easily access the systems and hence the likelihood of security breach is reduced. So, when patients observe robust physical protection measures, they perceive that the security of their information is protected. Hence, it can be hypothesized that:

H3. Patients' perceptions toward the robustness of physical protection mechanisms have a positive relationship with their perceived information security.

Physical protection, training, monitoring, technical protection and ethics lead to trust

There are two different types of trust: trust in technology and trust in the service/goods provider [24]. This research refers to trust as the later form. In this sense, trust is an attitude of confidence towards a party [29]. According to [30], one of the prerequisites of trust in an organization is perceived ethics (also called benevolence), which deals with the perception that the trustee cares about the benefits of the trusting party to protect the rights of the trusting party. Indeed, ethics refer to the belief about the goodwill of another party. Perceived ethics reduces perceived uncertainty by making the trusting party to ignore the trustee's undesirable behavior. According to [31], an ethical party tries to adjust to the trusting party needs. This can be achieved by the trusted party's observation and application of rules, procedures and policies to ensure the benefits of the trusting party. Johnson [32] illustrates that customers' belief in the ethical practices in an organization positively influence their trust in the organization. Indeed, individuals' perceptions about the extent of which a service provider adheres to ethical values and codes of ethics indicates the extent to which the service provider is willing to tolerate opportunistic behavior. Therefore, the more the service provider is perceived as an ethical party, the less would be the likelihood of unfair practices in the interaction, which reduces the perceived level of transaction uncertainty and risk. Some researchers have associated perceived ethics of the organization with individuals' trust in it [33, 34]. Hence, it can be suggested that:

H4. Patients' perceptions about the ethical practices in a hospital have a positive relationship with their trust in the hospital.

Belanger et al. [35] on the other hand have referred to institutional, structural-based trust as the belief that trust is likely because of regulations, promises, guarantees, legal recourse, contracts, processes or procedures. Likewise, [23] uses institutional-based trust as the belief of a trustor about the security of a situation based on the guaranteed safety procedures, policies and practices. Physical protection, training, monitoring, technical protection and ethics can be considered as the key factors in shaping patients' trust. Technical protection are the overall technical solutions and capabilities deployed by the information technology department to ensure the confidentiality of the transmitted information [8]. For instance, [5] found that perceived technical protection in the context of e-payment systems can significantly predict their trust in the system. Likewise, [6] found that technical protection can significantly predict customers' trust in the e-commerce context. According to [36], in the e-commerce context, customers' perceived technological trustworthiness of a website enhances their trust in the website. They maintain that the lack of technical reliability can end in users' loss of trust. In another research, [8] speculate that the overall technical capabilities of an organization to ensure the security of the exchanged information can lead to individuals' trust. Likewise, when an organization formulates and implements certain policies, such as the provision of training to its staff, deploying physical protection to deter a security breach and monitoring the staff to prevent their abuse, this can lead to individuals' trust in the service provider. It is in line with [29] who refer to trust as the attitude of confidence towards a party. It is applicable in the context of the health sector because patients believe that the hospital does not try to violate their rights and endanger them by improper policies and practices. Hence, it is suggested that:

H5. Patients' perceptions toward the physical protection capabilities has positive relationship with their trust in hospitals.
H6. Patients' perceptions toward the technical protection capabilities has positive relationship with their trust in hospitals.
H7. Patients' perceptions toward the staff training on security issues has positive relationship with their trust in hospitals.
H8. Patients' perceptions toward staff monitoring has positive relationship with their trust in hospitals.

Ethics leads to security

Organizations should build an effective culture among their employees to ensure data security [15]. Ruighaver et al. [17] speculate that organizations should encourage ethics in situations where information security is at risk. Adherence to ethics can become a culture amongst employees, which leads to the protection of data [15]. The ethical principles have been developed for health professionals to encourage them to take on responsibility of protecting information security [21]. Many of the security and privacy threats could be prevented if the computer users observed the ethical standards in the other interacting parties [20, 22]. D'Arcy et al. [11] suggest employees' ethical behavior as an important prerequisite for information security. Likewise, [13] state that employees may threaten the security of the information systems due to the lack of ethics. Therefore, it is suggested that:

H9. Patients' perceptions toward the ethical practices in a hospital has positive relationship with their perceived information security in the hospital.

Training leads to ethics

According to [22], organizations should provide training to their employees to promote their ethical practices. They speculate that many of the ethical violations could be prevented by training the employees. Employees' training programs can include the organization's expected code of conduct and ethics [37]. When the employees are made aware that their organization rewards good behavior and adherence to ethics, they are more likely to adhere to the ethical guidelines of the organization [13]. According to [19], training employees can form and enhance an ethical culture in the organization to influence personnel to act ethically and feel responsible for the protection of information. Hence, it is suggested that:

H10. Patients' perceptions about the employees' training has positive relationship with their perceptions about employees' ethics in the hospital.

Trust leads to security

While some researchers have found that individuals' perceptions about the security and privacy features of a technology lead to their trust in the technology [23, 24, 31, 38], others have found that individuals' trust is one of the antecedents of their perceived risk and security in online environment [27, 29, 39, 40, 41]. Likewise, [42] found that individuals' trust in the context of e-commerce could negatively influence their perceived risk. The higher the degree of trust, the lower the degree of uncertainty and perceived risk by customers [43]. This is because trust in an organization can reduce individuals' uncertainties in dealing with the organization. In other words, when individuals can trust in an organization, they perceive fewer risks in their relationship and interactions with the organization. This includes the risk on information security. Hence, it is hypothesized that:

H11. Patients' trust in a hospital has a positive relationship with their perceived information security in the hospital.

Technical protection leads to perceived security

Kim [5] argue that an acceptable level of data integrity and stability can enhance customers' perceived security in the e-payment context. Since it is difficult for individuals to assess the technical protection robustness from the technical perspective, they evaluate it based on their perceptions on the functionality of these mechanisms [6, 8]. Hence, this research also utilizes this approach to evaluate technical protection mechanisms in hospitals. In the context of e-commerce, [6, 8] found that customers' perceived technical protection can predict their perceived security. Hence, it is suggested that:

H12. Patients' perceived technical protection capabilities of the hospitals has positive relationship with their perceived information security.

Methods

This study used a quantitative, self-administered survey method and collected data by using a cross-sectional approach. The questionnaire was composed of 38 questions, which was expected to take less than 15 min on average for respondents to be filled out. As shown in Table 1, the questions were adopted and adapted from other sources. Apart from the demographic questions, the other questions used a 5-point Likert scale. Before collecting the data, the questionnaire was independently checked by three academics and three practitioners who were experts in the field of information security and the scale was revised according to their comments. This indicates the face and content validity of the scale. The

Table 1 Questionnaire Details

Variable	No. of Items	Sources	Reliability
Perceived Physical Protection	7	[71]	0.82
Perceived Security	3	[72]	0.89
Perceived Ethical Practice	6	[73–75]	0.87
Perceived Monitoring	7	[76, 77]	0.84
Perceived Training	5	[78]	0.85
Trust in Hospital	3	[39]	0.75
Technical Protection	4	[72]	0.82

questionnaire was then tested in a pre-test stage, with five respondents, testing the questionnaire separately.

After the process of content validity at the pilot study stage, a convenient sampling method was utilized. The target population was consisted of the patients of 9 educational hospitals in Isfahan. Since the population size was greater than 100,000 people; the sample size was 384 respondents, following the sample size table outlined by [44]. To meet this number, 450 questionnaires were distributed amongst the patients of the mentioned hospitals. The participation in the data collection process was voluntarily and the participants were ensured that their identification and answers will be kept confidential. After 1 month, 382 usable questionnaires were collected, which is very close to the 384 sample size outlined by [44] for large populations. One probable reason for such a high response rate was that the patients had sufficient time to complete the questionnaires between the time they had entered the hospital and the time they were admitted. However, we had a small portion of lost or incomplete questionnaires. After the collection of the questionnaires, descriptive statistics was carried out by SPSS 20; while partial least square (PLS) modeling technique, using SmartPLS 3.0 was utilized to assess the construct validity and examine the hypotheses.

Results

Demographic results

As shown in Table 2, most of the respondents were older than 50 years old (45.29%), followed by those between 41 and 50 years old (21.2%). Moreover, the analysis revealed that there was a fairly even split between male and female respondents (52% and 47.12% respectively) and almost half of the respondents had a diploma degree (46.86%).

Research model analysis

To analyze the model, the Partial Least Squares (PLS) analysis technique was utilized by the SmartPLS 3.0 software [45]. Following the two-stage analytical procedure recommended by some scholars [46–50], the measurement model was tested to confirm the validity and then the structural model were tested to examine the significance of the loadings and path coefficients.

Table 2 The Results of the Demographic Analysis

Demographics	Categories	Frequency	Percent
Age (years)	Less than 21	8	2.09
	21–30	53	13.87
	31–40	67	17.55
	41–50	81	21.20
	> 50	173	45.29
Gender	Female	180	47.12
	Male	202	52.88
Education	Under diploma	43	11.26
	Diploma	179	46.86
	B.A.	43	11.26
	B.Sc.	90	23.56
	M.Sc. and above	27	7.06

Validity and reliability

To evaluate the measurement model in PLS, construct validity was examined by confirmatory factor analysis approach. To test the construct validity, 2 types of validity test procedures were employed; the convergent and discriminant validity. The former is usually tested by examining the path loadings, average variance extracted (AVE) and also the composite reliability [24, 51]. As shown in Table 3, the path loadings were all higher than 0.5, the composite reliability (CR) values were all greater than 0.7 and the AVE values were also all higher than 0.5. The discriminant validity of the scale was examined by following the [52] criterion. As shown in Table 4, all the values on the square root of AVE were higher than the corresponding rows, which indicates the discriminant validity. Moreover, since all the CR and Cronbach's alpha values exceeded 0.7, it can be concluded that the questionnaire is reliable.

Structural model

To assess the structural model, [47, 48, 53] recommended looking at the beta, R^2 and the corresponding t-values by using a bootstrapping procedure with a resample of 5000. They also suggested that researchers should also evaluate the predictive relevance (Q^2).

First, the predictors of trust were examined and it was found that ethics ($P < 0.01$), physical protection ($P < 0.05$), technical protection ($P < 0.05$), staff training ($P < 0.01$) and staff monitoring ($P < 0.01$) had positive relationship with trust; explaining 39.8% of the variance in trust. Moreover, training had positive relationship with ethics ($P < 0.01$) with an R^2 of 0.212. Next, the relationship of the predictors with perceived information security was examined. The results of the analyses illustrated that staff training ($P < 0.01$) and staff monitoring ($P < 0.01$), ethics ($P < 0.01$), trust ($P < 0.1$)

Table 3 Assessment of Measurement Model

Construct	Items	Loadings	AVE	CR
Ethics	Ethics1	0.743	0.551	0.880
	Ethics2	0.727		
	Ethics3	0.730		
	Ethics4	0.753		
	Ethics5	0.741		
	Ethics6	0.759		
Monitoring	Monitor1	0.584	0.516	0.881
	Monitor2	0.616		
	Monitor3	0.722		
	Monitor4	0.768		
	Monitor5	0.820		
	Monitor6	0.751		
	Monitor7	0.737		
Physical	Physical2	0.686	0.549	0.859
	Physical3	0.736		
	Physical4	0.790		
	Physical6	0.743		
	Physical7	0.746		
Security	Security1	0.887	0.816	0.930
	Security2	0.915		
	Security3	0.908		
Technical	Technical1	0.865	0.659	0.884
	Technical2	0.873		
	Technical3	0.859		
	Technical4	0.624		
Training	Training1	0.801	0.630	0.895
	Training2	0.813		
	Training3	0.766		
	Training4	0.768		
	Training5	0.819		
Trust	Trust1	0.871	0.731	0.890
	Trust2	0.896		
	Trust3	0.793		

Note: Item Physical1 was deleted due to low loadings

and technical protection ($P < 0.01$) had positive relationship with perceived information security; explaining 45.7% of the variance in perceived information security while physical protection was not a significant predictor. All the R^2 values were above the 0.35 value as outlined by [54], indicating a substantial model. The results of the hypotheses have been illustrated in Table 5 and Fig. 1.

In the next step, the Q^2 was evaluated by running the blindfolding procedure in SmartPLS, which is a sample reuse procedure that deletes every d-th data point in the endogenous variable's indicators and estimates the parameters with the remaining data points [55–57]. If the Q^2 value is higher than 0, the model has sufficient predictive relevance for a certain endogenous variable and vice versa [48, 53, 58]. According to Hair et al. [47, 53] Q^2 values of 0.02, 0.15, and 0.35 imply that an exogenous variable has a small, medium or large predictive relevance for a certain endogenous construct. The Q^2 in this study was 0.282 (trust) and 0.363 (perceived security) which can be categorized as medium and large predictive relevance.

Discussion

Security breaches impose huge financial and reputational costs to the health sector. Hence, studying the factors that can reduce security concerns are necessary. While some researchers have employed an engineering (technical) approach to measure/develop the mechanisms of security protection in organizations [59–64], others have used a subjective approach and studied the issue from a subjective perspective [3, 5, 6, 8]. Considering the importance of disclosing sensitive and vital information by patients to health staff, to receive quality and necessary health services, patients should have minimal concern about the security of their information. Therefore, this research aims to employ the subjective perspective to study the clues that patients may look for to inform their concerns on the unauthorized disclosure of their sensitive information. While some researchers have employed a subjective method to study perceived information security, they suffer from numerous shortcomings in this regard. For instance, some [4, 15, 65–69] have neglected to study the factors that predict clients' perceptions about

Table 4 Discriminant Validity Assessment

	1	2	3	4	5	6	7
1. Ethics	**0.742**						
2. Monitoring	0.639	**0.718**					
3. Perceived Security	0.559	0.566	**0.903**				
4. Physical	0.433	0.463	0.411	**0.741**			
5. Technical	0.607	0.506	0.556	0.563	**0.812**		
6. Training	0.461	0.620	0.510	0.451	0.465	**0.794**	
7. Trust	0.507	0.570	0.445	0.270	0.426	0.495	**0.855**

Note: Values on the diagonal (bolded) are square root of the AVE while the off-diagonals are correlations

Table 5 Hypotheses Testing

Hypothesis		Std Beta	Std Error	t-value	Decision
H1	Training - > Perceived Security	0.160	0.068	2.350***	Supported
H2	Monitoring - > Perceived Security	0.186	0.065	2.862***	Supported
H3	Physical protection- > Perceived Security	0.024	0.042	0.587	Not Supported
H4	Ethics - > Trust	0.187	0.059	3.176***	Supported
H5	Physical protection- > Trust	0.121	0.052	2.317**	Supported
H6	Technical - > Trust	0.123	0.058	2.107**	Supported
H7	Training - > Trust	0.212	0.057	3.693***	Supported
H8	Monitoring - > Trust	0.313	0.067	4.638***	Supported
H9	Ethics - > Perceived Security	0.181	0.064	2.845***	Supported
H10	Training - > Ethics	0.461	0.052	8.914***	Supported
H11	Trust - > Perceived Security	0.060	0.042	1.420*	Supported
H12	Technical - > Perceived Security	0.238	0.068	3.526**	Supported

***$p < 0.01$, **$p < 0.05$, *$p < 0.1$

the security of their information in organizations and just focused on the factors preventing employees from violating the information security system and rules in organizations. Some, on the other hand, have focused on clients' perceptions about the factors that enhance their perceived security [3–8]; however their research had only considered the technical factors and was conducted with regards to customers' perceptions in online transactions. Hence, there were no studies which had examined the relationship of the organizational and human factors with patients' perceived security in an Asian country. Addressing this gap was the objective of this research.

To meet the above objective, 12 hypotheses were proposed. In order to collect data, a cross-sectional, self-administrative survey was utilized and after a pilot study, 450 questionnaires were distributed amongst the patients in 9 hospitals. After 1 month, 382 usable questionnaires were collected. Since it was found that the assumption of normal distribution is violated in this research, SmartPLS 3.0 was used to analyze the hypotheses. The results revealed that apart from the third hypothesis, other hypotheses were empirically supported. The details have been illustrated in Table 5. This has numerous implications and applications.

We found that staff's training had positive relationship with patients' trust in hospitals ($P < 0.01$) and perceived security threats ($P < 0.05$). This is in line with some researchers who stated that staff's training on security skills is expected to reduce the security risks in organizations [1, 11, 13, 15, 70]. This is a novel theoretical contribution in this regard, because none of the above researchers have empirically examined the relationship of patients' perceptions about employees' training with perceived security. The results of these two findings have numerous practical implications. First, health organizations should set policies to train their employees on information security issues such as potential threats and penetration techniques, employees' responsibilities on protecting the security of the information, required skills

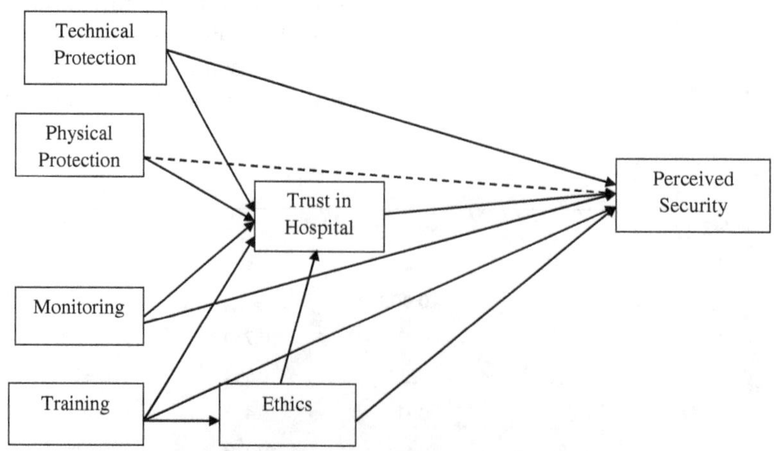

Fig. 1 Hypotheses Results (--->: Not Supported,➔: Supported)

to deal with security threats, legal issues, etc. Next step, in order to influence patients' perceptions about the extent of which their sensitive information is protected, hospitals need to communicate their policies on employees' training to their patients. This can help patients reduce their concern on the violation of their information security.

The results of the quantitative analysis found that patients' trust in hospitals can significantly predict their perceived security at a 0.10 significance level. This is to some extent consistent with [27, 29, 39, 40, 41], who had referred to individuals' trust as a predictor of their perceived risk and security. This is however, a novel theoretical finding of this research, because none of the above studies had empirically tested the relationship of patients' trust with their perceived security. Moreover, these findings can contribute to hospital practices, in the sense that if a hospital's management formulate and implement policies to enhance patients' trust in hospital, this can ultimately lead to their perceived security. The results, however, imply that this relationship is not as significant as the association of the other mentioned predictors of perceived security.

The results of the statistical analysis found no significant relationship between patients' physical protection mechanisms in the hospital and their perceived information security in a hospital. This is not consistent with [19], who speculated that implementing physical protection mechanisms are expected to lead to the reduction of security threats. This inconsistency can be explained from the point that although physical protection has been mentioned as one of the dimensions of information security management [18], patients may not believe that unauthorized parties can access their information physically and they may be more concern either about online security breach or insider breach.

The results, however, found that patients' perceptions about the physical protection mechanism of a hospital can significantly predict their trust in hospitals ($P < 0.05$). This is a novel finding since the researchers found no empirical papers, which have examined the relationship of perceived physical protection mechanisms with patients' trust in hospitals. This phenomenon can be explained by the institutional-based trust, which states that an individuals' trust can be guaranteed by safety procedures, policies and practices [23]. Since physical protection is considered as a safety procedure with regards to information security [19], patients' perceptions about the physical protection mechanisms can lead to their trust in hospitals. This is because the deployment of physical protection in hospital can make patients feel that the hospital cares about the benefits of its patients and hence they find the hospital trustworthy. According to this finding, hospitals should design and deploy robust physical protection mechanisms to limit unauthorized access to their information resources and then communicate such deployments to their patients. This enhances patients' trust in hospitals, which ultimately reduces patients' information security concerns.

The analysis also found that patients' perceptions about the monitoring of employees has positive significant relationship with their trust in hospitals ($P < 0.01$) and security violation concerns ($P < 0.01$). This is in line with some researchers who stated that monitoring employees' activities and behaviors [11, 15, 17] is expected to reduce the security risks in organizations. This is a novel theoretical contribution in this regard, because none of the past studies have empirically examined the relationship of employees' monitoring with patients' trust in hospital and perceived information security. While this research is one of the first, if not the only research, which has examined the relationship of perceived monitoring with patients' trust in hospitals, this novel finding can be explained by [23]. According to [23], trust can be predicted by individuals' perceptions on safety procedures, policies and practices. Monitoring employees can be one of the safety policies and practices in hospitals, which was found as a significant predictor of patients' trust in hospitals. Indeed, by monitoring employees' security behavior and actions, patients can be satisfied that the hospital tries to reduce the vulnerability in their relations with the hospital and hence, can trust in the hospital. These findings have numerous implications. Firstly, health organizations should formulate policies to monitor their employees' security related behavior and actions by using advanced network activity monitoring systems and system usage behavior by their employees. Secondly, in order to influence patients' trust and perceived security in hospitals, hospitals need to communicate their policies on employees' training and monitoring to their patients. This can help patients reduce their concern on the violation of their information security.

This research also found that patients' perceptions about staff ethics can predict their perceived information security and trust in hospitals at a 0.01 significance level. This is in line with some researchers who have speculated that patients' perceptions about staff's ethics can predict their perceptions about information security [13, 15, 17, 21, 22] and trust in hospitals [30, 31, 33, 34]. Moreover, this research found that patients' perceptions about staff's training can shape their perception in relation to the ethical behavior of staff in hospitals ($P < 0.01$); which is consistent with the past research [13, 19, 22, 37]. First, the relationship of perceived ethics with perceived security is theoretically a novel finding of this research. None of the past research in this field has empirically examined the relationship of patients' perceived ethics with their perceived security. Second, examining the relationship of patients' perception about staff's training with ethics is a new theoretical contribution by this paper as all of the mentioned papers [13, 19, 22, 37] have not provided any empirical results and analysis in this regard. Third, these findings have some practical implications as well. The results imply that health organizations need to formulate some policies and programs to promote ethical culture of dealing with patients' information amongst their employees and staff. One way to do so is by training their staff on the code of conduct and expected ethical behavior of the organization while dealing with patients' private and sensitive information in hospitals. Moreover, they need to communicate the existence of such programs cultural values amongst their staff to the patients. This practice can ultimately enhance patients' perceived information security in hospitals.

This research also found that patients' perception about technical protection can significantly predict their trust in a hospital ($P < 0.05$) and perception towards information security ($P < 0.01$). These findings are in line with some researchers, who found that perceived technical protection has positive relationship with individuals' trust [5, 36] and perceived security [5, 6, 8]. This finding, however, provides new theoretical contributions in this field. It is because none of the above research has been conducted in the context of hospital and health information, but in the context of online transactions. Hence, this research provides new insights in this regard compared to the past similar research, where the relationship of technical protection with trust and security has been examined. These findings also have some practical implications. These findings imply that hospitals should deploy robust technical mechanisms to protect patients' information security and then communicate these solutions to their patients. This can lead to patients' trust in hospitals and the improvement of perceived security.

Conclusions

Overall, this research provided numerous theoretical contributions and insights. This research is one of the few attempts to examine the interrelations among the antecedents of perceived information security from the patients' points of view, as the majority of the existing papers had either employed a technical approach to design a framework to protect information security or had concentrated on the relationship of mostly technical factors with individuals' perceived security in the online environment. Indeed, the past attempts had numerous shortcomings: firstly, they had mostly focused on technical aspects of information security mechanisms or technical antecedents of perceived security in online environment, and secondly, they had neglected to consider and examine the relationship of organizational and human factors with perceived security in the context of health and medical organizations. Moreover, a few studies only considered organizational and human factors, but mostly measured employees' perceptions on the predictors of their perceived security, in organizations other than health organizations. As discussed earlier, those studies which had examined organizational and human factors had neglected to examine factors such as employees' training, monitoring, technical and physical protection, ethics and trust in hospital in their model. Hence, this research was designed and developed to address these research gaps and examine the relationship of organizational and human factors with patients' perceived information security in hospitals.

This paper developed and empirically tested a model that contributes to the current knowledge regarding the predictors of patients' perceived information security, which helps both practitioners and academics better understand the clues that can predict patients' perceived information security in hospitals. The results of this study and the final model developed (as shown in Fig. 1) in this research can be used as a base-model for researchers to develop more comprehensive and complex models of patients' perceived security in health organizations. According to the findings of this research, as illustrated in Fig. 1, the factors: technical protection, physical protection and monitoring have a positive relationship with patients' trust; staff training is associated with both patients' trust and ethics. Moreover, according to the empirical analyses, the factors technical protection, staff training, ethics, patients' trust and monitoring can predict patients' perceived security in hospital.

In terms of practical implications, hospital managers and health policy makers can have better insights to the factors which can establish and enhance perceived information security among patients to practice and communicate such values to patients.

Despite its merits, this paper is not free from limitations. First, not all the organizational and human factors have been studied in this research. For instance, factors such as employees' commitment, culture, loyalty, or even employees' reaction towards probable penalties they may face in the case of security breach have not been considered in this research. Moreover, another set of factors which can play an important role in predicting patients' perceived security is patients' psychological characteristics such as risk-taking behavior, general optimism towards information technology, etc. This research also did not consider such factors as the moderators and predictors of patients' perceived information security. Hence, it is suggested that researchers consider these factors in developing and testing their models in future attempts. Another point, acknowledged by this research, is that this research considered patients' trust in hospitals as a predictor of patients' perceived security. It is suggested that future research examine the relationship of perceived security with patients' trust in hospitals and hospital information technology. Another point is that patients' perception of security does not reflect actual security, but it is important to reduce their concern and perceived risk of disclosure of sensitive information. Therefore, actual security of information systems in a hospital should be differentiated from patients' perception of the security.

Appendix

Table 6 Studies on the behavioural Security in Organizational Context

Study	Antecedents of Security	Dependent variable	Respondents
[79]	Mandatoriness	Precautions Taken	Employees (system Users)
[80]	Mimetic Pressure, Coercive Pressure, Normative Pressure	Level of information security control resources	Employees (system Users)
[81]	Perceived certainty and severity of sanctions, Attachment, Commitment, Involvement, Belief, Subjective Norm, Co-worker Behavior	IS security policyviolation Intention	Employees (system Users)
[11]	Perceived certainty of sanctions, PerceivedSeverity of sanctions,	IS misuse intention	Employees (system Users)
[82]	Self-Efficacy, Attitude, Normative Beliefs	Intention to resist social engineering	Employees (system Users)
[83]	Organizational Sanctions, Workgroup sanctions	intention to violate information security	Employees (system Users)
[67]	Organizational commitment, Self-Efficacy, Security Policy Attitude, Punishment Severity, Detection Certainty, Subjective Norm, Descriptive Norm.	Security Policy Compliance Intention	Employees (system Users)
[84]	Self-control	Information Security Violations	Undergraduate students
[85]	Perceived vulnerability, Perceived severity, Response efficacy, Response cost, Self-efficacy, Attitude towardcompliance with ISSP, Subjective norms	Information security compliancebehavioral intention	business managers and IS professionals
[68]	Attitude toward information security compliance, Subjective norms, self-efficacy, Locus of control	compliance behavioral intentions	Employees (system Users)
[86]	Perceived threat Severity and certainty, ResponseEfficacy, Self-Efficacy, Perceived Cost, Vendor support, IT Budget, Firm Size	Intention to Adopt Anti-malware by SME Executives	Information systems experts
[87]	Perceived susceptibility, Perceived severity, Perceived benefits, Perceived barriers, Cues to action, General security orientation, Self-efficacy,	Computer security behavior	Employees (system Users)
[88]	Conservative Behavior, Exposure to Offence, Risk Perception	IS users' risky behaviors threatening information security	IS users'
[89]	Self-Efficacy in Information Security	Security Practice Technology, Intention to Strengthen Security Effort, Security Practice Care Behavior	Business management students
[90]	Severity, Vulnerability, Response efficacy, Self-efficacy, Attitude, Normative beliefs, Rewards	Intention to comply with information security policies	Employees (system Users)
[91]	Intention, Trust, Organization Support,	Information security knowledge sharing	Employees (system Users)
[92]	Attitude, subjective norm, behavioral control, Threat appraisal, Self-Efficacy	Information security conscious care behavior	Employees (system Users)
[93]	Information security knowledge sharing, Information security collaboration, Information security intervention, Information security experience, Attachment, Commitment, Personal norms, Attitude	attitude towards compliance with information security policy compliance	Employees (system Users)
[94]	Perceived severity, Perceived vulnerability, Response efficacy, Self-efficacy, Perceived realism, Response cost, Rewards	Intention to IS security compliance	Employees (system Users)
[16]	Data Evaluation, Risk Analysis, Training, Integration, Policies, Legislation/Regulation, Architecture	Human Resource IS security	No data collection/No respondents

Abbreviations
AVE: Average variance extracted; CR: Composite reliability; PLS: Partial Least Squares; Q^2: Predictive relevance

Acknowledgements
None.

Funding
No funding was available for this research.

Authors' contributions

HRP developed the idea for the paper and led the development of the paper and collected the data; RT did the reviewing and finalizing of the structure and flow while MHS and MCL did the literature search and updates. All authors read and approved the final manuscript.

Competing interests

The authors declare that they have no competing interests.

Author details

[1]Department of Management, Isfahan (Khorasgan) Branch, Islamic Azad University, Isfahan, Iran. [2]School of Management, Universiti Sains Malaysia, Penang, Malaysia. [3]School of Strategy and Leadership, Coventry University, Coventry, UK. [4]Research & Innovation Management Centre (UNIMAS INNOVATION), Universiti Malaysia Sarawak (UNIMAS), 94300 Kota Samarahan, Sarawak, Malaysia.

References

1. Fernández-Alemán JL, Sánchez-Henarejos A, Toval A, Sánchez-García AB, Hernández-Hernández I, Fernandez-Luque L. Analysis of health professional security behaviors in a real clinical setting: an empirical study. Int J Med Inform. 2015;84(6):454–67.
2. Fernández-Alemán JL, Señor IC, Lozoya PÁO, Toval A. Security and privacy in electronic health records: a systematic literature review. J Biomed Inform. 2013;46(3):541–62.
3. Chellappa RK, Pavlou PA. Perceived information security, financial liability and consumer trust in electronic commerce transactions. Logist Inf Manag. 2002;15(5/6):358–68.
4. Hartono E, Holsapple CW, Kim KY, Na KS, Simpson JT. Measuring perceived security in B2C electronic commerce website usage: a respecification and validation. Decis Support Syst. 2014;62:11–21.
5. Kim C, Tao W, Shin N, Kim KS. An empirical study of customers' perceptions of security and trust in e-payment systems. Electron Commer Res Appl. 2010;9(1):84–95.
6. Peikari HR. Does nationality matter in the B2C environment? Results from a two nation study. In: Tenreiro de Magalhães S, Jahankhani H, Hessami AG, editors. Global security, safety, and sustainability. ICGS3 2010. Communications in computer and information science. Berlin, Heidelberg: Springer; 2010. p. 149–59.
7. Salisbury WD, Pearson RA, Pearson AW, Miller DW. Perceived security and world wide web purchase intention. Ind Manag Data Syst. 2001;101(4):165–77.
8. Shah MH, Peikari HR, Yasin NM. The determinants of individuals' perceived e-security: evidence from Malaysia. Int J Inf Manag. 2014;34(1):48–57.
9. Appari A, Johnson ME. Information security and privacy in healthcare: current state of research. Int J Internet Enterprise Manage. 2010;6(4):279–314.
10. Box D, Pottas D. A model for information security compliant behaviour in the healthcare context. Procedia Technol. 2014;16:1462–70.
11. D'Arcy J, Hovav A, Galletta D. User awareness of security countermeasures and its impact on information systems misuse: a deterrence approach. Inf Syst Res. 2009;20(1):79–98.
12. D'Arcy J, Herath T. A review and analysis of deterrence theory in the IS security literature: making sense of the disparate findings. Eur J Inf Syst. 2011;20(6):643–58.
13. Mohjel Eghdam A, Khameneh S, Hasankhni H, Moghadam S, Zamanzadeh V. Nurses' performance on Iranian nursing code of ethics from Patients' perspective. Iran J Nurs. 2013;26(84):1–11 (In Persian).
14. Colwill C. Human factors in information security: the insider threat–who can you trust these days? Inf Secur Tech Rep. 2009;14(4):186–96.
15. Farzandipour M, Sadoughi F, Ahmadi M, Karimi I. Security requirements and solutions in electronic health records: lessons learned from a comparative study. J Med Syst. 2010;34(4):629–42.
16. Veiga AD, Martins N. Improving the information security culture through monitoring and implementation actions illustrated through a case study. Comput Secur. 2015;49:162–76.
17. Zafar H. Human resource information systems: information security concerns for organizations. Hum Resour Manag Rev. 2013;23(1):105–13.
18. Ruighaver AB, Maynard SB, Warren M. Ethical decision making: improving the quality of acceptable use policies. Comput Secur. 2010;29(7):731–6.
19. Vellani K. Strategic security management: a risk assessment guide for decision makers. Oxford: Butterworth-Heinemann; 2006.
20. Zakariya NI, Kahn MTE. Safety, security and safeguard. Ann Nucl Energy. 2015;75:292–302.
21. Kluge EHW. Secure e-health: managing risks to patient health data. Int J Med Inform. 2007;76(5):402–6.
22. Lusignan SD, Chan T, Theadom A, Dhoul N. The roles of policy and professionalism in the protection of processed clinical data: a literature review. Int J Med Inform. 2007;76(4):261–8.
23. Taherdoost H, Sahibuddin S, Namayandeh M, Jalaliyoon N. Propose an educational plan for computer ethics and information security. Procedia Soc Behav Sci. 2011;28:815–9.
24. Rockville MD. Quality and Patient Safety. Agency for Healthcare Research and Quality. Available from: http://www.ahrq.gov/professionals/quality-patient-safety/index.html. [Last Visit: 2015 Jun 30].
25. Hsieh PJ. Healthcare professionals' use of health clouds: integrating technology acceptance and status quo bias perspectives. Int J Med Inform. 2015b;84(7):512–23.
26. Peikari HR, Yasina NM, Shah MH. Determinants of online trust: a system oriented view. Am J Sci Res. 2013;87:25–45.
27. Hu X, Wu G, Wu Y, Zhang H. The effects of web assurance seals on consumers' initial trust in an online vendor: a functional perspective. Decis Support Syst. 2010;48:407–18.
28. Baker J, Parasuraman A, Grewal D, Voss GB. The influence of multiple store environment cues on perceived merchandise value and patronage intentions. J Mark. 2002;66(2):120–41.
29. Chang HH, Chen SW. The impact of online store environment cues on purchase intention: trust and perceived risk as a mediator. Online Inf Rev. 2008;32(6):818–41.
30. Chang HH, Chen SW. Consumer perception of interface quality, security, and loyalty in electronic commerce. Inf Manag. 2009;46(7):411–7.
31. Connolly R, Bannister B. E-commerce trust beliefs: the influence of national culture. Proceedings of European and Mediterranean Conference on Information Systems (EMCIS 2007). 2007. doi:10.1.1.98.3780..
32. Gefen D, Straub DW. Consumer trust in B2C e-commerce and the importance of social presence: experiments in e-products and e-services. Omega. 2004;32(6):407–24.
33. Flavián C, Guinalíu M, Gurrea R. The role played by perceived usability, satisfaction and consumer trust on website loyalty. Inf Manag. 2006;43(1):1–14.
34. Johnson DS. Achieving customer value from electronic channels through identity commitment, calculative commitment, and trust in technology. J Interact Mark. 2007;21(4):2–22.
35. McCole P, Ramsey E, Williams J. Trust considerations on attitudes towards online purchasing: the moderating effect of privacy and security concerns. J Bus Res. 2010;63(9):1018–24.
36. Roca CJ, García JJ, Vega JJDL. The importance of perceived trust, security and privacy in online trading systems. Inf Manage Comput Secur. 2009;17(2):96–113.
37. McKnight DH, Chervany NL. What trust means in e-commerce customer relationships: an interdisciplinary conceptual typology. Int J Electron Commer. 2001;6(2):35–59.
38. Corbitt BJ, Thanasankit T, Yi H. Trust and e-commerce: a study of consumer perceptions. Electron Commer Res Appl. 2003;2(3):203–15.
39. Workman M, Gathegi J. Punishment and ethics deterrents: a study of insider security contravention. J Am Soc Inf Sci Technol. 2007;58(2):212–22.
40. Kim G, Shin B, Lee HG. Understanding dynamics between initial trust and usage intentions of mobile banking. Inf Syst J. 2009;19(3):283–311.
41. Bélanger F, Carter L. Trust and risk in e-government adoption. J Strateg Inf Syst. 2008;17(2):165–76.
42. Hsieh PJ. Physicians' acceptance of electronic medical records exchange: an extension of the decomposed TPB model with institutional trust and perceived risk. Int J Med Inform. 2015a;84(1):1–14.
43. Kim DJ, Ferrin DL. Rao HR. a trust-based consumer decision-making model in electronic commerce: the role of trust, perceived risk, and their antecedents. Decis Support Syst. 2008;44(2):544–64.
44. Teo TS, Liu J. Consumer trust in e-commerce in the United States. Singapore and China Omega. 2007;35(1):22–38.
45. Chen YH, Barnes S. Initial trust and online buyer behaviour. Ind Manag Data Syst. 2007;107(1):21–36.

46. Krejcie RV, Morgan DW. Determining sample size for research activities. Educ Psychol Meas. 1970;30(3):607–10.
47. Ringle CM, Wende S, Becker JM. SmartPLS 3. Hamburg: SmartPLS; 2015. http://www.smartpls.com
48. Anderson JC, Gerbing DW. Structural equation modeling in practice: a review and recommended two-step approach. Psychol Bull. 1988;103(3):411–23.
49. Hair JF, Ringle CM, Sarstedt M. PLS-SEM: indeed a silver bullet. J Mark Theory Pract. 2011;19(2):139–51.
50. Hair JF, Sarstedt M, Ringle CM, Mena JA. An assessment of the use of partial least squares structural equation modeling in marketing research. J Acad Mark Sci. 2012;40(3):414–33.
51. Ramayah T, Lee JWC, In JBC. Network collaboration and performance in the tourism sector. Serv Bus. 2011;5(4):411–28.
52. Ramayah T, Yeap JA, Ignatius J. An empirical inquiry on knowledge sharing among academicians in higher learning institutions. Minerva. 2013;51(2):131–54.
53. Gholami R, Sulaiman AB, Ramayah T, Molla A. Senior managers' perception on green information systems (IS) adoption and environmental performance: results from a field survey. Inf Manag. 2013;50(7):431–8.
54. Fornell C, Larcker DF. Evaluating structural equation models with unobservable variables and measurement error. J Mark Res. 1981;18(1):39–50.
55. Hair JF, Sarstedt M, Hopkins L, Kuppelwieser VG. Partial least squares structural equation modeling (PLS-SEM): an emerging tool in business research. Eur Bus Rev. 2014;26(2):106–21.
56. Cohen J. Statistical power analysis for the behavioral science. Mahwah, New Jersey: Lawrence Erlbaum; 1988.
57. Chin WW. The partial least squares approach for structural equation modeling. In: Marcoulides GA, editor. Modern methods for business research. Mahwah, NJ: Lawrence Erlbaum Associates; 1998. p. 295–358.
58. Henseler J, Ringle CM, Sinkovics RR. The use of partial least squares path modeling in international marketing. Adv Int Mark. 2009;20:277–319.
59. Tenenhaus M, Vinzi VE, Chatelin YM, Lauro C. PLS path modeling. Comput Stat Data Anal. 2005;48(1):159–205.
60. Fornell C, Cha J. Partial least squares. In: Bagozzi RP, editor. Advanced methods of marketing research. Cambridge, MA: Blackwell Business; 1994. p. 52–78.
61. Choe J, Yoo SK. Web-based secure access from multiple patient repositories. Int J Med Inform. 2008;77(4):242–8.
62. Jafari M, Safavi-Naini R, Saunders C, Sheppard NP. Using digital rights management for securing data in a medical research environment. Proceedings of the Tenth Annual ACM Workshop on Digital Rights Management. 2010. https://doi.org/10.1145/1866870.1866883.
63. Zhijun W, Zhihan C, Caiyun W, Jin L. Access control scheme with attribute revocation for SWIM. J China Univ Posts Telecommunications. 2017;24:49–54.
64. Khan FA, Ali A, Abbas H. Haldar NAH. A cloud-based healthcare framework for security and patients' data privacy using wireless body area networks. Procedia Comput Sci. 2014;34:511–7.
65. Mundy DP. Customer privacy on UK healthcare websites. Med Inform Internet Med. 2006;31(3):175–93.
66. Sucurovic S. An approach to access control in electronic health record. J Med Syst. 2010;34(4):659–66.
67. Cho J, Park I, Michel JW. How does leadership affect information systems success? The role of transformational leadership. Inf Manag. 2011;48(7):270–7.
68. Dhillon G, Syed R, Pedron C. Interpreting information security culture: an organizational transformation case study. Comput Secur. 2016;56:63–9.
69. Herath T, Rao HR. Encouraging information security behaviors in organizations: role of penalties, pressures and perceived effectiveness. Decis Support Syst. 2009;47(2):154–65.
70. Ifinedo P. Information systems security policy compliance: an empirical study of the effects of socialisation, influence, and cognition. Inf Manag. 2014;51(1):69–79.
71. Vaidyanathan G, Berhanu N. Impact of security countermeasures in organizational information convergence: a theoretical model. Issues Inform Syst. 2012;13(2):21–5.
72. Lluch M. Healthcare professionals' organisational barriers to health information technologies - a literature review. Int J Med Inform. 2011;80(12):849–62.
73. Arizona state university. IT-General controls questionnaire [Internet]. [cited 2008 January 31]. Available from: https://www.asu.edu/fs/documents/icq/IT_general_controls_icq.pdf
74. Hussain Shah M, Peikari HR, Yasin NM. The determinants of individuals' perceived e-security: evidence from Malaysia. Int J Inf Manag. 2014;34:48–57.
75. Ghobadei Far M, Mosalanejad L. Evaluation of staff adherence to professionalism in Jahrom University of Medical Sciences. J Educ Ethics Nurs. 2013;2(2):1–7 (In Persian).
76. Educational Managers. Questionnaire of patient security culture from nurses view; 2014 [cited 2014April 30]. Available from: http://eduadmin.ir
77. Financial Studies. Questionnaire of internal monitoring controls evaluation; 2014 [cited 2013April 26].Available from: http://tse.ir/cms/Portals/1/arzyabi_nezarat.pdf.(in Persian).
78. Beigi Khortabsara Y. Evaluation questionnaire of training system effectiveness;2014 [cited 2010 March 20] .Available from: http://yazdanmb.persianblog.ir/post/65 (in Persian).
79. Boss SR, Kirsch LJ, Angermeier I, Shingler RA, Boss RW. If someone is watching, I'll do what I'm asked: mandatoriness, control, and information security. Eur J Inf Syst. 2009;18(2):151–64.
80. Cavusoglu H, Cavusoglu H, Son JY, Benbasat I. Institutional pressures in security management: direct and indirect influence on organizational investment in information security control resources. Inf Manag. 2015;52: 385–400.
81. Cheng L, Li Y, Li W, Holm E, Zhai Q. Understanding the violation of IS security policy in organizations: an integrated model based on social control and deterrence theory. Comput Secur. 2013;39:447–59.
82. Flores WR, Ekstedt M. Shaping intention to resist social engineering through transformational leadership, information security culture and awareness. Comput Secur. 2016;59:26–44.
83. Guo KH, Yuan Y. The effects of multilevel sanctions on information security violations: a mediating model. Inf Manag. 2012;49:320–6.
84. Hu Q, West R, Smarandescu L. The role of self-control in information security violations: insights from a cognitive neuroscience perspective. J Manag Inf Syst. 2015;31(4):6–48.
85. Ifinedo P. Understanding information systems security policy compliance: an integration of the theory of planned behavior and the protection motivation theory. Comput Secur. 2012;31(1):83–95.
86. Lee Y, Larsen KR. Threat or coping appraisal: determinants of SMB executives' decision to adopt anti-malware software. Eur J Inf Syst. 2009; 18(2):177–87.
87. Ng BY, Kankanhalli A. Xu YC. Studying users' computer security behavior: a health belief perspective. Decis Support Syst. 2009;46(4):815–25.
88. Öğütçü G, Testik ÖM, Chouseinoglou O. Analysis of personal information security behavior and awareness. Comput Secur. 2016;56:83–93.
89. Rhee HS, Kim C, Ryu YU. Self-efficacy in information security: its influence on end users' information security practice behavior. Comput Secur. 2009;28(8): 816–26.
90. Siponen M, Mahmood MA, Pahnila S. Employees' adherence to information security policies: an exploratory field study. Inf Manag. 2014;51:217–24.
91. Safa NS, Von Solms R. An information security knowledge sharing model in organizations. Comput Hum Behav. 2016;57:442–51.
92. Safa NS, Sookhak M, Von Solms R, Furnell S, Ghani NA, Herawan T. Information security conscious care behaviour formation in organizations. Comput Secur. 2015;53:65–78.
93. Safa NS, Von Solms R, Furnell S. Information security policy compliance model in organizations. Comput Secur. 2016;56:70–82.
94. Vance A, Siponen M, Pahnila S. Motivating IS security compliance: insights from habit and protection motivation theory. Inf Manag. 2012;49(3):190–8.

Permissions

All chapters in this book were first published in MI&DM, by BioMed Central; hereby published with permission under the Creative Commons Attribution License or equivalent. Every chapter published in this book has been scrutinized by our experts. Their significance has been extensively debated. The topics covered herein carry significant findings which will fuel the growth of the discipline. They may even be implemented as practical applications or may be referred to as a beginning point for another development.

The contributors of this book come from diverse backgrounds, making this book a truly international effort. This book will bring forth new frontiers with its revolutionizing research information and detailed analysis of the nascent developments around the world.

We would like to thank all the contributing authors for lending their expertise to make the book truly unique. They have played a crucial role in the development of this book. Without their invaluable contributions this book wouldn't have been possible. They have made vital efforts to compile up to date information on the varied aspects of this subject to make this book a valuable addition to the collection of many professionals and students.

This book was conceptualized with the vision of imparting up-to-date information and advanced data in this field. To ensure the same, a matchless editorial board was set up. Every individual on the board went through rigorous rounds of assessment to prove their worth. After which they invested a large part of their time researching and compiling the most relevant data for our readers.

The editorial board has been involved in producing this book since its inception. They have spent rigorous hours researching and exploring the diverse topics which have resulted in the successful publishing of this book. They have passed on their knowledge of decades through this book. To expedite this challenging task, the publisher supported the team at every step. A small team of assistant editors was also appointed to further simplify the editing procedure and attain best results for the readers.

Apart from the editorial board, the designing team has also invested a significant amount of their time in understanding the subject and creating the most relevant covers. They scrutinized every image to scout for the most suitable representation of the subject and create an appropriate cover for the book.

The publishing team has been an ardent support to the editorial, designing and production team. Their endless efforts to recruit the best for this project, has resulted in the accomplishment of this book. They are a veteran in the field of academics and their pool of knowledge is as vast as their experience in printing. Their expertise and guidance has proved useful at every step. Their uncompromising quality standards have made this book an exceptional effort. Their encouragement from time to time has been an inspiration for everyone.

The publisher and the editorial board hope that this book will prove to be a valuable piece of knowledge for researchers, students, practitioners and scholars across the globe.

List of Contributors

Xiaoyi Pan and Zhiying Gu
School of Information Science and Technology, Guangdong University of Foreign Studies, Guangzhou, China

Tianyong Hao
School of Information Science and Technology, Guangdong University of Foreign Studies, Guangzhou, China
School of Computer, South China Normal University, Guangzhou, China

Yingying Qu
School of Business, Guangdong University of Foreign Studies, Guangzhou, China

Heng Weng
The Second Affiliated Hospital, Guangzhou University of Chinese Medicine, Guangzhou, China

Georgy Kopanitsa
Institute Cybernetic Center, Tomsk Polytechnic University, Lenina 30, 634050 Tomsk, Russia
Tomsk State University for Architecture and Building, Tomsk, Russia

Ilia Semenov
Medlinx LLC, Saint-Petersburg, Russia

Andrea C. Tricco
Li Ka Shing Knowledge Institute of St. Michael's Hospital, 209 Victoria Street, East Building, Toronto, ON M5B 1W8, Canada
Epidemiology Division, Dalla Lana School of Public Health, University of Toronto, 6th Floor, 155 College St, Toronto, ON M5T 3M7, Canada

Wasifa Zarin, Erin Lillie, Rachel Warren, Paul A. Khan, Reid Robson and Ba' Pham
Li Ka Shing Knowledge Institute of St. Michael's Hospital, 209 Victoria Street, East Building, Toronto, ON M5B 1W8, Canada

Serena Jeblee and Graeme Hirst
Department of Computer Science University of Toronto, 10 King's College Road, Toronto, ON M5S 3G4, Canada

Sharon E. Straus
Li Ka Shing Knowledge Institute of St. Michael's Hospital, 209 Victoria Street, East Building, Toronto, ON M5B 1W8, Canada
Department of Geriatric Medicine, Faculty of Medicine, University of Toronto, 27 Kings College Circle, Toronto, ON M5S 1A1, Canada

Hansi Zhang, Yi Guo, Qian Li, Elizabeth Shenkman, François Modave and Jiang Bian
Department of Health Outcomes and Biomedical Informatics, College of Medicine, University of Florida, Clinical and Translational Research Building Suite 3228, 2004 Mowry Road, Gainesville, FL 32610-0219, USA

Thomas J. George
Division of Hematology and Oncology, Department of Medicine, College of Medicine, University of Florida, Gainesville, Florida, USA

Mario Mariño
Centro de Investigación en Diseño Industrial de Productos Complejos (CIDI-FADU-UBA), Facultad de Arquitectura, Diseño y Urbanismo, Universidad de Buenos Aires, 2160 Intendente Güiraldes Ave, Buenos Aires, Argentina

Ignacio Ghersi and Mónica Teresita Miralles
Centro de Investigación en Diseño Industrial de Productos Complejos (CIDI-FADU-UBA), Facultad de Arquitectura, Diseño y Urbanismo, Universidad de Buenos Aires, 2160 Intendente Güiraldes Ave, Buenos Aires, Argentina
Laboratorio de Biomecánica e Ingeniería para la Salud (LaBIS-FI-UCA), Facultad de Ingeniería y Ciencias Agrarias, Pontificia Universidad Católica Argentina, 1600 Alicia Moreau de Justo Ave, Buenos Aires, Argentina

Jian-Xiang Wei
School of Internet of Things, Nanjing University of Posts and Telecommunications, Nanjing 210003, China

Jing Wang and Yun-Xia Zhu
School of Computer Science and Technology, School of Software, Nanjing University of Posts and Telecommunications, Nanjing 210023, China

Jun Sun, Hou-Ming Xu and Ming Li
Jiangsu Center for ADR Monitoring, Nanjing 210002, China

Shaker El-Sappagh
Information Systems Department, Faculty of Computers and Informatics, Benha University, Banha, Egypt
Department of Information and Communication Engineering, Inha University, Incheon, South Korea

Francesco Franda
Department of Philosophy, University at Buffalo, Buffalo, NY, USA

Farman Ali and Kyung-Sup Kwak
Department of Information and Communication Engineering, Inha University, Incheon, South Korea

Huiqin Chen, Xiaofeng Li and Ying Liang
Department of Pediatrics, The Third Affiliated Hospital, Sun Yat-sen University, Guangzhou, Guangdong, China

Dihua Zhang
Department of Nephrology, The First Affiliated Hospital, Sun Yat-sen University, Guangzhou, Guangdong, China

Guoping Zhang
Department of Oncology, Yuebei People's Hospital, Shaoguan, Guangdong, China

Mohan Vamsi Kasukurthi and Shengyu Li
School of Computing, University of South Alabama, Mobile, AL 36688, USA

Glen M. Borchert
College of Medicine, University of South Alabama, Mobile, AL 36688, USA

Jingshan Huang
School of Computing, University of South Alabama, Mobile, AL 36688, USA
College of Math and Computer Science, Fuzhou University, Fuzhou, Fujian, China
School of Information, Qilu University of Technology (Shandong Academy of Sciences), Jinan, Shandong, China

Sooyoung Yoo, Seok Kim, Eunhye Kim, Kee-Hyuck Lee and Hee Hwang
Office of eHealth Research and Businesses, Seoul National University Bundang Hospital, 166, Gumi-ro, Bundang-gu, Seongnam-si 436-707, South Korea

Eunja Jung
Nursing Department, Seoul National University Bundang Hospital, 166, Gumi-ro, Bundang-gu, Seongnam-si 436-707, South Korea

Stuart Speedie
Institute for Health Informatics, University of Minnesota, Minneapolis, MN, USA

Rui Zhang
Institute for Health Informatics, University of Minnesota, Minneapolis, MN, USA
College of Pharmacy, University of Minnesota, Minneapolis, MN, USA

Sisi Ma
Institute for Health Informatics, University of Minnesota, Minneapolis, MN, USA
Department of Medicine, University of Minnesota, Minneapolis, MN, USA

Liesa Shanahan, Jessica Munroe and Sarah Horn
Medtronic, Inc., Minneapolis, MN, USA

Yue-Shu Zhao
The Third Affiliated Hospital of Zhengzhou University, Kangfu Road, Zhengzhou, Henan 450072, China

Kun-Li Zhang, Hong-Chao Ma and Kun Li
School of Information Engineering, Zhengzhou University, Science Avenue, Zhengzhou, Henan 450001, China

Erik Berglund, Ragnar Westerling and Per Lytsy
Department of Public Health and Caring Sciences, Uppsala University, SE-751 22 UPPSALA, Sweden

Johan Sundström
Department of Medical Sciences, Uppsala University, Uppsala, Sweden

Jingcheng Du, Yaoyun Zhang, Qiang Wei, Cui Tao and Hua Xu
The University of Texas School of Biomedical Informatics, 7000 Fannin St Suite 600, Houston, TX 77030, USA

Jianhong Luo
The University of Texas School of Biomedical Informatics, 7000 Fannin St Suite 600, Houston, TX 77030, USA
Department of Management Science and Engineering, Zhejiang Sci-Tech University, Hangzhou 310018, China

Yuxi Jia
The University of Texas School of Biomedical Informatics, 7000 Fannin St Suite 600, Houston, TX 77030, USA
Department of Medical Informatics, School of Public Health, Jilin University, Changchun 130021, Jilin, China

Jeongeun Lee
Interdisciplinary Program for Bioengineering, Graduate School, Seoul National Universty, Seoul, Republic of Korea

Hyun-Je Song and Seong-Bae Park
School of Computer Science and Engineering, Kyungpook National University, Daegu, Republic of Korea

Eunsil Yoon
PAS1 team, TmaxSoft, Gyeonggi-do, Republic of Korea

Sung-Hye Park and Jeong-Wook Seo
Department of Pathology, College of Medicine, Seoul National University, Seoul, Republic of Korea

Jinwook Choi
Interdisciplinary Program for Bioengineering, Graduate School, Seoul National Universty, Seoul, Republic of Korea
Department of Biomedical Engineering, College of Medicine, Seoul National University, Seoul, Republic of Korea

Peom Park
Department of Industrial Engineering, Ajou University, Suwon, Republic of Korea

Iona Crumley, Lisa Blom, Lucie Laflamme and Helle Mölsted Alvesson
Department of Public Health Sciences, Karolinska Institutet, Tomtebodavägen 18A, SE-171 77 Stockholm, Sweden

Sara Bersche Golas and Jennifer Felsted
Partners Connected Health Innovation, Partners HealthCare, 25 New Chardon St., Suite 300, Boston, MA 02114, USA

Stephen Agboola, Sujay Kakarmath, Joseph Kvedar and Kamal Jethwani
Partners Connected Health Innovation, Partners HealthCare, 25 New Chardon St., Suite 300, Boston, MA 02114, USA
Massachusetts General Hospital, Boston, MA, USA
Harvard Medical School, Boston, MA, USA

Takuma Shibahara, Hiroko Otaki, Jumpei Sato, Tatsuya Nakae, Toru Hisamitsu and Go Kojima
Research and Development Group, Hitachi, Ltd, Tokyo, Japan

Franziska Singer, Nora C. Toussaint, Linda Grob and Daniel J. Stekhoven
NEXUS Personalized Health Technologies, ETH Zurich, Otto-Stern-Weg 7, 8093 Zurich, Switzerland
SIB Swiss Institute of Bioinformatics, 4058 Basel, Switzerland

Anja Irmisch, Mitchell P. Levesque and Reinhard Dummer
Department of Dermatology, University Hospital Zurich, 8091 Zurich, Switzerland

Jochen Singer, Thomas Thurnherr and Niko Beerenwinkel
SIB Swiss Institute of Bioinformatics, 4058 Basel, Switzerland
Department of Biosystems Science and Engineering, ETH Zurich, 4058 Basel, Switzerland

Christian Beisel
Department of Biosystems Science and Engineering, ETH Zurich, 4058 Basel, Switzerland

Sacha I. Rothschild and Andreas Wicki
Division of Oncology, Department of Biomedicine, University Hospital Basel, Petersgraben 4, 4031 Basel, Switzerland

Luca Quagliata
Department of Pathology, University Hospital Basel, Schönbeinstrasse 40, 4056 Basel, Switzerland

Carol E. Adair
Community Health Sciences, University of Calgary, Calgary, Canada

Shawn X. Dodd
University of Alberta, Edmonton, Canada

Stacey Page
Community Health Sciences, University of Calgary, Calgary, Canada
Conjoint Health Research Ethics Board, University of Calgary, Calgary, Canada

Nicole Letourneau
University of Calgary, Calgary, Canada

Xinjie Cui
PolicyWise for Children & Families, Edmonton, AB, Canada

Suzanne C. Tough
PolicyWise for Children & Families, Calgary, Canada
Pediatrics & Community Health Sciences, University of Calgary, Calgary, Canada

Kiran Pohar Manhas
Community Health Sciences, University of Calgary, Calgary, Canada
University of Alberta, Edmonton, Canada
Alberta Health Services, Calgary, Canada

Hamid Reza Peikari
Department of Management, Isfahan (Khorasgan) Branch, Islamic Azad University, Isfahan, Iran

Ramayah T.
School of Management, Universiti Sains Malaysia, Penang, Malaysia

Mahmood Hussain Shah
School of Strategy and Leadership, Coventry University, Coventry, UK

May Chiun Lo
Research & Innovation Management Centre (UNIMAS INNOVATION), Universiti Malaysia Sarawak (UNIMAS), 94300 Kota Samarahan, Sarawak, Malaysia

Index

www.ingramcontent.com/pod-product-compliance
Lightning Source LLC
LaVergne TN
LVHW080903210926
848485LV00004B/584
* 9 7 8 1 6 3 2 4 2 8 7 8 3 *